Geographical aspects
of health

Geographical aspects of health

Essays in honour of Andrew Learmonth

edited by

Neil D. McGlashan

Department of Geography,
University of Tasmania,
Hobart, Australia

John R. Blunden

Faculty of Social Sciences,
The Open University,
Milton Keynes, England

1983

Academic Press
A Subsidiary of Harcourt Brace Jovanovich, Publishers
London · New York · Paris · San Diego · San Francisco · São Paulo ·
Sydney · Tokyo · Toronto

ACADEMIC PRESS INC. (LONDON) LTD
24/28 Oval Road, London NW1 7DX

United States Edition published by
ACADEMIC PRESS INC.
111 Fifth Avenue, New York, New York, 10003

British Library Cataloguing in Publication Data

McGlashan, N.
  Geographical aspects of health.
  1. Medical geography—History
  I. Title   II. Blunden, J. R.
  614.4′2   RA792

ISBN 0-12-483780-8

Photoset by Paston Press, Norwich
and printed in Great Britain by
Galliard (Printers) Ltd., Great Yarmouth

Contributors

Sheila M. Bain
Department of Geography
University of Aberdeen
Aberdeen AB9 1FK
Scotland

John R. Blunden
Faculty of Social Sciences
The Open University
Walton Hall
Milton Keynes MK7 6AA
England

Andrew D. Cliff
Department of Geography
University of Cambridge
Downing Place
Cambridge CB2 3EN
England

John A. Giggs
Department of Geography
University of Nottingham
University Park
Nottingham NG7 2RD
England

Graham G. Giles
Department of Community Health
University of Tasmania
Royal Hobart Hospital Clinical School
43 Collins Street
Hobart, Tasmania
Australia 7000

Michael R. Greenberg
Department of Community
  Development
Rutgers University
Livingston College
New Brunswick
New Jersey 08903
USA

Peter Haggett
Department of Geography
University of Bristol
University Road
Bristol BS8 1SS
England

L. D. Brian Heenan
Department of Geography
University of Otago
Box 56, Dunedin
New Zealand

J. Anthony Hellen
Department of Geography
University of Newcastle upon Tyne
Newcastle upon Tyne NE1 7RU
England

G. Melvyn Howe
Department of Geography
University of Strathclyde
Livingstone Tower
26 Richmond Street
Glasgow G1 1XH
Scotland

Helmut J. Jusatz
Heidelberger Akademie der
  Wissenschaften
Geomedizinische Forschungsstelle
6900 Heidelberg 1
Karlstrasse 4
Postfach 10 27 69
West Germany

Melinda S. Meade
Department of Geography
The University of North Carolina at
  Chapel Hill
203 Saunders Hall
Chapel Hill
North Carolina 27514
USA

Neil D. McGlashan
Department of Geography
University of Tasmania
Box 252C, GPO,
Hobart, Tasmania,
Australia 58150

Ted Nawalinski
Smith Kline Animal Health Products
West Chester
Pennsylvania
USA

David R. Phillips
Department of Geography
University of Exeter
Amory Building
Rennes Drive
Exeter, Devon EX4 4RJ
England

R. Mansell Prothero
Department of Geography
University of Liverpool
Roxby Building
P.O. Box 147
Liverpool L69 3BX
England

Gerald F. Pyle
Department of Geography and Earth
    Sciences
University of North Carolina at
    Charlotte
UNCC Station, Charlotte
North Carolina 28223
USA

Attur Ramesh
Department of Geography
University of Madras
Madras 600005
India

Lynn M. Roundy
John F. Kennedy Medical Center
Edison, New Jersey
USA

Robert W. Roundy
Department of Human Ecology
Rutgers University
Cook College
New Brunswick
New Jersey 08903
USA

Robert J. Stimson
School of Social Sciences
Flinders University
Adelaide
South Australia
Australia

Jean-Pierre Thouez
Department of Geography
University of Montreal
Case Postale 6128
Succursale "A"
Montreal, P.Q. H3C 3J7
Quebec
Canada

Yola Verhasselt
Geografisch Instituut
Vrije Universiteit Brussel
Pleinlaan 2
1050 Brussel
Belgium

Hella Wellmer
Heidelberger Akademie der
    Wissenschaften
Geomedizinische Forschungsstelle
6900 Heidelberg 1
Karlstrasse 4
Postfach 10 27 69
West Germany

Preface

Two basic ideas lie behind the planning of this book. In the one instance, it seemed evident that medical geography as a field of study had, in the period from the end of the Second World War to the early 1980s, ultimately reached a maturity which was reflected in the nature of the research undertaken by its practitioners and the methods employed by them and it was thought perhaps appropriate that a publication should appear which would not only review how it had developed regionally but should be illustrative of the kinds of work now being undertaken at its frontiers. In the other, it was felt by the geography discipline at the Open University that some fitting means should be found of marking the retirement of its professor, Andrew Learmonth, a distinguished scholar whose research work over a period of 30 years had been devoted almost entirely to aspects of medical geography.

What could be more appropriate than that these two ideas should fuse and become a reality in the production of this volume, particularly when, as one leading medical geographer has put it, "Andrew and medical geography are virtually synonymous". Thus it is to Andrew Learmonth that his colleagues at the Open University, the contributors to this volume and many others working in the field of medical geography, dedicate this book.

Hobart and Milton Keynes
February 1983

Neil D. McGlashan
John R. Blunden

Acknowledgements

The editors would like to thank all those who have in so many ways helped with the preparation of this book through the useful advice they have proffered or the information they have passed on. Of those who have otherwise made formal contributions we would particularly like to thank Dr J. A. Hellen, Professor G. M. Howe, Professor R. M. Prothero and Dr David Phillips. Others who have played a valuable role and who deserve our gratitude include Dr J. Chappell, Professor C. D. Deshpande, Professor J. N. Jennings, J. A. Leslie, Dr N. McDonald, Professor A. J. Rose and last but by no means least, Nancy Learmonth, who proved an indefatigable archivist in the documentation of her husband's career.

We are also much indebted to John Hunt, Research Cartographer in the Faculty of Social Science at the Open University, for his co-ordination and realization of much of the graphic material; to Pat Cooke in Milton Keynes for her liaison work on behalf of two editors 11,000 miles apart; to Paul Smith of the Open University Library for his generous help in checking many of the references cited in the text; and to Mrs. T. Hughes at the University of Tasmania who carried the main burden of typing and retyping the manuscripts.

Contents

Part Two

Part Three

Introduction

N. D. McGlashan and J. R. Blunden

The period since the end of the Second World War has been one of unparalleled change in medical geography as in geography itself, a major parent discipline. These years—approximately one man's working lifetime—have seen more change than many centuries before and more scientists are now employed in medical geography all round the world than ever before. In choosing 1983 as a year to review progress in the subject it is necessary to step back a little, to distance oneself to try to recognize major features, perhaps minor numerically, which may develop usefully in the future.

The dominant paradigm of medical geography is the vision of man as a creature of and within an environment which is not only affected by him but also affects him personally and collectively in health-related ways. Man's relationship with the surroundings which cocoon him from cradle to grave implies that that relationship may be positive, that is stimulating and healthful or, alternatively, negative, that is noxious or harmful.

In some senses the environmental relationships of Man have always been of concern to geographers. However, a major paradox is that, until recently, little more than lip-service had been paid to what might be claimed to be the prime (among many) parts of that relationship—those related to overt good health; that is Man's physical, mental and spiritual well-being.

Whilst, as we shall see later, there were some important earlier figures, two men dominated the English-speaking world of medical geography just after the war; Jacques May in the United States and Sir Dudley Stamp in England. The intention here is not to review their extensive and very different work but to pay tribute to their role as initiators. Some of their work reads today as truism, some is severely dated by the advances of later knowledge. None the less for students in the 1950s and even into the

GEOGRAPHICAL ASPECTS OF HEALTH
ISBN 0 12 483780 8

1960s there was little else devoted directly to human health in a spatial context.

These founding fathers handed down two principal themes. The major methodological concept of medical geography had regard to the place of risk in which some hazard of environment might be passively experienced by man. Secondly, they envisaged the concept, difficult to come to terms with, of total ecological risk. By this was meant study of man's active role in an environmental web which would vary minutely even at the micro scale from place to place.

Whilst such ideas seem simplistic today they formed, we believe, the beginnings of modern medical geography. It is not hard to see the line from Stamp's apparent determinism to possibilism which takes account of man's free will and then, later, to stochastic approaches which allow for the operation of chance in which only certain individuals of many at risk suffer actual ill-health.

Of course these lines of thought would in any case have led in many, widely different directions. That they arose contemporaneously with the quantitative revolution in geography and the arrival for scientific purposes of the first generation of computers vastly broadened their scope. It was only too natural that, in the absence of any particular unifying theme, medical geographers through the 1960s and 1970s developed their interests in a great variety of health-related directions.

Place of risk may be firstly concerned with the home but it obviously additionally subsumes place of work and place of recreation. It extends on all those fronts with changing family status as each place of risk varies through the Seven Ages of Man; from cradle, to school, to work-place and so on. Place of risk extends even more dramatically with travel, either as a tourist or as a migrant and, with ever-rising mobility, the numbers of people on the move are constantly and rapidly increasing. Thus the variety of separable personal environments occupied *seriatim* by any modern man leads to serious methodological and data problems.

Place of risk further subsumes both physical and social exposure to risk. The former has led to searches for optima in human physical environments, certainly most often recognized by their absence. The relationships between goitre and naturally occurring iodine from the geology of the parent rock, soil or water have been discussed by Learmonth (1978). A similar concept, often ascribed to Huntington (1945), from another physical science is that of optimum climate for human endeavour. Thermal stress implies fairly extreme temperature conditions deviating beyond the normal bodily tolerance of man. Yet there are still doubts about optimum conditions for his activities, doubts which stem from intra-species variation as well as from questions about symptoms acceptable as indicating thermal stress. Only when such questions have been answered can environmental conditions in artificially-controlled situations be selected on a basis of logic.

A second broad field of study of health-related interest is concerned with nutrition at either the physico-chemical level of what certain peoples eat or at the social awareness level of why we choose certain constituents to consider as food. Patterns of staple foodstuffs vary most evidently across our world and there is a coarse relationship in most cases with local agriculture—a point well made by May (1961). Again it is often extreme conditions which can be most easily recognized to produce overt ill-health, the endemic kwashiorkor and marasmus of many under-developed tropical lands. As well as basic deficiencies there are, of course, food-related dangers. These include hepatoxic substances like the naturally-occurring, mould-related aflatoxin of south-east Africa (McGlashan, 1982) as well as chemical carcinogens actually added to foods for colouring or preservative functions. Overall and given the ideal dietary situation, we still have little quantitative understanding of the relationships of bodily nutrient energy intake and output of labour. This deficiency has incalculable importance for estimating world needs for food (Edmundson, 1980) and has wide political and geo-political implications for man's future on earth.

The physical intake of particular chemicals in drinking water or potatoes is a further part of medical geographers' concern for human nutrition.

The asbestos industry illustrates many of these points. Reduced lung function from asbestosis or mesothelioma (diffuse malignant tumour formation in the chest cavity) may result from breathing even small quantities of crocidolite fibres (Bogovski et al., 1973). The miners are at first risk; so are their wives and families in homes where fibre-laden overalls are laundered. Then the residents of accommodation, shops or services down-wind of the mineral workings are at risk. Next come transportation workers by rail or ship and next the distant industrial workers in the consumer nations. Next in risk are the telephone linesmen or dockyard engineers who apply blue asbestos in lagging and fire-proofing installations. Finally in the chain of risk, is the ship's stoker or council house tenant who, all unsuspecting, lives and breathes in proximity to asbestos products. Although dangers to health from asbestos fibre were documented in the 1930s, legal restrictions on its use were generally not imposed until the 1960s and may still not be entirely effective. The peak of use, however, was probably during the years of the Second World War and, with a latent period of up to 40 years from exposure until clinical disease (by which time mesothelioma is invariably fatal), cases of asbestos-induced malignancy from those years are still on the increase (Jones *et al.*, 1976).

Social exposure is therefore not merely a question of person-to-person spread of infection but also of the groups of people liable to particular risks, whether schoolchildren, gaolbirds or factory workers confined together.

All of this adds up to very great internal diversity within medical geography. Variety arises in the disease of interest, in the region of study and in the scale, whether trans-regional, national, local or individual.

In attempting to portray the subject in 1983 we have therefore divided our approach into three parts. We begin with a number of review studies of the achievements of national groups of workers in the field, selected on the basis of representing endogenous streams of work major in terms of numbers involved and variety of work output. The rationale is that here is opportunity for the authors to trace and account for the development of the subject as it has occurred in specific national environments with each its particular needs and problems. This part of the book also lays claim to presenting a comprehensive cover not possible if only selected research areas were quoted. These selections become the second part.

The whole work opens with a biographical sketch of Andrew Learmonth by John Blunden who has been closely associated with Learmonth for some 12 years. Two facets of the chapter stand out. The charm and quiet friendliness of a man totally devoid of "side" has made him the acknowledged *guru* of medical geographers across the world. Secondly he has, over a lifetime in the field himself, the breadth which allows him to have useful comments to offer from his own experience on almost any medical geographical study under discussion.

Melvyn Howe and David Phillips give us the first national review, the United Kingdom from 1945 to 1982. Much that they say is, of course, common ground at world scale for they comment on both the values and the necessary limitations of a cartographic approach to health-related problems. Data is, contrariwise, related to ill-health or death more usually than to positive good health. The development of a sound medical diagnosis and recording system (see Kupka, 1978) was of crucial importance to the development in Britain of sophisticated means of defining and portraying spatial patterns of death and it is this which has tended to be thought of as the major British contribution to the subject. Whilst its influence has been great, Howe and Phillips show that other areas have not been neglected. They have interesting comments on both the theoretical and actual role of the National Health Service in a welfare framework.

Geomedicine in the German-speaking realm has, in contrast, in Professor Jusatz' chapter, a greater emphasis on an ecological holism. Paramount have been German scientists working abroad to build up the superb series of national geomedical monographs for countries in Africa and south-west Asia. In these volumes scholarship based on detailed local knowledge from real boot-leather geographical study and technology of colour cartographic presentation complement each other along lines going back over one hundred years.

Yola Verhasselt reviews for us the work of French and Benelux scientists in medical geography. Each of these metropolitan countries has also retained research interests in the tropics but perhaps the dominant theme (among many, very varied ones) has been the place of regional studies of ill-health, both in rural and in urban areas. In France especially it is tempting to perceive such studies as continuing the elegant form and tradition of Vidal de la Blache!

Gerald Pyle provides the next review, that for the United States, and it is of such scale as to be nearer continental than national in its coverage. Of course mortality studies are not neglected but there is no doubt that the major American thrust in medical geography has been in health care studies. De Vise' 1969 study of Chicago's "apartheid" system of care characterizes the inequity by which the poor have been under-served at every level; geographical access, freedom of choice, quality of care. Because the problems are on so vast a scale the medical geographer in the US has perforce become political apologist for those deprived within the world's richest nation.

Canada as a neighbour has been much influenced by US developments in medical geography. She has in addition received streams of thought directly from Britain and France. Thouez convincingly demonstrates an emerging Canadian identity, especially in academic courses and teaching, with disproportionately strong numbers of well-qualified young workers coming forward.

Indian work in medical geography has recently been displayed at two major meetings—the IGU Congress at New Delhi in 1968 and the IGU Regional Symposium in Madras in 1981. In his chapter, Professor Ramesh brings these and other indigenous works together into a coherent form. The dominant impression is of Indian scientists, usually young, underfunded and often on individual initiatives, trying to put their spatial training to work in the service of a desperately poor country. Many of these studies descend directly in terms of method from the British spatial distribution school and, in India, what may be lost in diagnostic or recording accuracy is made up for by the vast scale of case numbers.

Finally in the review section Mansell Prothero, considering medical geography in tropical Africa, demonstrates the combination of an ecological with a spatial definitional approach needed for tropical disease amelioration. At the same time, where finance is endemically in short supply, geographical rationalization of health services is even more than usually important.

We had hoped to include in this review part of the volume a chapter from the Soviet Union. Unfortunately invitations to several Soviet and Comecon scholars have not been taken up and one can feel only sadness that open contacts so promisingly begun in Moscow at the IGU congress in 1976 are not being here maintained. Whilst one cannot here do justice to the scale and breadth of Soviet efforts in medical geography as revealed at that meeting, certain emphases can be noted.

Medical geography in the USSR has had a long and distinguished role in the service of the State. Human health has long been regarded there as intrinsic to studies of population and this has been allied with an ecological approach to disease vector distribution and with an economic, even industrial, slant far removed from simple determinism. The subject has been far more development oriented. Given particular conditions of environment, including naturally occurring disease vectors, what use can be made by man of this place? One clear example of the approach comes from far-east Asia where it was proposed to re-route a railway alignment. Geographical studies of the health implications for construction workers and for travellers on the line were carried out prior to any building at all. Health-planning in this sense of foreseeing potential environmental risks seems to be a field in which the West has (still) much to learn—especially perhaps in instances of major irrigation development proposals.

Soviet geographers at the Moscow meeting were clearly out of sympathy with, for example, the North Americans with regard to mechanistic studies of health facility locations at local level where, in America at least, uneven opportunity is overtly displayed. In Russia this falls within the realm of State Planning and consequently offers no potential for academic study or improvement.

A second country omitted from the reviews is Australia on the quite different grounds that a close equivalent has already and recently been published. At quite the opposite pole for population numbers from the USSR, in Australia the growth of interest in health geography is both recent and varied. A 1980 collection of work from Australia and New Zealand (McGlashan, 1980) illustrates the dual flows of ideas into these countries. There is a group of British-type distributional-cum-correlational approaches to ill-health with, for example, a study of the relationship between trachoma among Aborigines and their outrageous living conditions. Secondly, the American-type facility maldistribution group of studies includes national policy issues in New Zealand both with regard to emphases on different parts of the facilities spectrum and questions of future supply of medical staff. Thirdly, there are signs of a distinctly practical down-to-earth truly Australian approach which may be caricatured from Brownlea's tub-thumping, "Well, what are we going to *do* about demonstrable inequity?" (Brownlea, 1981).

It is not the intention to imply that other countries have produced no work in the geography of health. However, it is probably fair to suggest that up to date—and the position is changing rapidly—involvement has been limited. For example, Mme Momiyama-Sakamoto at Tokyo's Institute of Meteorology has had a lifetime's interest in seasonal variations of mortality both in her own country and abroad, culminating in a major treatment of the subject (Momiyama-Sakamoto, 1977). Her work has, moreover, sparked energetic interest in a number of younger Japanese scientists of a variety of disciplines whose papers were read at the Tokyo meetings of the International Geographic Union in 1980 (Learmonth, 1981). Examples of work from Latin America too can already be quoted both on parasite ecology (Ward, 1972) and on mathematical modelling of smallpox outbreaks (Angulo *et al.*, 1977) and no doubt more will be published from the IGU regional meetings in Brazil in 1982.

South Africa has had a geographical approach to its medical research dating from before the Second World War. Öettlé's (1964) and Robertson's (1971) endeavours offer typical examples. Besides Japanese atlases of disease mortality (1980 and Shigematsu, 1981) China too has published an atlas of cancer mortality (1981). Two points about the latter atlas can be made which illustrate the general value of such geographical publications. Each cancer had its own distribution with implied relationships varying over the vast land mass and enormous population. Secondly, each map "shows that the trends of cancer mortality in neighbouring regions between provinces were not influenced by the man-made boundaries of administrative units, organizations of the survey, or differences in diagnosis and treatment". More specifically this atlas clearly defines the extraordinary and fascinating patterns of oesophageal cancer in China (see also McGlashan, 1982).

Examples of geographical studies could be quoted from many other lands and it is frequently difficult—and probably immaterial—to distinguish between indigenous workers and overseas scientists visiting or assisting in projects.

Part Two of this volume is concerned with discrete studies of some of the major health problems of our world today. Each is chosen to show the relevance of a geographical approach. Michael Greenberg opens the section with a consideration of environmental toxicology. Whilst his chapter concentrates upon the US experience of the problems of waste disposal, occupational exposure to toxic substances is on the increase worldwide and, of course, many of the harmful effects are covert, insidious and irreversible. The author draws largely on his own wide experience of planning to minimize toxic hazards in a high risk industrial area and outlines appropriate roles for geographers in designing programmes to counter these environmental hazards.

In the next chapter Melinda Meade takes up at a local scale the geographical question of spatially varying patterns of cardiovascular disease. As with other geographical studies which "home in" on a particular area of disease anomaly, the answers have wider relevance if general "laws" can be recognized from them. Meade develops a model to take account of the myriad of factors which co-vary with heart disease. This leads to her recognition in Savannah city of typical housing areas of high risk.

There are some similarities with John Giggs' approach to schizophrenia in Nottingham. As a contribution to ecological psychiatry, the author is able to define a spatial framework within the city with strong statistical links with the disorder. His argument relates to the "breeder" hypothesis implying environmental influence upon ill-health rather than the "drift" of already affected individuals into specific environmental circumstances.

From a completely contrasted, because rural, environment comes Sheila Bain's study of health care problems in far north-west Scotland. She demonstrates the close interweave between facilities and transportation, the measure so often glossed over as "access", but also points out the very real expenditure difficulties faced by socialized medicine even with the best will to serve thinly scattered small communities of people.

Whilst there is no direct change from developed to less-developed realm in health matters the next two chapters are a contrast in looking at behaviour patterns in those two zones. Brian Heenan considers the smoking habits of New Zealanders and demonstrates not only the significant variations within the nation but also the considerable opportunities for intervention which this definition provides. Robert Roundy, on the other hand, provides a comparative study of behaviour as it relates to parasite infestation loads in villagers in Malaysia. The central question is whether particular community habits with regard to water use and hygiene do or do not increase the disease burden. Here the author demonstrates the value of varying scales of study—down to the individual—to assess such matters.

Hella Wellmer continues this picture of the disease spectrum in the less developed world with an account of geographical efforts to define the space–time spread of dengue haemorrhagic fever in Thailand. The utility of computer mapping over time sequences and the role of man himself in the ecology of the mosquito vector are convincingly exemplified.

Lastly in this section, and in a sense, pulling together several disparate threads from the less developed world, Tony Hellen gives us a study of Nepal. The background of the epidemiological transition is sketched within that spatial context and the implications especially for health but also for development planning generally are drawn out. Analogies with other developing countries are implicit and the chapter sums up much of the health-related dilemma of the world—better health care and improved survival leads to increasing proportions of elderly and consequently to greater personal and national economic dependency.

Part Three is slightly different in kind. A small group of chapters, each deliberately brief, suggest some thinking ahead in this subject. In general terms each has, as its objective, emphasis on the creative use of statistical approaches to solving health-related environmental problems. Robert Stimson evaluates for us the methods, statistics and pitfalls encountered in medical geography to date. He provides a rational do-it-yourself kit of "do's and dont's" and makes a plea for greater unity of approach within the subject. Whether such internal unity is valuable *per se* is not debated but, at least, the subject would be more clearly distinguishable and recognizable by other scientists.

Andrew Cliff and Peter Haggett next offer a concise and readable account which summarises much of their work on the spatial diffusion of epidemic waves. The understanding of such phenomena has important potential for the erection of public health barriers to disease spread and the theoretical background is of far wider relevance than to only the specific disease, measles, studied in the specific spatial context, Iceland.

Neil McGlashan and Graham Giles both suggest greater use of methods not much employed in medical geography to date and each employs a chosen method with conviction upon real data sets. McGlashan employs cluster analysis to seek similarities between geographical patterns of ill-health, predominantly cancers. The implication is that certain environments will contain risk factors affecting more than one bodily site—perhaps, for example, an ingested substance affecting several parts of the total digestive tract. Particular areas too may exhibit similarities or contrasts between the overall constellations of their disease patterns. Giles urges greater use of the relative risk calculation based on case-control individual questionnaires rather than community-wide data. He then uses this method to evaluate Hodgkin's Disease in Tasmania. His message is perhaps that medical geographers should be alert to possibilities of learning or developing methods by analogy from other disciplines. By coincidence (rather than collusion!) one such study using relative risk appeared as he wrote and in time to reinforce his plea (McGlashan *et al.*, 1982). In their study these authors demonstrate the gradients of relative risk in the use of alcohol and especially of tobacco (especially if used in pipes) among regions of Transkei with previously defined and significant differences of oesophageal cancer incidence.

The theme of implacable environmental retribution for human mis-use recurs in many individual chapters without, we hope, giving a hopeless or fatalist flavour to the whole. Rather let us recognize that we ourselves have a duty to exert ourselves not to be indifferent to the environment which, in so many ways, nurtures the human race.

References

Angulo, J. J., Haggett, P., Megale, P. and Pederneiras, C. A. A. (1977). Variola Minor in Braganca Paulista County, 1956: A trend surface analysis. *American J. Epidemiology* **105**, 272–280.

Atlas of Cancer Mortality in the People's Republic of China (1981). Peking.

Atlas of Lung and Liver Disease Mortality in Japan, 1969–74 (1980). Daiwa Health Foundation, Tokyo.

Bogovski, P., Gilson, J. C., Timbrell, V. and Wagner, J. C. (1973). Biological effects of asbestos. IARC Scientific Publication No. 8, Lyon, 1973.

Brownlea, A. A. (1981). From public health to political epidemiology *Soc. Sci. Med.* **15D**, 57–68.

De Vise, P. (1969). Slum Medicine: Chicago's Apartheid Health System. Report No. 6. InterUniversity Social Research Committee, University of Chicago.

Edmundson, W. (1980). Adaption to undernutrition. *Soc. Sci. Med.* **14D**, 119–126.

Huntington, E. (1945). *Mainsprings of Civilization*. Wiley, New York.

Jones, J. S. P., Pooley, F. D. and Smith, P. G. (1976). Factory populations exposed to crocidolite asbestos. *INSERM* **52**, 117–120.

Kupka, K. (1978). International classification of diseases, ninth revision. *WHO Chronicle* **32**, 219–225.

Learmonth, A. T. A. (1978). *Patterns of Disease and Hunger*. David and Charles, Newton Abbot.

Learmonth, A. T. A. (Ed.) (1981). The geography of health. *Soc. Sci. Med.* **15D**, 1–262.

May, J. M. (1958). *The Ecology of Human Disease*. M.D. Publications, New York.

May, J. M. (Ed.) (1961). *Studies in the Ecology of Malnutrition*. Hafner, New York.

McGlashan, N. D. (Ed.) (1980). Health problems in Australia and New Zealand. *Soc. Sci. Med.* **14D**, 81–269.

McGlashan, N. D. (1982). Environmental detectives probe riddle of cancer. *Geogrl. Mag.* **54**, 263–267.

McGlashan, N. D. (1982). Primary liver cancer and food-based toxins: A Swaziland review. *Ecology of Disease* **1**, 37–44.

McGlashan, N. D., Bradshaw, E. and Harington, J. S. (1982). Cancer of the oesophagus and the use of tobacco and alcoholic beverages in Transkei, 1975–76. *Int. J. Cancer* **29**, 249–256.

Öettlé, A. G. (1964). Cancer in Africa, especially in regions south of the Sahara. *J. nat. Cancer Inst.* **33**, 383, 439.

Robertson, M. A., Harington, J. S. and Bradshaw, E. (1971). Observations on cancer patterns among Africans in South Africa. *Brit. J. Cancer* **25**, 377–402.

Sakamoto-Momiyama, M. (1977). *Seasonality in Human Mortality*. University of Tokyo Press, Tokyo.

Shigematsu, I. (1981). *National Atlas of Major Disease Mortalities in Japan*. Japan Health Promotion Foundation, Tokyo.

Stamp, L. D. (1964). *The Geography of Life and Death*. London.

Ward, J. S. (1972). Yellow Fever in Latin America: A Geographical Study. Centre for Latin America Studies Monograph No. 3. University of Liverpool.

Part One

Andrew Learmonth and the evolution of medical geography—A personal memoir of a career

John R. Blunden

Faculty of Social Sciences, The Open University,
Milton Keynes, England

Andrew Thomas Amos Learmonth was born in Edinburgh in 1916, the second son of a father who was a solicitor practising in that city and a mother of hardy, colourful lowland stock.

At Boroughmuir School he had the usual secondary school education current in Scotland between the Wars, built as it was on a broad academic base and designed to imbue those who embraced it with a sound cultural background and the wherewithal to enter one of the safer, more secure professions. Although it would be convenient to believe that it was this background that led him to comprehend the value of a career in banking, it would be wide of the mark. The truth is that he would have liked to emulate the academic success of his elder brother George at university where his first class homours degree in chemistry had taken him on to complete his PhD. Andrew's particular proclivities would have undoubtedly led him in the direction of the medical profession. But the training was long, unemployment high and the future uncertain. With his brother unable to find work, in spite of his training, his parents decided that irrespective of his own wishes, Andrew should seize the offer of a bank apprenticeship without even remaining at school long enough to take his Higher Leaving Certificate. Accordingly, he left school in 1933 to enter the service of the Bank of Scotland at the South Morningside branch in Edinburgh for the handsome salary of £40 per year. During his four-year apprenticeship Andrew moved to a number of branches—all in the Edinburgh area—because it was the Bank's policy, having regard to the limited salary paid to its young trainees, to keep them near their own

GEOGRAPHICAL ASPECTS OF HEALTH
ISBN 0 12 483780 8

homes! At this time he also embarked upon evening classes at Heriot Watt College leading to the examination for the membership of the Institute of Bankers in Scotland. Apart from an early taste of the pains and pleasures of part-time higher education which would ultimately feed back into his later career, the Institute's examination also provided him with his first real opportunity to study geography, though largely of the George Chisholm commercial variety. In this class alone he gained top marks and a medal, ultimately being awarded "honours" for his overall results.

However, having now clearly and successfully established a certain bent for work of a more academic kind he immediately looked for further fields of study but related to his imposed career. In those days, practically the only graduates in the employment of Scottish Banks were a handful of officials who had taken the degree of Bachelor of Law at one or other of the Scottish Universities concurrently with their work in the Bank's Legal Departments. Not surprisingly, and perhaps particularly in view of his fathers' vocation, this was the course on which he set his sights, but as attendance at the University law classes did to some extent cut across the working day, the Bank's permission had to be obtained—and this was not just a matter of form. However, after a long spell of persistent pressure on the appropriate department, he was at last authorized, in the light of his earlier outstanding results, to go ahead. But the 1939–45 War was imminent and instead of beginning his studies at Edinburgh University, he joined the Territorial Army choosing to serve with a local Field Ambulance Unit of the Royal Army Medical Corps, certainly a response to his long standing interest in all matters medical as well as his deep humanitarian concerns.

His six years of war service began in earnest with a number of UK postings and a short spell in France immediately prior to Dunkirk. By 1941 he had become a sergeant and was posted to India to serve for nearly four years in hospitals in Ranchi and Calcutta as a chief clerk. The work was hard and made more onerous by both a rebellion of the Indian forces in August 1942 and, a year later, a famine in Bengal. By the time he reached the second of his postings, he was in charge of the administration of five separate hospitals. Yet he also combined this immense task with the role of chief organizer of welfare, entertainment and educational facilities for the Indian and British troops in Calcutta and the editorship of his Unit's newspaper. Although he finished the war as a Quartermaster Sergeant (a much deserved commission had been impossible because of the rules prevailing in India at the time), his stay there had proved personally hugely satisfying. Apart from his work he had made several life-long friends, had undertaken two treks through the Himalayas and was able to say that he "enjoyed the war far more than anyone had a right to". Though his sojourn in India can best be described as the result of pure chance, from it there emerged two key strands in his subsequent life—a deep and abiding fascination for that sub-continent and the beginnings of an interest in the spatial aspects of disease.

With his return to Edinburgh in 1946, the world that he had known had changed markedly. Now there were opportunities in abundance for ex-servicemen to undertake university courses on a full-time basis, and so instead of returning to banking and the possibility of a long slow haul towards a legal qualification, he decided to become a full-time student. In the light of his banking experience it seemed logical to offer himself for a course in economics, but after discussions with the Director of Studies at Edinburgh University who persuaded him that he was far too old at 30 to commence studies in an area of such erudition, he was pushed uncere-moniously in the direction of that "soft option", geography. It was only after an interview with Professor A. G. Ogilvie that Andrew began to see that geography was not just about "capes and bays" as he had thought at school, or "the geographical facts relating to commerce" as his experience at Heriot Watt might have persuaded him, but a discipline which he could study with a real sense of enthusiastic intellectual conviction.

This decision was particularly fortunate in that he was not only an undergraduate with Mansell Prothero who subsequently became a close friend and a colleague at Liverpool University (where he is now Professor and head of the Department of Geography), but he became a student of the inimitable (and some would say impossible) Arthur Geddes. It was the latter who undoubtedly further stimulated and extended Andrew's latent interests in the human and regional geography of India. Few students could, or were prepared to make much of Geddes, whose genetic inheritance from the great Patrick Geddes was combined with exposure to Celtic mysticism and the mystique of India. Andrew, with his greater maturity and what his professor was to later describe as "a critical comprehension considerably in advance of even most ex-service students", proved to be a notable exception and although Geddes did not specifically teach medical geography (there were no such specialisms taught at that time), his mentor's concern for the people of India and his interests in the regional change and variability of population in the sub-continent undoubtedly involved a regard for health and disease among other influencing factors.

By the time Andrew graduated in 1949, and graduated with first class honours, he had fully embraced the undoubted freedom and intellectual stimulation that academic life could offer. Apart from the fact that for the first time he had begun to stretch his mental capabilities to the full, the possibility of pursuing a career in commerce was now far from attractive. The ultra-conservative Scottish banking system had steadfastly adhered to its pre-war traditions; staff could not marry without their employer's permission and that was not willingly given to persons until their late twenties. Moreover, with little chance to prove oneself before the age of 30, the total prospect was indeed quite unpallatable. So he would marry Nancy, the girl he had come to know as President of the Edinburgh University Geographical Society whilst he had been Secretary and look around for an academic post at an university. The latter he found in Liverpool and was appointed as an assistant lecturer in 1950.

Although this move was ultimately to bring him back into a working relationship with his undergraduate friend Mansell Prothero, there were other aspects of that university that would prove crucial in the development of Andrew's interests—most notably the Liverpool School of Tropical Medicine both through its academic staff and its very fine library. Perhaps most significant of all was the fact that the Chair in Tropical Hygiene at the Liverpool School was then held by the late Professor T. H. Davey. Davey was a man of wide perspectives, particularly for a medical man of his generation, who in his work in the tropics had come to appreciate the complex man–environment interrelationships in health and disease. He recognized the contribution that other disciplines might make to the understanding of these relationships and encouraged Andrew who was more than willing to work on the medical geography of the Indian sub-continent, which with the completion of his PhD (a regional study of survival, mortality and disease in India), had by then become the major imperative of his academic research. Indeed, it was at this time that Andrew was co-opted as a corresponding member by the IGU Commission on Medical Geography to join with his Edinburgh mentor, Arthur Geddes, in the development of work relating to the medical geography of Asia. This was to be part of an agreed approach to the problems of stimulating research in the field on a continental basis amongst what was then a relatively small and dispersed population of medical geographers.

Davey apart, there were, on his home ground, other encouraging contacts with members of the Liverpool School, among them Professor Brian Megraith, now Dean Emeritus. But whilst the fructifying inter-change of ideas between a burgeoning medical geographer and the medical staff of the School became increasingly worthwhile and easy at a personal level, it was difficult for him to move beyond this in terms of the formal recognition of his professional skills. Even after publishing part of his research work in the School's Annals of Tropical Medicine and Parasitology in 1954, Andrew was not accorded the true accolade of being asked to lecture in the School. A similar experience befell Mansell Prothero who in 1955 returned from Nigeria to work at Liverpool. Mansell's increasing interest in medical geography, largely a product of Andrew's influence, eventually led him in the 1960s to undertake a number of consultancies for the World Health Organization. In spite of such prestigious activities and his efforts to build and develop the contacts initiated by Andrew within the School, he was equally spurned by it in this one respect. However, in spite of this disappointing aspect of the relationship, undoubtedly the School was for Andrew an enormously positive force in the development of his career as a medical geographer in the 1950s and its ultimate flowering. The excellence of his work of this period, and in particular the monograph based on his doctoral thesis and papers related to the Indian sub-continent, bear witness to this.

Indeed the 1958 publication of an edition of the Indian Geographical Journal devoted entirely to his regional study of survival, mortality and disease in Indo-Pakistan over the period 1921–1940 has been described as a milestone in the development of medical geography as a recognized branch of the discipline. Such distinction was achieved not only as a result of its presentation of maps which were statistically and carto-graphically advanced, but also because as a generalized regionalization of health and disease, it was derived in an imaginative and novel format. From the start this work is redolent of his clear understanding of the value of the subject in practical and human terms; it is no mere exercise in data manipulation but the thoughtful interpretation of distributions and trends which can result in a better comprehension of diseases and related phenomena, and lead ultimately to the relief of human suffering. As one of Andrew's younger colleagues in the field has said of this work

> when he discusses the limitations of the data, the reader obtains an inspiring picture of the problems and prospects of working in medical geography at such an early and exciting stage of its 'modern' development and can appreciate the advances to the subject brought about by this research.

But if the very nature of the quantitative data available to Andrew as a medical geographer had led him towards a practical concern for the use of statistical techniques in his own research, it had also led him to realize their value in the wider field of human geography and to the student of the discipline. Thus with Stan Gregory, a Liverpool colleague, he began to develop one of the first undergraduate courses in a geography depart-ment which aimed at providing "a grounding in a variety of basic methods, all of which were developed, and applied in terms of geographi-cal problems". Not surprisingly Gregory later paid generous tribute to Andrew in the preface to his book *Statistical Methods and the Geographer* in the realization that this work, later to become classic in the field, owed much to their course and their many valuable exchanges about its content and its teaching.

Towards the end of this decade Andrew's association with India in terms of his research as a medical geographer and his on-going concern for regional studies, took him, one day, to hear a discussion at the Royal Geographical Society in which Professor P. C. Mahalanobis, head of the Indian Statistical Institute was a participant. Andrew was immediately impressed with his personality and his towering intellect and sought him out afterwards. There followed a late night meeting at the hotel at which Mahalanobis was staying in which it is said that Andrew could do no more than listen with awe, and occasionally interject "yes", "no" or "I don't believe it". However, he must have impressed the great man for that meeting led to an invitation to spend two years in the sub-continent working at the Indian Statistical Institute under the auspices of the Colombo Plan and to contribute towards India's Third Five Year Plan. Andrew accepted with alacrity but not merely because of the likely congeniality of the work he had been offered. Following the untimely death of the distinguished economic geographer Wilfred Smith with whom he had enjoyed a close rapport, his professional life in the Department of Geography at Liverpool had lost some of its zest.

Andrew's particular brief at the Institute in Calcutta was to inject a geographical component into the activities of the Institute with particular emphasis upon the task of developing work in the field of regional planning. With the aid of a small but powerful team to assist him, including his wife, V. L. S. Prakash Rao (now a professor at the Indian Institute of Management) and L. S. Bhat, he began a regional survey of Mysore State (now part of Karnatak) with special reference to its most backward area of Malnadu. The recommendations of the team were accepted by the State Government but more importantly, with the experience gained from this task force behind him, Andrew set about establishing a permanent body within the Institute to undertake work of a similar kind, the Regional Survey Unit. Now very much an established force under the highly effective direction of L. S. Bhat, it works in close association with the Planning Commission of the Government of India.

But in spite of his commitment during this stay in India to work of an essentially regional planning kind, Andrew did not neglect his concern for his specialism, medical geography. Concurrent with his work in India he prepared a number of papers largely dealing with the sub-continent, the most significant of which was his already referred to spatial study of 20 years data pertaining to health matters in what he termed Indo-Pakistan. At the same time (and since) he was doing much to stimulate a greater interest and concern for his own special interest amongst Indian academics. As Professor C. D. Deshpande of the Centre for Regional Development at Jawaharlal Nehru University puts it:

> He has greatly advanced our knowledge of diseases and epidemics of the sub-continent over the pioneer work of Ross and others. Besides encouraging medical geography in Rajputana, Uttar Pradesh and South India Universities, his bibliography of the contributions to the medical geography of the sub-continent has become a basic source of reference.

At the time of his initial stay in India under the Colombo Plan and during his subsequent visits, Andrew's contacts with Indian geographers have been "wide and deeply sustaining". Indeed, another distinguished ex-colleague of Andrew's speaking about his association with India has expressed the view that the quality of theses in medical geography emanating from that country "owes not a little to Andrew's pioneering efforts".

On his return to Liverpool after a happy and fulfilling two years, Andrew's contacts with India remained strong and in 1962 he was appointed honorary consultant to the Indian Statistical Institute. Although he was quickly promoted from lecturer to senior lecturer and soon established as Professor Robert Steel's "No. 2" in the department, Andrew's stay in north-west England was to be short-lived, for in the late summer of that same year an invitation came to accept the foundation chair in geography in the School of General Studies of the Australian National University in Canberra, an invitation which arrived whilst he was recovering from a vaguely defined tropical disease collected on an International Geographic Union regional conference in Malaysia! Although acceptance in itself would mean a heavy burden of administration and teaching perhaps over a wide range within the boundaries of an ever expanding discipline, the challenge was irresistible. In the five week voyage by sea to Australia with his family, Andrew therefore recreated himself each day in the officer's dining room by reading volumes on regional science and what his wife has cryptically described as "a monumental work by Isard".

Both Andrew and his family quickly settled into their new country and its society, their liking for which was evident from the beginning. That they seemed able to understand Australia and its people in an amazingly short time is surely reflected in the books which Andrew, in collaboration with his wife Nancy, quickly began to work upon, most notably *Regional Landscapes of Australia*. Much less easy was the task which faced Andrew at Canberra in his professional role. To begin with the Geography Department turned out to be housed in temporary buildings, a warren of war-time Nissen huts on the edge of the campus which suffered from seasonal extremes of temperature plus the additional hazard of "big, noisy, muscular blowflies" throughout the summers. Not surprisingly a good deal of his early period at the Australian National University was involved in the planning of the purpose-built premises to which they would ultimately move. This he did through the long, hot summers with the manifest ease of a desert campaigner dressed in "baggy shorts and a blue T-shirt". However, one irksome problem for a man devoted to high standards of teaching and research lay in the fact that there always seemed to be funds available for the physical and tangible accoutrements of academic endeavour though much less for meaningful projects and personnel.

But perhaps the real problems which confronted Andrew throughout his period of tenure stemmed from the history of the School of General Studies, because this was the successor to the Canberra University College of the University of Melbourne. Its attachment to the Australian National University at the time of Andrew's appearance on the scene, had been described as a shot-gun marriage. The relationship between the School of General Studies and the Australian National University, which had hitherto consisted of relatively prestigious but loose collections of research schools, frequently reflected the resentments inevitably inherent in such a union. The latter viewed the former as somewhat poor relatives—which is indeed what they were in terms of access to power and therefore to resources. Andrew really did disapprove strongly of this antagonism between the two parts of the University, and, from his own Indian experience, the suggestion of a caste-distinction which he seemed to detect in the local atmosphere. Indeed he often referred to the Institute of Advanced Studies as the Taj Mahal and no doubt thought of his own more modest area as the Bustees!

Characteristically Andrew drew what satisfaction he could from his relationship with his students at all levels. His approach in taking up his new and first professorial appointment was clearly influenced by his recollections of his own professor at Edinburgh, A. G. Ogilvie. One very significant aspect of his attitude was that students should, from their first days at university, be taught by their professor. Andrew emulated this policy, though when combined with the desire to teach in informal seminar groups rather than in conventional lectures, it led to a very heavy teaching commitment.

As at Liverpool, Andrew again tried to build bridges to other disciplines and faculties, particularly at the research level where experience had taught him more success might accrue. Indeed, at this time he was never more convinced of the value of bringing to specific research topics a wide range of inter-disciplinary expertise. Thus it was at post-graduate level rather than undergraduate course work, that links were achieved, mainly with the Geology Department and some of the Research Schools. At the same time, with the agreement of Oskar Spate, his opposite number in the National Institution and with whom he had been associated during his work with the Indian Statistical Institute, he also encouraged the presentation of short courses by Spate's post-graduates in his own new department. On a more personal basis he ultimately played an essential part in the preparation of the third revised edition of Spate's regional geography of *India and Pakistan*.

Certainly the most rewarding aspect of his work at the Australian National University was his contact with a very sizeable body of part-time adult students, whose presence within the University student body in the 1960s was very characteristic of higher education in Australia. Perhaps his rapport with them was to some extent the result of his own late entry into academic geography. Those with whom he came into contact, often in the Government service in Canberra and working for a degree in their own time, impressed him with their maturity of approach and strong dedication to learning. The tutorials he had with such people, "the old men's tea parties" as he affectionately called them, gave him a good deal of stimulus and satisfaction and foreshadowed his subsequent attraction and commitment to the Open University.

Towards the end of the Canberra period, yet more administrative duties fell to Andrew; in 1966 he assumed the mantle of Convenor for the National Committee for Geography of the Australian Academy of Sciences and then a year later his essential fair mindedness and lack of "side" was recognized by his peers in his election to Dean of the Faculty of Arts, a task which he undertook with credit. Yet throughout he maintained and strengthened his research in the field of medical geography. This could not have been other than fostered by his involvement with the International Geographical Union Commission on Medical Geography which had commenced in 1954, and of which he had become chairman in 1964, and by his six months study leave taken at the Liverpool School of Tropical Medicine where he renewed his interests in malaria. But perhaps most notably during his period at the Australian National University he worked for several years on Australian mortality data, ultimately publishing work in 1965 concerning the mapping of standardized mortality ratios for the country over the period 1959–1963. Four years later he published a similar study covering the years 1965–1966 in which he was not only able to make methodological improvements, but by re-examining the earlier mortality ratios he introduced a comparative element to demonstrate spatial changes. At the same time further publications on health and disease in the Indian sub-continent appeared along with review articles on statistical sampling in relation to geographical studies, fresh versions of the regional geography of India and Pakistan written with Oskar Spate, and at a less academic level, the two volumes on Australia written with his wife Nancy.

By 1969 we find Andrew at the peak of his academic powers, in middle age and with a wealth of senior administrative experience behind him, an excellent research record and a clear penchant for adult students, perhaps looking for one more challenging experience to round off a career. It was perhaps a happy coincidence that the newly appointed Vice Chancellor of the Open University, Dr. Walter Perry (now Lord Perry of Walton), should have met Andrew at a Vice Chancellor's Conference in Australia and realized that here was a man ideally qualified and suited for appointment to a senior position in a new university whose aims were related entirely to the education of mature students. The post of Professor of Geography in the Faculty of Social Science was therefore offered and accepted. On his departure his department in Canberra presented him with the volume *The Voyage of Governor Philip to Botany Bay* in which was aptly inscribed the following: "To Professor, who with unmatched success, came and founded an establishment in the colonies and leaves with our affection and best wishes". Certainly the consensus view amongst his colleagues at Canberra was that by the time of his return to Britain, despite the difficulties inherent in the ANU situation, he had created an admirably staffed and cohesively structured Geography Department.

Although it was no part of Andrew's new task to found a department as such—indeed his role in the egalitarian hot house of the Open University as a geographer may best be described as a disciplinary *primus inter pares*—none the less the 1970s can surely be considered as the most testing of all his career. This is because, as a senior appointment, he was looked to for the demonstration of powers of imagination, inventiveness, entrepreneurial skill and leadership in the formulation and articulation of the aims and objectives of a complete Faculty of Social Science. It was a Faculty whose credibility would be tested in the quality and the range of its disciplinary and interdisciplinary courses, all of which would be placed on open view before the world and published as teaching texts and television and radio programmes for anyone to appraise favourably or otherwise. It was an environment where there were no precedents— merely a collection of youngish academics determined to succeed in their task, if only to prove the academic establishment wrong in viewing the University as a brash six-day wonder which would, comet-like fade and die as rapidly as it had appeared in the academic firmament.

That Andrew was equal to the challenge is beyond doubt. He played a

major role in evolving and producing the first inter-disciplinary foundation course, the basis for all other studies within the Faculty, and
eventually took on the responsibilities of chairman of the academic team
preparing its replacement. Then after the initial but exhausting period of
creative activity the first Dean of the Faculty of Social Science decided to
stand down and Andrew was prevailed upon to take over the reins from
1972 to 1974. In the preparation of teaching texts he was to be active in the
first two geography courses offered by the Faculty at second and third
levels of study as well as contributing to the first replacement of its second
level offering. The renewal of its third level course has been very much in
Andrew's hands with one of the three projects on offer to the students by
the course designed to reflect his own interest in spatial variations in the
provision of health care. But not least has been his concern for the
development of part-time post-graduate research at the University. Here
he has, by example, encouraged other members of his discipline to have
a full commitment in this direction. Apart from giving his time fully and
freely to the supervision of his students, he has played a leading role in
annual seminars designed to assist in the solution of the problems that
the part-time research worker may face.

However, in spite of all the demands made upon an academic within a
university essentially creating its own teaching materials and making its
own very distinctive imprint on higher education, Andrew's research
and publications record has remained undiminished. During the 1970s
he has shown an increasing concern with the resurgence of malaria,
especially in India, and the characteristics of its spatial diffusion and a
number of papers have appeared reflecting this. In 1978 he had published
a major work *Patterns of Disease and Hunger*, a book primarily concerned
with examining and accounting for significant differences in health
patterns in both the developed and developing countries and has edited
others including *The Geography of Health*, arising from the papers presented in Tokyo at the IGU symposium of 1980. But as if to bring the
wheel full circle, he has recently played a major part in the preparation for
publication of a text on which his undergraduate tutor at Edinburgh,
Arthur Geddes, was working at the time of his death in 1967. Together
with his wife and his former Indian colleagues C. D. Deshpande and L. S.
Bhat, he has been responsible for selecting and assembling material
which under the title *Man and Land in South Asia* considers the inter-
relationship between the natural environment and the people in the
Indian sub-continent. Much of the rest of his output has involved him in
the preparation of broad reviews of main currents in the developing tide
of medical geography, contributions which he somewhat dismissively
describes as "elder statesman efforts". In this he is being less than fair to

his own wealth of experience and to those who naturally see him as a key figure in the evolution of medical geography, not only because of his academic work but also because of the leadership he has shown in the development and sponsorship of research through the IGU Commission on Medical Geography. Indeed, in his 12 years as chairman he put his authority behind the identification of a specific range of tasks to be undertaken by the Commission, relating first to the preparation of atlases based on standardized mortality ratios and with an increasing concern for morbidity mapping, studies of single disease aimed at in-depth causal analysis, studies of the geography of genes, the use of modelling as a technique, and the promotion of work involving regional synthesis.

In more recent years he has backed work upon the geography of nutrition, the achievement of a composite index of community health, the preparation of a syllabus for the training of medical geographers and the geographical aspects of pollution. He has also been active in the promotion of regional congresses outside the meetings of the Union and perhaps most significant of all, he has been the motive force behind the initiation of a newsletter, published three times a year, aimed at promoting exchanges of ideas and methodological approaches between research workers in the field, the dissemination of selected bibliographical material, exchanges on the nature and role of medical geography and the purposeful instruction of its practitioners.

To his credit he has appreciated the dangers of prematurely attempting to achieve a coherent programme of collaborative research on a worldwide basis in spite of the fact that there are "a number of pockets of intense activity" with "increasing powers of problem solving" and "a sophistication in methodology". For him whilst "many workers in this still small field, particularly in under-developed countries are rather isolated", the value of the Commission as a forum of liaison and information exchange has been paramount. It is no small wonder then that one of his senior colleagues, Professor Melvyn Howe, has been aptly able to say of him as his career reaches its end "Andrew and medical geography are virtually synonymous".

But if his writings and his work with the IGU Commission remain a testament to his contribution to medical geography (though those with whom he has worked in this field know that they only tell part of the story), how shall we remember his 12 years with the Open University? Certainly for much more than the mere record of courses chaired, administrative tasks conducted, unit texts written. We shall recall his positive virtues—his capacity to see some ray of hope in the most desperate situations, his ability to listen and give support to his colleagues at both a personal and professional level ("never to push, but always there to lend a helping hand"), his gentle humour, and his capacity to assuage the cut and thrust of course team or disciplinary meetings with the timely uncorking of a bottle of wine or sherry or even the suggestion that it was time we all adjourned for "a wee dram". These qualities are not just the ones that we were privileged to share here at the Open University because they are referred to again and again by all those he came into contact with whether in Liverpool, India or Australia.

Perhaps in many ways his personal qualities and his professional attitudes are well illustrated by two stories. The first comes from a former student in his department at ANU, now an academic working in New Zealand. "When I came to the University as a green research student", he told me,

> I had intended to work in physical geography but I met with an uncompromising reception from a staff member under whom it was intended that I should carry out my studies. He maintained that I was inadequately trained to work in the field and unless I took drastic steps to remedy this, he would refuse to have me. This was a pretty upsetting response to one's first day at the place which had already granted me a scholarship. As I walked back to college I noticed a car reversing the full length of the street. It mounted the footpath in front of me and Andrew got out to say that he had heard what I had been told, that I should not take his colleague's view of a narrowly confined approach and consider building on other strengths in my previous training, particularly to go and talk to people in prehistory and anthropology. In 1964 such cross-disciplinary notions were quite novel. So I was impressed by his concern for a new student whom he had met only briefly in a courtesy call the day before, and his concern to promote broadly based cross-disciplinary research. He started me on a research field of human ecology/cultural geography that I am still primarily concerned with today. Incidentally, his driving also impresses most of those who ever get to ride with him!

Geographers are probably unusual in that they frequently work with their colleagues in circumstances that are not always academic, taking them away from the formality of offices and corridors and out into the field. Indeed, such field trips can be revealing in terms of true character and I am reminded by a former colleague of Andrew's, John Chappell, of a second story which speaks eloquently of his practicality and his gentle humour. "We were", he says,

> once camped on low ground beside a swollen river with a large group of students. Night fell and rain continued to inflate the river which overflowed its banks towards midnight. Another lecturer and I continued to sit at a table arguing about some microscopic intellectual matter and quite oblivious of the welfare of the students. We discerned Andrew off in the dark, moving about with a torch. Ultimately he approached and said mildly, "It doesn't seem much good here". (There was by now a foot of water swirling under the table.) "I've got the vehicles on the road with all safe and sound. Would you care to join us?"

Of his Australian days a former colleague, A. J. Rose, now Professor of Geography at Macquarie University, remembers well Andrew's dislike of the high summer temperatures at Canberra which, he averred, exceeded those of South India. But, Professor Rose concludes, "whilst Andrew's own recollections of his Australian years may be dominated by the memory of excessive heat, we who were his colleagues hold memories of his own gentle warmth".

Whatever Andrew may bring to mind of those turbulent but exciting years that made up the first decade of the Open University, his colleagues here will be equally able quickly to summon up Rose-like recollections. At one time on his desk, so it is said, Andrew had a cartoon (a momento from his student days in Edinburgh) of a figure seated small astride an exceptionally large elephant in the process of galloping off into the jungle in a cloud of dust. Perhaps we may now think, with affection, of Andrew as that figure, for the caption read "After Geddes—and not too far behind!"

The publications of Andrew Learmonth

The population of Skye (Newbigin Prize Essay, 1949). *Scottish Geog. Mag.* **66**, 2, 77–103 (1950).

The Floods of 12th August, 1948, in South-east Scotland. A monograph circulated privately in mimeographed form (1950). Note: A pecuniary grant from the Carnegie Trust for the Universities of Scotland assisted with the expense of the field work of the investigation. A hundred copies of the *typescript* version were prepared, each 45 pages in length. (See also *Scottish Geog. Mag.* **66**, 3–4, 147–153 (1950).)

Regional differences in natality and in mortality in the sub-continent of Indo-Pakistan, 1921–1940. *Proc. 8th General Assembly & 17th International Geographical Congress, Washington D.C., 8–15 August, 1952,* pp. 195–205. The United States National Committee of the International Geographical Union, National Academy of Sciences—National Research Council (1952).

The medical geography of India: an approach to the problem. In *The Indian Geographical Society, The Silver Jubilee Volume: N. Subramanyam Memorial Volume* (Ed. K. Kuriyan), pp. 201–202. The Indian Geographical Society, Madras (1952).

Variability in population change in India and regional variations therein, 1921–40. *Indian Geog. J.* **28**, 3–4, 69–73 (1953) (with A. Geddes).

The middle Mersey and the chemical area. In *A Scientific Survey of Merseyside*, pp. 251–267. Liverpool University Press for the British Association (1953) (with S. Gregory and R. Lawton).

A method of plotting on the same map health data on both intensity and variability of incidence, illustrated by three maps of cholera in Indo-Pakistan. *Annals Trop. Med. & Paras.* **48**, 4, 345–348 (1954).

Malaria—some implications of recent revolutionary progress. In "This Changing World", *Geography* **39/1**, 183 (1954).

Aspects of village life in Indo-Pakistan. *Geography* **40/3**, 189, 145–160 (1955) (with A. M. Learmonth).

Le Kwashiorkor, exemple de carence de protéines au cours de sevrage. *Annales de Géog.* **64**, 343, 202–208 (1955).

Kwashiorkor: social and geographical relationships of a malnutrition of the under-developed areas. In "This Changing World", *Geography* **41**, 1, 61–63 (1956).

Some contrasts in the regional geography of malaria in India and Pakistan. *Trans. Inst. British Geog.* **23**, 37–59 (1957).

A map of calories and proteins in poor Indian diets. *Nat. Geog. J. India* **2/4**, 211–212 (1956).

Landscapes of New Mysore. *The Indian Geographer* **2/2**, 356–368 (1957) (with A. M. Learmonth).

The regional concept and national development. *The Economic Weekly (Annual Number)* **10**, (Nos 4, 5 and 6), 153–156. Bombay, January 1958 (with A. M. Learmonth).

Medical geography in Indo-Pakistan: A study of twenty years' data. *Indian Geog. J.* **33**, 1–2, 1–59 (1958).

The Eastern Lands: Asia except the USSR. Oxford University Press, Oxford (1958, 1964) (with A. M. Learmonth).

Prelude to a national atlas. *The Economic Weekly.* July, 839–840 (1958). A review of the *National Atlas of India* (Ed. S. P. Chatterjee). Preliminary Hindi edition (with L. S. Bhat).

Geography and health in the tropical forest zone. In *Geographical Essays in Memory of Alan G. Ogilvie* (Eds R. Miller and J. W. Watson), pp. 195–220. Nelson, Edinburgh (1959).

A method of plotting two variables (such as mean incidence and variability from year to year) on the same map, using isopleths. *Erdkunde* **13**, 145–150 (1959) (with M. N. Pal).

Report of the Regional Survey Unit, Indian Statistical Institute, Mysore State. Indian Statistical Institute, Calcutta (1960) (with L. S. Bhat).

Aspects of the medical geography of Liverpool—a study prompted by a mass radiography campaign in the city. *Abstr. Proc. 19th International Geographical Congress, Norden,* pp. 169–170 (1960) (with M. C. Endall).

Sample survey and national planning in India: a geographer's contribution to sample design. Paper given at the Institute of British Geographers Annual Conference, Southampton, 2 January (1960).

Regional planning in India: now or never? *The Economic Weekly (Annual Number)* **11**, 241–244. Bombay, January (1960).

Mysore State, Vol. I: *An Atlas of Resources.* Indian Statistical Series No. 13. Statistical Publishing Society, Calcutta. Asia Publishing House, Bombay and London (1961) (with L. S. Bhat as joint editor).

Mysore State, Vol. II: *A Regional Synthesis.* Indian Statistical Series No. 16. Statistical Publishing Society, Calcutta. Asia Publishing House, Bombay and London (1962) (as joint editor).

Medical geography in India and Pakistan. *Geog. J.* **127/1**, 10–26 (1961).

Sample villages in Mysore State, India: a geographical study. University of Liverpool, Department of Geography Research Paper No. 1, vi, 155 (August 1962).

Retrospect on a project in applied regional geography in Mysore State, India. In *Geographers and the Tropics, Liverpool Essays* (Eds R. W. Steel and R. M. Prothero), pp. 323–348. Longmans, London (1964).

The Vegetation of the Indian Sub-Continent: A geographical review of works by Spate, Champion, Puri, Whyte and others. Department of Geography, ANU School of General Studies, Occasional Paper No. 1 (December 1964).

Health in the Indian Sub-Continent 1955–64: A geographer's review of some medical literature. Department of Geography, ANU School of General Studies, Occasional Paper No. 2 (April 1965).

Maps of some Standardised Mortality Ratios for Australia 1959–63. Department of Geography, ANU School of General Studies, Occasional Paper No. 3 (July 1965) (with Christine Nichols).

Applications of Statistical Sampling to Geographical Studies, with Special Reference to Cartographic Representation of Sampling Error. Department of Geography, ANU School of General Studies, Occasional Paper No. 5 (July 1966) (with I. D. Reid).

India and Pakistan, 3rd edition. Methuen, London (1967) (with O. K. Spate).

Selected aspects of India's population geography. The Australian Journal of Politics and History, Vol. XII, No. 2, pp. 146–154 (August 1966).

Geografia Medica: tendencias y perspectivas. In Reunion Especial de la Comision de Geografia Medica, pp. 1–10. Edicion de la Sociedad Mexicana de Geografia y Estadistica, Vol. 6. Proc. Conferencia Regional Latina-Americana, Mexico City (1966) (meeting chaired and introduced by Professor Learmonth).

Two laboratory exercises in areal sampling. Contribution to the Principal C.B. Joshi Memorial Volume of the Bombay Geographical Magazine 13/1, 61–74 (December 1965).

Models and medical geography. Abstr. Proc. 21st International Geographical Congress, New Delhi, p. 21. National Committee for Geography, Calcutta (1968).

An Encyclopaedia of Australia. Frederick Warne & Co., London (1968, 1973) (with A. M. Learmonth).

A million enumerators: some census of India publications and other relevant material. Australian Geographer 10/5, 425–427 (March 1968).

Maps of some Standardised Mortality Ratios for Australia 1964–1968. Department of Geography, ANU School of General Studies, Occasional Paper No. 8 (1969) (with R. Grau).

Regional Landscapes of Australia: Form, Function and Change. Angus and Robertson, Sydney and Heinemann Educational, London (1971) (with A. M. Learmonth).

Applied geography in undergraduate studies. In Studies in Applied and Regional Geography (Eds M. Shafi and M. Raza), pp. 34–44. Department of Geography, Aligarh Muslim University (1971).

Geography at the Open University (UK). Papers submitted to the 22nd International Geographical Congress, Toronto, p. 1055. University of Toronto Press on behalf of the 22nd International Geographical Congress, Montreal (1972).

Commission on medical geography. In "Reports of the IGU Commissions 1968–1972", Bulletin U.G.I. 23, 1, 1–71 (1972).

Macro- and micro- in rural–urban studies: a possible role for nested samples? Bombay Geographical Magazine 20–21, 1, 1–22 (1972–1973).

Atlases in medical geography, pp. 133–152 and Medicine and medical geography, pp. 17–42. In Medical Geography: Techniques and Field Studies (Ed. N. D. McGlashan). Methuen, London (1972).

Geographical models and geomedicine. In Forschritte der Geomedizinischen Forschung; Beiträge zur Geoökologie der Infektionskrankheiten (Ed. H. J. Jusatz), pp. 115–125. Franz Steiner, Wiesbaden.

Ecological medical geography. In *Progress in Geography* (Ed. C. Board), Vol. VII, pp. 201–226. Edward Arnold, London (1975).

The I.G.U. Commission on medical geography, 1972–76. In *General Problems of Geography and Geosystems Modelling*. Volume 11 of Proceedings of Papers Submitted to the *23rd International Geographical Congress, Moscow*, pp. 14–17. Published in Moscow and distributed by Pergamon Press, London (1976).

Models and medical geography. In *Essays in Applied Geography in Memory of the Late Professor S. Muzafer Ali* (Eds V. C. Misra, N. P. Ayyar and P. Kumar), pp. 17–38. Saugar University Press, Sagar, Madhya Pradesh, India (1976).

So you want to be a medical geographer? An open letter to students. In *The Indian Geographical Society, Golden Jubilee Volume, Madras* (Eds V. L. S. Prakasa Rao *et al.*), pp. 280–288. The Indian Geographical Society, Madras (1976).

The International Geographical Union Commission on medical geography 1972–76. *Geoforum* **7/2**, 152–157 (1976).

Malaria. In *A World Geography of Human Diseases* (Ed. G. M. Howe), pp. 61–108. Academic Press, London and New York (1977).

The resurgence of malaria in India 1965–76. *GeoJournal* **1/5**, 69–79 (1977) (with R. Akhtar).

Medicine and medical geography before the Second World War. *Geographia Medica* **8**, 67–102 (1978).

Patterns of Disease and Hunger. David and Charles, Newton Abbot (1978).

Arthur Geddes, 1895–1968. In *Geographers: Bibliographical Studies* (Eds W. Freeman and P. Pinchemel), pp. 45–51. Mansell, London (1978).

India's malaria resurgence, 1965–1978. In "This Changing World", *Geography* **64/3**, 221–223 (June 1979) (with R. Akhtar).

Malarial Annual Parasite Index Maps of India by Malaria Control Unit Areas, 1965–1976. Faculty Research Paper No. 3. Open University, Milton Keynes (June 1979) (with R. Akhtar).

The resurgence of malaria in India 1965–1976. In *Geomedizin in Forschung und Lehre; Beiträge zur Geoökologie der Menschen* (Ed. H. J. Jusatz), pp. 29–41. Franz Steiner, Wiesbaden (1977).

Reflections on the regional geography of disease in late colonial South Asia. *Soc. Sci. Med.* **14D**, 3, 271–276 (1980). (Special issue on "Contemporary Perspectives on the Medical Geography of South and South-east Asia".)

Probabilities in the malaria cycle: a graphic presentation. *Geographia Medica* **10**, 12–19 (1980) (with J. Hunt).

The Geography of Health (Ed.). Selected papers from the 24th International Geographical Congress, Tokyo, August 1980. Pergamon Press, Oxford (1981). (Special issue of *Soc. Sci. Med.* **15D**.)

Geographers and health and disease studies, 1972–80. In *The Geography of Health* (Ed. A. T. A. Learmonth), pp. 9–19. Pergamon Press, Oxford (1981). (Special issue of *Soc. Sci. Med.* **15D**.)

Man and Land in South Asia (Eds A. T. A. Learmonth *et al.*). Concept Publishing Company, New Delhi (1982).

Open University Teaching Texts

1971   Unit 4. Societies and Environments.
        Unit 23. Frontiers and Boundaries.
        Unit 33. Demographic regions in the Indian Sub-continent.
        In *Understanding Society*. The Open University Press, Milton Keynes.

Regional disparities in the health sector, pp. 23–76. In Block V (Parts 1–5) Health.
        Decision Making in Britain. The Open University Press, Milton Keynes.

1972   Unit 1. Continuity and Change.
        Parts of Unit 13. Scale in Political Geography, Macro and Micro.
        Parts of Unit 15. Regional Geography to Regional Analysis.
        In *New Trends in Geography*. The Open University Press, Milton Keynes.

1973   Unit 3. Towards a Model of the South Asian City. In *Urban Development*.
        The Open University Press, Milton Keynes.

1974   Unit 7. Economic and Social Surfaces.
        Unit 11. Economic Complexes.
        In *Regional Analysis and Development*. The Open University Press, Milton
        Keynes.

1975   Introduction to Block 2 with Dennis Mills.
        Unit 5, Demographic Tools and Social Science Viewpoints, pp. 43–71 with
        Brendan Connors.
        Unit 6. Does Technology Control Population Numbers?, pp. 73–101 with
        Brendan Connors.
        Block 9, 2. Geography in the Social Sciences, pp. 29–52.
        In *Making Sense of Society*. The Open University Press, Milton Keynes.

1977   Unit 8. Man–Environment Relationships as Complex Ecosystems, with
        Ian Simmons. In *Fundamentals of Human Geography*. The Open Univer-
        sity Press, Milton Keynes.

1978   Unit 29. Values, Ideology and Neutrality in Geography: A Revision Guide.
        In *Fundamentals of Human Geography*. The Open University Press,
        Milton Keynes.

1981   Module 3. Access to Primary Health Care, with David Phillips. In *A Guided
        Project Course in Human Geography*. The Open University Press, Milton
        Keynes.

Medical geography in the United Kingdom, 1945–1982

G. Melvyn Howe and David R. Phillips

*Department of Geography, University of Strathclyde, Glasgow, Scotland
and Department of Geography, University of Exeter, England*

Major themes

The purpose of this chapter is to review the development of medical geography within the United Kingdom since the end of the Second World War. Worthy work in medical geography undertaken by British geographers but conducted outside the UK is not included. During the period of the review medical geography has developed into a dynamic and robust sub-branch of geography in which geographical concepts and techniques are applied to a wide range of health-related problems. From a somewhat specialized focus in the immediate post-war years it has expanded into a multi-stranded discipline ranging across the broad spectrum of physical, social, economic and urban geography and strongly committed to inter-disciplinary activity in concepts, substance and techniques.

A major theme of medical geography during the last 35 years has been the analysis of spatial variations in human health (or, as Howe (1980) points out, more often the *lack* of health) and the search for the environmental and social conditions which may be causally related to these variations. In the UK as in most other developed countries of the world the acute, infectious, life-threatening conditions of the past have been largely controlled by enlightened environmental changes, health legislation and therapeutic advances, particularly since 1945 with the general advent of antibiotic treatments. The disorders which now shorten life are of a more chronic kind and include cardiovascular diseases, cancer, bronchitis and mental and occupational disorders. Such disorders have in common the fact that their prevention is still very much in its infancy.

GEOGRAPHICAL ASPECTS OF HEALTH
ISBN 0 12 483780 8

Medical geographical research in the geopathological field has endeavoured to demonstrate high risk communities and areas and propose appropriate social and environmental management for their control.

Introduced into the UK in 1948 the National Health Service (NHS) aimed to provide all citizens with equal opportunities for health care. However, 25 years later, there is still much evidence of inequality, and certainly of differences in use of the Service by the different social groups. Such inequalities have provided the focus and thrust for more recent medico-geographical studies into the national and local availability of health services, their accessibility, their use by consumers and into the general functioning of the NHS. Hopefully, and in due time, such studies of health care provision (health service delivery) will be related to those in geographical pathology (disease ecology) and the two main research avenues of medical geography will become co-ordinated and unified.

The concept of health is varied and complex. The World Health Organization (WHO) defines health as "a state of complete physical, mental and social well-being and not merely the absence of disease or infirmity" (WHO, 1965). This represents a state of adjustment or harmony between man (his living tissues, cells and components of cells) and his physical, biological and socio-cultural environment. Health equates with ecological equilibrium. Ill-health, on the other hand, may be considered to be a state of maladjustment, *dis*harmony or ecological disequilibrium. The health of a human being may be measured in physical terms but, in the light of the WHO definition, mental health also requires attention (whether this is the result of physical, social or other factors) because this, too, represents a type of disequilibrium. The environment is viewed as a reservoir of physical, chemical, biological and socio-cultural forces which either support or threaten health. Such a concept might be judged as equating with the environmental determinism paradigm of early geography except in so far as man is able to use his intelligence in order to adapt or adjust to variations in the various physical and human environments. In which case it is more realistic to invoke the possibilist school of thought with its emphasis on man and the way in which he adapts his surroundings rather than the way in which the physical environment conditions his activities. Analytically, the forces or factors which place man's health in jeopardy may be regarded as *stimuli* and the behaviour or reaction of man when exposed to them as *responses*. An analysis of stimuli and responses provides a basis for the understanding of environmental maladjustment and provides underpinnings for much of the earlier or traditional orientation of medical geography in both the UK and elsewhere in the world.

It is a generally accepted, though incorrect, view that the level of health of both the individual and the community is related to the quality of medicine and with the health-care system generally. Such a view is inadequate because health care is but one facet of the total health field. It might be argued that the underlying provocative factors (stimuli) of sickness and death (responses) are as important if not more important than the quality of the health-care system. This would suggest that the goal of medical geography should embrace both disease ecology (geographical pathology: spatial variations in disease and their environmental relationships) and health care geography (spatial variations in availability, quality, and use of health-care facilities). Shannon (1980), Phillips (1981) and others have written to this effect. If health-care geography is regarded as a more recent development in medical geography and ecological medical geography (Learmonth, 1975) an earlier and more traditional approach this is not to imply that the one has superseded the other. Rather they should be viewed as being potentially complementary.

It is in the development of such an orientation that the future of medical geography must surely lie. Possibly, the "two medical geographies rather than one" identified by Learmonth (1978) will continue into the 1980s, but more mutual support and convergence may occur, even if specialized research continues into each of the identifiable avenues of the subject.

Early emphases in medical geography and medical cartography

Much interesting and often pioneering work in the more traditional media of medical geography—the mapping of occurrence of diseases and deaths—was performed in the middle and late years of the nineteenth century and up to the Second World War. The term "geographical pathology" explains a proportion of the early work and readers may be referred to the summary by Gilbert (1958) of the cartographic development by Victorian pioneers in medical geography.

The great value of cartographic presentations of medical data for purposes of description, analysis and aetiological enquiry has long been recognized. However, cartographic techniques were previously descriptive and suggestive of associations rather than being analytical of variables under consideration. It will emerge later that the map is still often a major medium of medical geographical research and, in recent years, cartographic techniques have been used to illustrate diffusion of diseases, probabilities of contracting ailments, and varying availabilities and usage of services. It is important, however, that their limitations and total dependence on the quality of data be realized (Howe, 1980) lest an impression of totally spurious reliability may be conveyed. As all cartographers know, the interpretation of maps can often be assisted or confounded by such technical matters as scale, class intervals, shadings, etc. This problem is even greater in medical geography because there is no single index which completely characterizes the impact of a disease in a community. Attack or incidence rates, prevalence rates, mortality rates and case fatality rates are all subject to different problems of interpretation and the derivation of reliable indices in medical geography is a matter to which useful research may still be applied.

Medical geography in the immediate post-war years

In the immediate post-war years and until the early 1960s, it seems that the majority of studies by geographers of medical topics (or of geographical topics by medical scientists) were either of the locational features and environmental associations of specific diseases or were concerned with the relationships between mortality and specific environmental features. It was mainly the medical geography of chronic, apparently non-infectious, diseases such as the cancers, coronary artery disease, cerebrovascular disease and bronchitis which received early and continuing attention.

Spatial variations in the distribution of cancers in Britain have been long recognized (Clemow, 1903) and when advances in medical science enabled data to be available of sufficient quality to differentiate amongst types of cancers, geographical work became more refined. This research was often conducted initially by geographically-inclined medical scientists and is reported in the medical literature. Legon (1951) indicated spatial variations of gastric cancer mortality in Wales, and more general aetiological aspects of geographical variations in mortality (Legon, 1952). As Learmonth (1978) points out, this work was not immediately capitalized upon, although the influence of specific agents such as cigarette smoke and atmospheric deposits in the causation of cancer and bronchitis received a degree of geographical attention in the late 1950s (Doll and Hill, 1956; Stocks, 1959). Other environmental influences on health such as background radiation (Court-Brown et al., 1960) and types of water supply (Allen-Price, 1960) have been studied and also have distinct geographical aspects. Many of these have been followed up in Britain in later years as, for example, the study of mortality and hardness of water by Crawford et al. (1968) and the general distributional features of mortality from a variety of causes by Howe (1959, 1963, 1971, 1972, 1976, 1979).

Recent developments in medical geography

Maps of mortality and morbidity for individual localities or even nationally for certain ailments were more frequently being produced by the early 1960s. A major development was the publication of a *National Atlas of Disease Mortality* with maps of the distribution of mortality for numerous causes of death (Howe, 1963). The nature of available data for mapping became crucial in this exercise. The most satisfactory single-figure comparison of the mortality in each local area with that of the UK as a whole is the Standardized Mortality Ratio (SMR) calculated for each sex separately. The SMR makes allowance for variations in age structure of local populations compared with the national populations (regarded as having a standard structure of age groups). Local SMRs are expressed in terms of the UK standard national rate, taken as 100. Therefore, a range of SMRs around 100 is found although some may doubtless occur by chance. It is therefore important for statistical tests to be applied to indicate the significance of findings and this interest in statistical accuracy is indicative of the more positivist leanings of scientifically-trained geographers in recent years. Giggs *et al.* (1980) emphasize the importance of such statistical testing if medical geographical research is to have credence and, unfortunately, relatively few cartographic examples using such tests are to be found in the British literature, notable exceptions being by Howe (1970), White (1972) and Giggs *et al.* (1980).

The different ways in which SMRs are represented on maps suggest different patterns and associations. As descriptive devices, choropleth maps are useful although used uncritically they suggest an impression of even spread of population across spatial units. Thus too much weight is given to extensive but sparsely or unevenly populated areas, whilst insufficient prominence is given to localized concentrations of population such as are found in towns or cities. An incorrect visual impression of the regional patterning of mortality may thus be created. A variety of techniques, such as demographic mapping on which an area assigned to a locality is proportional to its population, has been adopted in an attempt to overcome this limitation (Forster, 1966; Howe, 1963, 1969, 1970). However, demographic maps distort geographical reality and problems arise when contiguity of neighbouring areas is lost. This shortcoming tends to be highlighted when the spatial diffusion of an ailment is being studied.

More recently, several cartographic methods have been used to demonstrate patterns of mortality at a variety of spatial scales (see, for example, Howe, 1970, 1980). As Howe (1980) explains, maps or cartograms by themselves explain nothing, but all pose the question regarding spatial distributions, "Why?". This leads to a search for explanations of the spatial patterns revealed. To date fairly elementary statistical techniques have been employed although increasingly sophisticated techniques are being introduced and a range of possible causal factors are being investigated. Rarely is the search simple or straightforward and the researcher has to be prepared to examine many possible and tentative correlations and be willing to reject preconceived hypotheses. The search for causation in the field of health is rarely simple and medical geographers have to recognize that they cannot hope to find definitive answers. Their contribution must be to prevention through social and environmental management rather than with disease aetiology and its management.

Statistical techniques of increasing sophistication have been brought into the armoury of methods of analysing human health problems. In particular, multivariate techniques developed in geography as a whole have been used to explore social and physical environmental associations with diseases. These are usually ecological analyses, relying on aggregate data of incidence rates of ailments in populations which are related to variables representing aspects of the physical and social environments. Physical conditions of housing, for example, may be one influence on the physical and mental health of occupants (Girt, 1972; Giggs, 1979) but a complete explanation is more likely to involve a wide range of social and environmental characteristics.

Within Britain, a number of city-wide surveys have found that socio-economic status can have a strong bearing on health differentials and use of services in particular. This has long been recognized by medical sociologists and medical writers (Titmuss, 1968; Rein, 1969; Alderson, 1970; Blaxter, 1976; Cartwright and O'Brien, 1976; Forster, 1976; Stacey, 1977; Walters, 1979) and has been formally investigated by the Department of Health and Social Security in the recently published "Black Report" (Department of Health and Social Security, 1980). A number of geographical studies lend support to this idea that in the UK mortality and morbidity rates generally exhibit a strong inverse relationship with social class (Castle and Gittus, 1957; Griffiths, 1971; Taylor, 1974). For some specific diseases, however, such a relationship may either disappear or even be reversed. Mental illnesses in particular have proved difficult to examine due to the lack of adequate definitions and diagnostic problems associated with many conditions. Even so geographers have made a number of useful environmental and ecological studies within the field of mental ill-health (Bain, 1971, 1974; Giggs, 1977, 1979; Dean, 1979).

Notable amongst such studies is that by Giggs (1973) employing the multivariate statistical technique, factor analysis.* This statistical technique relates a number of variables to each other and picks out any specific groupings in the data. It was used to investigate the spatial distribution of schizophrenics in Nottingham and to highlight possible social and environmental associations of the ailment. Although the analysis proved rather controversial at the time, the statistical technique employed proved valuable in that it showed the incidence of schizophrenia to be related to a range of unfavourable life circumstances. A causal relationship could not be established. The same technique has been employed to analyse the admission to hospital of child medical emergency cases in West Glamorgan (Thomas and Phillips, 1978). In this study, high rates of child admissions were related to both poor physical housing conditions and certain life-styles associated with residence in particular local authority housing estates. Results from aggregate, ecological analyses are usually heavily qualified but they are useful in indicating the kinds of relationships which may justify further detailed research.

A variety of statistical techniques have been used to investigate the behaviour of diseases in populations. Theoretical models have been used but, as with many modelling attempts, results have little practical value and are usually too complex for use in general settings. Even so, some academically important work has evolved, often from the ecological-associative types of study; some of the more statistically sophisticated have been models of diffusion of diseases. A knowledge of the historical progression of diseases, such as the epidemics of cholera in the nineteenth century, can contribute to an understanding of disease progression at the current time (Howe, 1972, 1980) and certain of the more recent studies of diseases may be used to predict future outbreaks. Haggett (1976),† for example, has examined the multiple diffusion of measles within an industrial culture and proposed a hybrid model from seven alternative versions of an epidemic diffusion model. Murray and Cliff (1977)† have produced a regionally-based stochastic model for the diffusion of measles in a multi-region setting, using data from the Registrar General's Weekly Return for England and Wales over a 222-week period. This model avoids one of the main problems of modelling infectious diseases, i.e. the assumption that all infected people spread the disease at a steady rate. Such an assumption is not realistic because the degree of infectiousness varies. In particular it varies with time from initial contact because the different diseases have differing incubation

---

* See also pp. 197–222.   † See also pp. 335–348.

periods. The Murray–Cliff model attempts to overcome this by subdividing the infected population into two categories, viz., "latent" and "contagious", and is potentially a useful technique for the study of other similar contagious conditions.

The more general principles of spatial diffusion have been recognized as valuable for studying the spread of disease (Haggett, 1972) and Hunter and Young (1971) have revealed that the diffusion of the specific ailment influenza displays a relationship with population potential. However, perhaps the most celebrated detailed epidemiological study of disease diffusion in the period of this review is that by Pickles (1948). This study concerned the spread of several infectious conditions in a small rural area, Wensleydale (Yorkshire), around the time of the Second World War. Despite the fact that the cases are presented in almost anecdotal fashion, the opportunity taken to estimate the incubation period of certain infectious diseases was of considerable novelty at the time and the report makes interesting reading.

Whilst the disease diffusion approach can be of value, this may be diminished if too rigid a concern is adopted for mathematical sophistication. Practical utility is all important and, of course, not all conditions are suitable for diffusion study. The same may be said of some other modelling and simulation studies which have been conducted elsewhere both for diseases and for health-care facilities. In the UK there are, as yet, relatively few instances where central place models or spatial interaction formulations have been used to study diseases. There are a limited number of studies which attempt to simulate visits to general practitioners or to estimate the effects of various spatial location strategies on the usage of community hospitals (Moyes, 1977; Haynes and Bentham, 1979). Location–allocation models and models based on variants of central place theory have been suggested to assist in the planning of locations for various health and social facilities (e.g. Robertson, 1977, 1978; Parr, 1980) but such models have yet to receive general attention in the UK. A weakness of many of the spatial interaction type models is that the demand side of the service, involving consumer perceptions and characteristics, is largely neglected. Their use as planning tools may therefore be called into question (Kivell and Shaw, 1980; Phillips, 1981).

Normative behavioural assumptions, such as the rational or economic man premise, underpin most theoretical models. Stipulated norms or assumptions underlie the development of optimal aggregate patterns of spatial behaviour. The fact that personal differences and consumer awareness are excluded makes the explanatory and predictive use of such models limited (Thomas, 1976; Phillips, 1981). Random or stochastic elements could be built into many models yet it remains doubtful as to how realistically this can be achieved. Furthermore, policy implications or practical application have been neglected in many models.

Because some models considered focus on diseases and disease behaviour, some depend on human behaviour to spread contagion and others study the distributional features of health service provision, it would seem that models provide a useful and meaningful link between the two main themes of medical geography (i.e. between disease ecology and health-care delivery).

In an ideal world service provision should bear some relationship with diseases, their behaviour, human behaviour and contagion. In which case it would seem convenient at this point to examine the development in the UK of the study of what Shannon and Dever (1974) term the geography of health care or what may also be called medical–social geography (Phillips, 1981), the main foci of which are the spatial characteristics of health-care systems and their utilization.

The geography of health care

Research in medical geography in Britain has previously focused upon the ecological approach to the study of the spatial distribution of diseases and their possible causes. This was the main emphasis until the early or mid-1970s. Thus, until almost the end of the period under review, relatively little attention had been paid to the spatial analysis of health-care services and planning and health behaviour. This important component of medical geography often strays into the territory of the health or social service planner and administrator, fields which are unfamiliar to most geographers. Giggs (1979) sees this field of study as comprising three main components. The first is summarized as the structure and spatial patterning of the sources which make up the health-care system in any given country (hospitals, clinics and physicians). A second component is concerned with identifying patterns of inequity in the supply and use of services and in planning "optimal" structural and spatial health-care systems. A third perspective focuses on patient utilization of various medical and welfare services and the factors which influence their behaviour. Because no single discipline can possess the information and knowledge necessary to make the "best" decisions in the face of the known facts, interdisciplinary understanding is essential in such studies. Until the mid-1970s virtually all research into the geography of health care had been undertaken outside the UK but within the last decade a substantial and growing body of research has developed.

An awareness of the need to study health care can be related to the development of the "welfare" approach in human geography (Smith, 1977, 1979) and to the recognition of the importance of health and welfare services in improving the quality of life for people. In the UK, since 1948, residents have been fortunate to have had available the facilities of the National Health Service (NHS). The existence of this Service did not, however, remove all inequalities in health either socially or spatially (Howe, 1963, 1970; Coates and Rawstron, 1971; Learmonth, 1972; Carter and Peel, 1976).

The NHS removed some of the more obvious inequalities in health-care provision while the welfare state in general improved the lot of the needy. This doubtless inhibited interest or enthusiasm for research into health care in the UK such as that which took place in the 1960s in North America. There, it would seem, the deficiencies of free enterprise in providing for the health and welfare needs of the nation were more obvious than they were in the UK. Probably for this reason the early research in health-care geography mainly developed outside the UK. Impetus in this field in the UK has been gained in recent years, partly with the realization by certain researchers that behavioural matters in the use of services were worthy of geographical research. In addition, such features as health service planning and health-care provision (aspects of the managerial approach) and questions concerning the "strategic" importance attached to matters such as social and health policy nationally (which may be dubbed the political economy approach) are also recognized as worthy of study if a full appreciation and understanding of social problems and their amelioration are to be achieved.

The spatial structure of health care in Britain

The first theme identified by Giggs (1979) examines structural features of health-care provision to meet the needs of the population in the country. As such, it is somewhat analogous to disease mapping discussed earlier in ecological medical geography. The basic "facts and figures" are sought in this approach, which can be conducted at scales ranging from the national (at which to date most research has been conducted) to that of the local health district.

In geographical terms, the study by Coates and Rawstron (1971) of aggregate regional disparities in Britain over a range of characteristics is a convenient starting place. This study confirmed certain prejudices about regional living conditions in Britain and dispelled others. The material by Coates and Rawstron has been used in conjunction with

Howe's (1963) *Atlas of Disease Mortality* to provide a basis for examining regional disparities in the health sector in Britain (Learmonth, 1972). With regard to need for services (if morbidity or mortality are good indicators of need) and actual levels of provision, many inequalities were revealed. The findings of such research (e.g. that there are too few doctors or hospitals in one region and too many in another) have been of value to health service planners. In this respect, a major evaluation of financial inducements to encourage more general practitioners to move to areas which are in need of doctors has been conducted. This has clear geographical implications for those areas of the country which are regarded as deficient in health and other services (Butler and Knight, 1974).

The changing organization and location of specific factors of the health service have been examined. Sumner (1971) has studied the national distribution of general practitioners, and the distribution of health-care facilities in a local area has been examined by Heller (1976). Community hospitals, their numbers nationally (While, 1978) and their potential locally (Haynes and Bentham, 1979), have been the subjects of research, as have specific locational and organizational developments within local general practice, e.g. the growth of group practices and health centres (Phillips, 1981; Phillips and Learmonth, 1981).

Patterns of inequity in health services

A more obvious development from the welfare approach has focused on unequal or inequitable availability or use of health services (Smith, 1977, 1979). Health administrators have a natural concern for the regional distribution of financial resources in the NHS (Noyce *et al.*, 1974), a theme which has been extensively discussed by the Resource Allocation Working Party (RAWP) of the Department of Health and Social Security (DHSS, 1976).

Access to health care facilities has been the concern of doctors and allied researchers for many years, focusing on matters such as surgery attendance methods (Sowerby, 1969) and the number of patients per doctor and their distribution in general practice (Vaughan, 1967; Richardson and Ding.wall-Fordyce, 1968). Access to primary care in particular was a concern of the Royal Commission on the National Health Service (1979). The question of "social" access to health care, referred to earlier, forms an important debate within the social sciences. One of the best known generalizations regarding access and availability of medical care is that by Hart (1971), who refers to the "inverse law of care", according to which, the availability of good care tends to vary inversely with the need for it in the population served. This observation by Hart prompted geographers to initiate inquiries to test its validity, both nationally and locally, within the UK.

Geographically, these matters are linked to health-care planning policy. Mohan (1981) discusses those aspects of the decision-making process which give rise to (sometimes inequitable) patterns of hospital and medical facility provision in an attempt to illustrate the criteria used in the planning process. At the primary level "on the ground", aggregate accessibility levels of neighbourhoods in certain Scottish cities have been examined by Knox (1978, 1979a). He notes that if the socio-economic status of their residents is taken into account some neighbourhoods may be disadvantaged in terms of their provision of services or access to services. Locational disparities of doctors may also be related to more general features of multiple social deprivation and Knox (1979b) calls for a concerted response from public policy makers to recognize this fact if inter-dependent problems of localized medical and social deprivation are to be effectively improved. Factors such as the locational preferences of doctors need also to be considered when attempting to devise policy to redistribute medical manpower to "needy" areas (Knox and Pacione 1980). Differential availability and access to services is important because, to quote but one example, the use of dental services and dental health has been shown to vary with the availability of, and access to, treatment facilities (O'Mullane and Robinson, 1977; Taylor and Carmichael, 1980). Such evidence suggests that geographical efforts should continue to be directed into researching levels of accessibility and provision of services. This is a major theme in which the more traditional disease ecology studies may be employed to highlight areas which appear to be in greater "need" of medical services.

Medical service utilization

Research into the patterns and determinants of patient use of physicians and hospitals is, as Giggs (1979) points out, a fairly well-established facet of medical geography. Until the mid-1970s however work was confined almost exclusively to the United States. Many of the studies outside the UK attempted only to establish travel patterns and demands for services. In the UK this topic has been recognized as rather more complex. It may be questioned whether utilization reflects need or merely reflects service availability. This problem has yet to be resolved and is worthy of considerable attention.

The utilization of services may be made amenable to theoretical modelling although the shortcomings concerning models as research and planning tools should be borne in mind. In the UK most research into health-care utilization has avoided modelling in general terms. Instead, attention has focused on the identification of the variables which influence utilization. This embodies the behavioural approach to human geography. Some early work along these lines related to a single medical practice in which the relationship between the age, sex and distance of patients from surgery to the usage made of the general practitioner has been discussed (Hopkins *et al.*, 1968). Further studies by other social scientists, including many referred to earlier, relate to social class variations in use of medical services.

There are very few explicit geographical studies in the UK of the use of medical services although their number is increasing. The study by Haynes and Bentham (1979) includes the utilization aspects of community hospitals, whilst that by Parkin (1979) shows that distance from facilities can have a negative effect on utilization for most age groups of the population, an observation noted in some other countries. Phillips (1979a, 1981) indicates how certain intangible factors, including the attitudes of patients to their general practitioners, can influence utilization behaviour. Less favourable attitudes towards general practitioner services displayed by lower status groups may indicate that a social inverse care law exists as well as the availability inverse care law proposed by Hart (1971). When it comes to the choice of which general practitioner to visit, it appears that factors such as inertia and location of previous residence may be as important as proximity (Phillips, 1979b, 1980). Such information enables planners to modify notions that consumers will attend the nearest available facility determined on a "central place" basis. In practice, however, complete freedom of choice of "family doctor" is not available to potential patients.

Utilization data of a different kind have been generated in the course of research into the behaviour of specific sectors of the population, such as the elderly (Herbert and Peace, 1980). This helps highlight the fact that certain sectors of the community have special needs over and above those of the majority, needs which should be incorporated into the planning process wherever possible. Behavioural studies have been criticized as being reductionist and have been eclipsed to some extent by other developments in human geography (Herbert, 1979; Phillips, 1981). Even so, they are of value when the lower levels of resource allocation and consumer uptake of services are being considered.

An interdisciplinary perspective for British medical geography?

This chapter has tended to further the idea that there are two distinct medical geographies, rather than one (Learmonth, 1978). This may appear to be the case at present and there are certainly problems in combining the two branches of the subject to gain optimum benefits for the community. Arguably, any such conjunction should not take place solely within the sphere of medical geography and should retain broad cross-disciplinary linkages. Medical geographers of all persuasions have, in the past, been progressive in their attempts to forge interdisciplinary links. Indeed, the subjects with which linkages have been made have actually been useful in defining the two fields of medical geography, as Learmonth (1978, p. 240) writes:

> the medical ecology workers tend to have their interdisciplinary links with the biomedical sciences, the health care geographers with demographers and economists, and possibly sociologists and social ecologists, and also to maintain strong links with current concerns in geography in general in quantitative, theoretical and applied aspects.

This was possibly true in the past and, to that extent, one might agree with Shannon (1980) when he says that "disciplinary" approaches have been one hindrance in health services research. Indeed the nature of their subject of study is such that medical geographers have long been accustomed to venturing beyond traditional disciplinary boundaries (Fig. 1). There is now the possibility of unity developing between studies in geographical pathology and the geography of health care due, in part, to impetus given by developments outside geography. Equally, epidemiologists, community physicians and health service planners and administrators appear to be becoming increasingly aware of the advantages of a spatial perspective to their work and of the possibilities of using geographical methodologies in planning (Scott-Samuel, 1977; E. G. Knox, 1979; Parry, 1979; Acheson, 1980).

It is appropriate in concluding this chapter to acknowledge the role played by the Institute of British Geographers in furthering this branch of the main discipline. The Medical Geography Study Group of the Institute has long fostered interdisciplinary links and is active in encouraging the conjunction and cooperation of the two aspects of this specialism in geography. In 1980 the Study Group hosted a joint symposium with the Society for Social Medicine and, at each recent annual conference of the Institute of British Geographers, it has convened meetings on a variety of medical geography themes. By such ventures geographical pathologists gain expertise in the techniques of health-care geographers, while the latter become experienced in the approach and methodologies of the disease ecologist. The task of conjoining the two main branches of the subject will not be an easy one but, with a concerted effort, the horizons of medical geography in the UK should continue to expand during and beyond the 1980s.

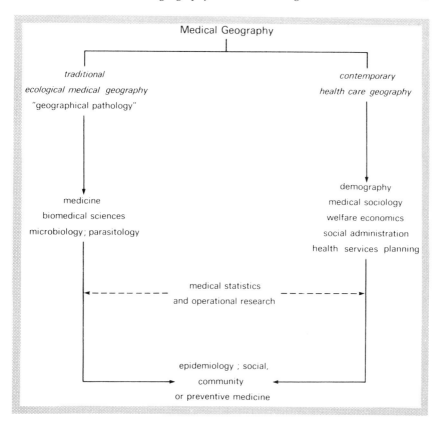

Figure 1. Some interdisciplinary linkages of medical geography. From Phillips (1981).

References

Acheson, R. M. (1980). Community medicine: discipline or topic? Profession or endeavour? *Community Medicine* 2, 2–6.

Alderson, M. R. (1970). Social class and the health service. *The Medical Officer* **CXXIV**, (3) 50–52.

Allen-Price, E. D. (1960). Uneven distribution of cancer in west Devon, with particular reference to the divers water supplies. *Lancet* 1, 1235–1238.

Bain, S. M. (1971). The geographical distribution of psychiatric disorders in the north-east region of Scotland. *Geographica Medica* 2, 84–108.

Bain, S. M. (1974). A geographer's approach in the epidemiology pf psychiatric disorder. *Journal of Biosocial Science* 6, 195–220.

Blaxter, M. (1976). Social class and health inequalities. In *Equalities and Inequalities in Health* (Eds. C. O. Carter and J. Peel), pp. 111–125. Academic Press, London and New York.

Butler, J. R. and Knight, R. (1974). The designated areas project study of medical practice areas—final report. Health Services Research Unit, Centre for Research in the Social Sciences, University of Kent at Canterbury.

Carter, C. O. and Peel, J. (Eds) (1976). *Equalities and Inequalities in Health.* Academic Press, London and New York.

Cartwright, A. and O'Brien, M. (1976). Social class variations in health care and in the nature of general practitioner consultations. In *The Sociology of the NHS* (Ed. M. Stacey), pp. 77–98. Sociological Review Monograph No. 22. University of Keele, Keele.

Castle, I. M. and Gittus, E. (1957). The distribution of social defects in Liverpool. *Sociological Review* 5, 43–64.

Clemow, F. G. (1903). *The Geography of Disease.* Cambridge University Press, Cambridge.

Coates, B. E. and Rawstron, E. M. (1971). *Regional Variations in Britain.* Batsford, London.

Court-Brown, W. M., Spiers, F. W. *et al.* (1960). Geographical variations in leukaemia mortality in relation to background radiation and other factors. *British Medical Journal* 1, 1753–1759.

Crawford, M. D., Gardner, M. J. and Morris, J. N. (1968). Mortality and hardness of local water supplies. *Lancet* 1, 827–8.

Dean, K. G. (1979). The geographical study of psychiatric illness: the case of depressive illness in Plymouth. *Area* 11, 167–171.

Department of Health and Social Security (1976). *Sharing Resources for Health in England.* Report of the Resource Allocation Working Party. HMSO, London.

Department of Health and Social Security (1980). *Inequalities in Health.* Report of a Research Working Group. HMSO, London.

Doll, R. and Hill, A. B. (1956). Lung cancer and other causes of death in relation to smoking. *British Medical Journal* 2, 1071–1081.

Forster, D. P. (1976). Social class differences in sickness and general practitioner consultations. *Health Trends* 8, 29–32.

Forster, F. (1966). Use of a demographic base map for the presentation of areal data in epidemiology. *British Journal of Preventive and Social Medicine* 20, 165–171.

Giggs, J. A. (1973). The distribution of schizophrenics in Nottingham. *Transactions of the Institute of British Geographers* 59, 55–76.

Giggs, J. A. (1977). Mental disorders and mental subnormality. In *A World Geography of Human Diseases* (Ed. G. M. Howe). Academic Press, London and New York.

Giggs, J. A. (1979). Human health problems in urban areas. In *Social Problems and the City* (Eds, D. T. Herbert and D. M. Smith), pp. 84–116. Oxford University Press, Oxford.

Giggs, J. A., Ebdon, D. S. and Bourke, J. B. (1980). The epidemiology of primary acute pancreatitis in the Nottingham Defined Population Area. *Transactions of the Institute of British Geographers* 5, 229–242.

Gilbert, E. W. (1958). Pioneer maps of health and diseases in England. *Geographical Journal* 124, 172–183.

Girt, J. L. (1972). Simple chronic bronchitis and urban ecological structure. In *Medical Geography: Techniques and Field Studies* (Ed. N. D. McGlashan), pp. 219–231. Methuen, London.

Griffiths, M. (1971). A geographical study of mortality in an urban area. *Urban Studies* **8**, 111–120

Haggett, P. (1972). Contagious processes in a planar graph: an epidemiological application. In *Medical Geography: Techniques and Field Studies* (Ed. N. D. McGlashan), pp. 307–324. Methuen, London.

Haggett, P. (1976)., Hybridizing alternative models of an epidemic diffusion process. *Economic Geography* **52**, 134–146.

Hart, J. T. (1971). The inverse care law. *Lancet* **1**, 405–412.

Haynes, R. M. and Bentham, C. G. (1979). *Community Hospitals and Rural Accessibility*. Saxon House, Farnborough.

Heller, T. (1976). The distribution of caring facilities: a case-study of East Anglia. *Development Studies Discussion Paper No. 12*. University of East Anglia, Norwich.

Herbert, D. T. (1979). Geographical perspectives and urban problems. In *Social Problems and the City* (Eds D. T. Herbert and D. M. Smith), pp. 1–9. Oxford University Press, Oxford.

Herbert, D. T. and Peace, S. M. (1980). The elderly in an urban environment. In *Geography and the Urban Environment* (Eds. D. T. Herbert and R. J. Johnston), pp. 223–255. Wiley, London.

Hopkins, E. J., Pye, A. M., Solomon, M. and Solomon, S. (1968). The relation of patients' age, sex and distance from surgery to the demand on the family doctor. *Journal of the Royal College of General Practitioners* **16**, 368–378.

Howe, G. M. (1959). The geographical distribution of disease with special reference to cancer of the lungs and stomach in Wales. *Journal of Preventive and Social Medicine* **13**, 204–210.

Howe, G. M. (1963). *National Atlas of Disease Mortality in the United Kingdom*. Nelson, London. Second edition, 1970.

Howe, G. M. (1969). Putting disease on a map. *Nature* **223**, 891.

Howe, G. M. (1970). Some recent developments in disease mapping. *Royal Society of Health* **90**, 16–20.

Howe, G. M. (1971). The geography of lung-bronchus and stomach cancer in the United Kingdom. *Scottish Geographical Magazine* **87**, 202–220.

Howe, G. M. (1972). *Man, Environment and Disease in Britain: A Medical Geography through the Ages*. David and Charles, Newton Abbot; Pelican, Harmondsworth, 1976.

Howe, G. M. (1976). The geography of disease. In *Equalities and Inequalities in Health* (Eds C. O. Carter and J. Peel), pp. 45–64. Academic Press, London and New York.

Howe, G. M. (1979). Mortality from selected malignant neoplasms in the British Isles: the spatial perspective. *The Geographical Journal* **145**, 401–415.

Howe, G. M. (1980). Medical geography. In *Geography Yesterday and Tomorrow* (Ed. E. H. Brown), pp. 280–291. Oxford University Press, Oxford.

Hunter, J. M. and Young, J. (1971). Diffusion of influenza in England and Wales. *Annals of the Association of American Geographers* **61**, 637–653.

Kivell, P. T. and Shaw, G. (1980). The study of retail location. In *Essays in Retail Geography* (Ed. J. Dawson), pp. 95–155. Croom Helm, London.

Knox, E. G. (Ed.) (1979). *Epidemiology in Health Care Planning*. Oxford University Press, Oxford.

Knox, P. L. (1978). The intraurban ecology of primary medical care: patterns of accessibility and their policy implications. *Environment and Planning A* **10**, 415–435.

Knox, P. L. (1979a). The accessibility of primary care to urban patients: a geographical analysis. *Journal of the Royal College of General Practitioners* **29**, 160–168.

Knox, P. L. (1979b). Medical deprivation, area deprivation and and public policy. *Social Science and Medicine*, **13D**, 111–121.

Knox, P. L. and Pacione, M. (1980). Locational behaviour, place preference and the inverse care law in the distribution of primary medical care. *Geoforum* **11**, 43–55.

Learmonth, A. T. A. (1972). Regional disparities in the health sector. *Decision Making in Britain*, D203, Block 5, pp. 19–76. The Open University Press, Milton Keynes.

Learmonth, A. T. A. (1975). Ecological medical geography. *Progress in Geography* **7**, 201–226.

Learmonth, A. T. A. (1978). *Patterns of Disease and Hunger*. David and Charles, Newton Abbot.

Legon, C. D. (1951). A note on geographical variations in cancer mortality, with special reference to gastric cancers in Wales. *British Journal of Cancer* **5**, 175–179.

Legon, C. D. (1952). The aetiological significance of geographical variations in cancer mortality. *British Medical Journal* **2**, 700–702.

Mohan, J. (1981). Hospital planning in north east England. Paper presented to Institute of British Geographers Meeting, Leicester, January.

Moyes, A. (1977). Accessibility to general practitioner service on Anglesey: some trip-making implications. Paper presented to Institute of British Geographers Meeting, Newcastle-upon-Tyne, January.

Murray, G. D. and Cliff, A. D. (1977). A stochastic model for measles epidemics in a multi-region setting. *Transactions of the Institute of British Geographers* **2**, 158–174.

Noyce, J., Snaith, A. H. and Trickey, A. J. (1974). Regional variations in the allocation of financial resources to the community health services. *Lancet* **1**, 554–557.

O'Mullane, D. M. and Robinson, M. E. (1977). The distribution of dentists and the uptake of dental treatment by schoolchildren in England. *Community Dentistry and Oral Epidemiology* **5**, 156–159.

Parkin, D. (1979). Distance as an influence on demand in general practice. *Epidemiology and Community Health* **33**, 96–99.

Parr, J. B. (1980). Health care facility planning: some developmental considerations. *Socio-Economic Planning Sciences* **14**, 121–127.

Parry, W. H. (1979). *Communicable Diseases*. Hodder and Stoughton, London.

Phillips, D. R. (1979a). Public attitudes to general practitioner services: a reflection of an inverse care law in intra-urban primary medical care? *Environment and Planning A* **11**, 815–824.

Phillips, D. R. (1979b). Spatial variations in attendance at general practitioner services. *Social Science and Medicine* **13D**, 169–181.

Phillips, D. R. (1980). Spatial patterns of surgery attendance: some implications for the provision of primary health care. *Journal of the Royal College of General Practitioners* **30**, 688–695.

Phillips, D. R. (1981). *Contemporary Issues in the Geography of Health Care*. Geo Books, Norwich.

Phillips, D. R. and Learmonth, A. T. A. (1981). Access to primary health care. *A Guided Project Course in Human Geography*, D306, Module 3. The Open University Press, Milton Keynes.

Pickles, W. N. (1948). Epidemiology in country practice. *New England Journal of Medicine* **239**, 419–427.

Rein, M. (1969). Social class and the health service. *New Society* **14**, 807–810.

Richardson, I. N. and Dingwall-Fordyce, I. (1968). Patient geography in general practice. *Lancet* **2**, 1290–1293.

Robertson, I. M. L. (1977). An automated approach to locating social facilities. *Town Planning Review* **48**, 149–156.

Robertson, I. M. L. (1978). Planning the location of recreational centres in an urban area: a case study of Glasgow. *Regional Studies* **12**, 419–427.

Royal Commission on the National Health Service (1979). *Access to Primary Care*. Research Paper No. 6. HMSO, London.

Scott-Samuel, A. (1977). Social area analysis in community medicine. *British Journal of Preventive and Social Medicine* **31**, 199–204.

Shannon, G. W. (1980). The utility of medical geography research. *Social Science and Medicine* **14D**, 1–2.

Shannon, G. W. and Dever, G. E. A. (1974). *Health Care Delivery: Spatial Perspectives*. McGraw-Hill, New York.

Smith, D. M. (1977). *Human Geography—a Welfare Approach*. Edward Arnold, London.

Smith, D. M. (1979). *Where the Grass is Greener*. Penguin, Harmondsworth.

Sowerby, P. R. (1969). The use of transport in a rural practice. *Journal of the Royal College of General Practitioners* **17**, 131–133.

Stacey, M. (1977). People who are affected by the inverse law of care. *Health and Social Services Journal* **3**, 898–902.

Stocks, P. (1959). Cancer and bronchitis mortality in relation to atmospheric deposit and smoke. *British Medical Journal* **1**, 74–79.

Sumner, G. (1971). Trends in the location of primary medical care in Britain: some social implications. *Antipode* **3**, 46–53.

Taylor, P. J. and Carmichael, C. L. (1980). Dental health and the application of geographical methodology. *Community Dentistry and Oral Epidemiology* **8**, 117–122.

Taylor, S. D. (1974). The geography and epidemiology of psychiatric disorders in Southampton. Unpublished Ph.D. Thesis, University of Southampton.

Thomas, C. J. (1976). Sociospatial differentiation and the use of services. In *Social Areas in Cities* (Eds. D. T. Herbert and R. J. Johnston), Vol. II, pp. 17–63. Wiley, London.

Thomas, C. J. and Phillips, D. R. (1978). An ecological analysis of child medical emergency admissions to hospitals in West Glamorgan. *Social Science and Medicine* **12D**, 183–192.

Titmuss, R. M. (1968). *Commitment to Welfare*. Allen and Unwin, London.

Vaughan, D. H. (1967). Dispersion of patients in urban general practice. *The Medical Officer* **117**, 337–340.

Walters, V. (1979). *Class Inequalities and Health Care*. Croom Helm, London.

While, A. E. (1978). The vital role of the cottage-community hospital. *Journal of the Royal College of General Practitioners* **28**, 485–491.

White, R. R. (1972). Probability maps of leukaemia mortalities in England and Wales. In *Medical Geography: Techniques and Field Studies* (Ed. N. D. McGlashan), pp. 173–185. Methuen, London.

World Health Organization (1965). *Basic Documents*, 16th edition, 1. WHO, Geneva.

Geomedicine in Germany, 1952–1982

Helmut J. Jusatz

Heidelberger Akademie der Wissenschaften.
Geomedizinische Forschungsstelle,
Heidelberg, West Germany

The early years

From the publication of Finke's *Bersuch einer allgemeinen medicinischprak-tischen Geographie* at the end of the eighteenth century to the conclusion of the second edition of August Hirsch's presentation of all the then known diseases in his *Handbook of Historical-Geographical Pathology* in 1862, medical geography in the German-speaking realm had produced inventories of diseases according to continents and countries. It had, with only a few exceptions, succeeded neither in taking into account the geographical factors for the established or varying occurrences of dis-eases in individual countries, nor in drawing conclusions from these facts.

Even the *Seuchen-Atlas* (Zeiss, 1942–1945), published during the Second World War between 1942 and 1945, only presented different epidemic diseases on the basis of physical maps of Europe, the Mediter-ranean and the Near East. Progress consisted solely of the addition of maps concerning the occurrence of vectors with data on climate and population statistics and so remained within the range of traditional medical geography.

New directions

As so often happens in the sciences, what was needed was an example capable of giving a fresh impetus to medical geography in Germany. This impulse was provided by the publication of the *World Atlas of Epidemic Diseases* (Jusatz, 1961) which appeared in ten parts over the period

GEOGRAPHICAL ASPECTS OF HEALTH
ISBN 0 12 483780 8

1952–1961 and comprised 120 maps of the world and of individual continents. Then as now, this work constituted an essential step forward in the field of mapping disease occurrence. In this work the cartographic presentation was restricted to single diseases on world or continental maps one at a time. The usual topographic information on hydrology, terrain and communications was supplemented by other data on climatic conditions, vegetation, distribution of animal reservoirs and the vectors of infectious disease agents according to epidemiological research of the time on the aetiological role of these physical and biogeographical components as environmental factors in the distribution of a disease.

In a 1953 review in *Erdkunde*, Carl Troll, later president of the IGU, described the publication of the *World Atlas of Epidemic Diseases* as a milestone in the history of medical geography. In his appreciation of this first truly geomedical atlas, Troll—himself the pioneer of the modern landscape-ecological approach in geography—particularly stressed the fact that these maps constituted the first-ever attempt to present medical facts about disease occurrence or the distribution of epidemic disease on a single map, associating each with the geographical conditions of the environment. Although this principle of co-ordinating evidence from two different disciplines was not then entirely successful in every one of the atlas's sheets, the multi-coloured maps of this publication did give a new direction to the medical geography of that time. Furthermore, the work constituted a milestone along the difficult road leading to recognition and respect for medical geography.

The most significant consequence for a fresh start in German medical geography in the post-war period—and this applies to both disciplines alike, medicine and geography—was the exemplary cooperation of geographers and medical scientists of the most diverse specialisms with cartographers working together on the *World Atlas* in their own purpose-built and generously equipped workplace. This common purpose awakened and promoted an understanding of the significance of space in the investigation and the control of diseases and epidemics.

The Heidelberg Academy of Sciences was the first scientific institution in the Federal Republic of Germany to take up the suggestion of one of its members, Professor Ernst Rodenwaldt (1878–1965), by establishing a department under the aegis of its Mathematics and Natural Sciences Division with the title of Centre for Geomedical Research (CGR) in 1952. It was charged with the task of continuing and advancing the cartographic presentation of all problems in the border area between geography and medicine.

After the completion of the *World Atlas of Epidemic Diseases* the CGR enlisted the services of 40 specialists and continued to produce cartographic publications of geomedical relevance; the *World Maps of Climatology* (Rodenwaldt and Jusatz, 1952–1961), for example. These were followed by maps on poliomyelitis, on the advance of rabies in Europe, by maps of brucellosis distribution in Europe, Africa and South America, and others on schistosomiasis in Africa and on tick-borne encephalitis in southern Germany.

At the same time attempts were made to restrict the cartographic presentation of disease distribution in each area to an exclusively numerical-statistical approach. This had the result that the term "medical geography" as then applied was considered to be too static in its implications. It was therefore replaced in Germany by the new term "geomedicine".

The concept of *Geomedizin*

The word *Geomedizin* had first appeared in German scientific literature in 1931 and had subsequently been developed as a separate branch of research from medical geography. Used in this more narrowly defined meaning of the world, geomedicine, whilst paying due regard to the findings of microbiology, parasitology and immunology, is regarded as the investigation of the *causes* involved in the correlation of disease processes in space and time with phenomena in the geosphere. That is it concerns the earth's surface as well as the factors of man's physical and biological environment, together with the biotropic forces and effects of the atmosphere. In this sense geomedicine, as a pure science, distances itself from socio-economic factors which may also influence disease processes.

By stressing this natural scientific aspect of research, geomedicine seeks to make a contribution both to the *general* geo-ecology of man as the ubiquitous inhabitant of the earth, as well as to the *special* geo-ecology of man's diseases. It also considers geofactors in regions at the micro-, meso- and macro-scales which affect the health status and diseases of the inhabitants of different regions; for example, in tropical and sub-tropical zones.

In the Federal Republic of Germany investigations of this sort have been undertaken into the spread of new diseases in central Europe, and the evidence presented in geomedical maps. In this connection observations of more general significance were made, which led to establishing the fact that certain regularly recurring conditions must be met if the effect of geofactors on a disease process in a particular region is to be discussed. Of these the first is the regularity of occurrence in the region, and the second the consistency with other regions of the same or similar qualities.

In an example of geomedical analysis Jusatz (1955) established that in the case of tularaemia (an epidemic disease affecting field-mice, ground squirrels, lemmings, hares and wild rabbits), there are permanent foci in Europe. These can be characterized by the same or similar conditions, making it possible to speak of accordant ecosystems and *isozoonoses*. These foci exhibited a constancy of occurrence in the same regions over more than ten years. On the world-scale map of tularaemia occurrence, the author was also able to show that the disease distribution is closely limited to the holo-arctic faunal region (Jusatz, 1961).

After investigating a focus in the Steigerwald area of Germany it was possible to prove its geographical accordance with another centre on the sunny limestone slopes of the Pontic Hills in the Côte d'Or of eastern France and also with that in the Marchfeld north of Vienna in lower Austria. Here in the remnants of steppe grassland, an infected tick population acts as a perennial source of infection and has kept the epidemic going for decades.

In the case of tick-borne encephalitis, another infectious disease new to central Europe which occurs in early summer, it was possible to establish and record on a map the geo-ecological conditions as well as the repeated infection of specific regions by infected ticks (Jusatz and Wellmer, 1979). In this case too it was proved possible to recognize a consistent recurrence over more than ten years of a disease which affects man in southern Germany only when he enters regions where ticks are infected. The accordance with affected regions in Slovakia and Austria was cartographically defined by the 8°C annual isotherm around areas which are distinguished by a warmth-loving vegetation in a region formerly covered by oak and beech forests (Wellmer and Jusatz, 1981).

That a geomedical approach does not have to be based exclusively upon the results and statistical data of a single special branch of science, but is achieved by interdisciplinary cooperation, is demonstrated by these examples. The researcher is forced to leave his desk or laboratory in order to study different disciplines each concerned with separate aspects of the possible influences of environmental factors. Without needing to become a specialist in another discipline, he thus comes into contact with other sciences and has to establish relations with botany, zoology, geology and climatology. This is a major attraction of modern geomedical research into environmental questions which have, to quote Erich Martini's words (1955), the prospect of discovery of "phenomena conditional upon the laws of nature". Of these laws the co-determinants of disease outbreaks are one aspect.

Standortraum—a multi-factor delineation

Initially, the common task of both the sciences is to establish if and where there is a local limitation of disease occurrence, or of the extent of an epidemic in a geographically delimitable region. In this the region is not merely a two-dimensional area on a map, but rather it is a highly complicated interplay akin, for example, to the concept of landscape (Jusatz, 1958). In each such region geofactors, both physico-abiotic and biotic, operate functionally and causally, directly and indirectly, upon the organisms of disease, upon the disease vectors and upon the recep- tivity of the inhabitants. If the correlation of all these phenomena can be ecologically proved, the affected area may be termed a *Standortraum* (location space) or *Naturherd* (natural focus).

The quality of each region can be described and compared with others on the basis of the occurrence of a single disease. An instance of this is the case of malaria distribution in a tropical country, where it is possible to qualify its occurrence as being hypo-, meso- or hyper-endemic or as malaria-free directly because of climatic conditions unfavourable to the development of anopheline mosquitos in areas above 2000 m. In most instances, however, the evaluation of a region on the basis of one factor alone is not sufficient; a monocausal approach can lead to false conclu- sions, which should be avoided from the very outset. In the case of a locally restricted disease occurrence a geomedical analysis demands the understanding of this network, together with the linking of geographical and medical viewpoints. An uninterrupted causal chain must be found.

As was to be expected, the promotion of mutual understanding be- tween members of the two principal disciplines involved required the establishment of a new basis for dialogue and the development of joint investigations. An ideal venue for such meetings at international level proved to be the Institute for International Scientific Cooperation at Schloss Reisensburg, a Bavarian castle on the river Danube near Ulm. Over the period 1972–1977 three symposia were held there, the results of which were published in three reports in the serial *Erdkundliches Wissen* as supplements to the *Geographische Zeitschrift*. In these reports are to be found a host of suggestions for the investigation of medico-geographical problems which range over the field of the geo-ecology of infectious diseases, as well as the state of geographical research into non-infectious and chronic morbidity. These included diseases of the circulatory organs and their links with differences in the quality of drinking water. The cancers and psychiatric diseases were also considered. Fundamental discussions on the principles, aims and methods of geomedicine were pursued, as were cartographic questions arising from an exhibition of geomedical maps.

These symposia have demonstrated that contemporary geomedical research in the proper and original sense of the word *geomedicine* is capable of giving a new direction to the formulation of a geo-ecology of man and his diseases and to investigations once considered as belonging to medical geography.

During the first symposium at Schloss Reisenburg a Working Group for Medical Geography, under the aegis of the Central Association of German Geographers was formed; subsequently this received formal recognition by the Central Association, and in conjunction with the Heidelberg research centre it has so far convened seven working colloquia. At the 39th German *Geographentag* in Kassel, Jusatz (1974) spoke on the principles of "Geomedicine in landscape-ecological research". These links have already led to the acceptance of geomedical topics in dissertations formally examined as part of the final degree by some universities. In recent years, Schweinfurth has given several lectures about geomedicine at the University of Heidelberg.

Geomedizin—methodological developments

The methodology of analytical geomedicine was developed further by Diesfeld (1973) when he produced the "disease panorama" of an East African region (the Lake Victoria sheet) for the *Afrika-Kartenwerk*, a programme supported by the German Research Council. For this purpose he used biostatistical methods to evaluate the reported figures for 27 infectious diseases supplied by 50 hospitals over several years. He then applied the disease panorama derived therefrom to the population of the catchment area defined in terms of Christaller's (1933) central place theory. Working throughout in close association with a geographer, H. Hecklau, and taking into account the geomedically relevant factors of the orographic situation, the agro-geographical and climatological conditions, they succeeded in identifying 17 groups of *nosochoretic types*. With the aid of computer evaluation of the field data collected by Hecklau the "disease pattern", that is the total composition in terms of frequency and intensity, was related to each hospital catchment area. In this manner areas with different degrees of disease frequency could be quite precisely distinguished from each other in a spatial sense and geomedically important correlations became apparent, even though these could not always be represented in map form.

The environmental dependence of human diseases can be conditional upon a multitude of geofactors, which become effective in association with the ecological conditions varying over time and space (Jusatz, 1966). These include:

Biotic factors:	influences on viruses and vectors.
Edaphic factors:	the effect of soil type or minerals in the soil (the field of geo-pedo-medicine).
Orographic factors:	the effects of landforms, for example, in valleys with foehn winds.
Climatic factors:	atmospheric effects as investigated by biometeorologists.

In accordance with these principles, Hinz (1983) has published a synoptic geomedical map for a section of Africa comprising southern Nigeria and western Cameroon.

The way forward

The next task of geomedical research will be measurement of the different operative geofactors and their arrangement in rank order. Here it is appropriate to recall that ecology operates on the *minimum rule* according to Thienemann's law (1939) on the effectiveness of environmental factors. This accords a key position to those vital factors of which a minimum number are present. This rule applies particularly to the role of animal vectors of disease organisms in maintaining a permanent natural focus. In the case of tick-borne encephalitis, for example, a density of only one virus-infected tick per thousand ticks is required in order to maintain a natural focus.

Another and very important task of geomedicine is the recording of changes in man's environment caused by his economic activities in so far as these changes may impair health conditions and give rise to epidemic diseases. More descriptions are required of geographical facts which man, acting formatively upon the earth, elicits by altering the natural environment. Also, investigations are needed into dynamic changes in health status and disease of the population. As Rodenwaldt (1957) stressed, in the geomedical significance of human actions upon the surface form of the earth, there are medical geographical facts about which the medical scientist needs to know if he wishes to practice the geomedical approach.

The geomedical consequences of environmental change formed the topic discussed at a special session of the 43rd German *Geographentag* in 1981, the overall theme of which was "Space and Environment—Tasks for

Geography". At this meeting geographers and physicians from different parts of the world expressed concern over man's own effects on changing human health. This offers a warning that greater attention should be devoted to such questions.

Apart from the *nosological* principle in the description of a disease in a particular country or area of the world, medical geography also applies the *geographical* principle of the description of a country with regard to the occurrence of various diseases. As a pre-condition for the writing of a medical regional study the same working method should be applied as in geomedicine: the analysis of a country's disease panorama requires investigations of geographical and ecological prerequisites for the occurrence and intensity of certain diseases.

The public health services have also attempted to revive this form of description of an administrative district, but the lack of researchers showing sufficient interest has meant that these efforts have so far found no response.

In Heidelberg, however, a great number of ideas have been put forward on how to produce a comprehensive presentation of the state of knowledge about the disease situation allied with the health services of a region taking into account its geographical structures. As early as 1963 the Heidelberg Academy of Sciences had arranged a symposium of geographers and physicians called *Medizinische Länderkunde*. The Mathematics and Natural Sciences Division of the Heidelberg Academy of Sciences has also resumed the tradition of medical topographies— descriptions of places and countries—in their editions of the *Medizinische Länderkunde—Geomedical Monograph Series* (1968–1980). This series now comprises six volumes, on Libya, Afghanistan, Ethiopia, Kuwait, Kenya and Korea, with three more (on Sri Lanka, Thailand and Nigeria) in preparation.

Apart from these the Academy has sought to provide an outlet for monographic treatments of particular diseases as part of its series of reports under the title *Sitzungsberichte*: in recent years maps and accompanying texts have been published on anthrax, rabies, tick-borne encephalitis, schistosoma intercalatum, dengue haemorrhagic fever and brucellosis.

Wherever possible these modern regional descriptions should be written as cooperative works by a physician and a geographer. They should include a description of the area under review, its inhabitants and their socio-economic and cultural conditions because these are almost bound to be significant contributory factors in the investigation of disease causation.

This expansion of medical geography into the socio-economic sphere can undoubtedly be explained in terms of changed environmental conditions. In this regard the Federal Republic of Germany has not yet gone as far as the United States of America, where investigations of health-care delivery problems, behavioural research and health planning have far exceeded the traditional bounds of geography. In Germany these subjects have for some considerable time been associated with the research areas of medical sociology, social medicine, social hygiene and health-care planning. However, according to the concepts of human geography, they do have a place in a geomedical monograph. Such a view can be defended in the words of Paffen (1969) who has written:

> an exact division of man's natural and cultural make-up is not possible. Due to the necessity of disaggregating the material, we cannot start other than by considering man separately in the geographical space of countries and regions, on the one hand in respect to biological phenomena and reactions, and on the other hand to his social groupings and actions.

Conclusion

This account of the contribution to the field of research by German geographers and medical scientists over the past 30 years aims at recognizing that a complementary role exists between that kind of medical geography which Andrew Learmonth has served for a great deal of his scientific life and that which he has, in the final words of his book *Patterns of Disease and Hunger* (1978), called "ecological medical geography", freely translatable into German as *Geomedizin*.

References

Christaller, W. (1933). *Die zentralen Ortin Südwestdeutschlands*. Fischer Verlag, Jena.

Diesfeld, H. J. (1973). *Internat. J. Epidem.* 2, 47–54, 55–61.

Finke, L. L. (1791–1793). *Versuch einer allgemeinen medizinisch-praktischen Geographie*. Leipzig.

Erdkundliches Wissen—Supplements to *Geographische Zeitschrifte*. No. 35 (1974): *Fortschritte der geomedizinischen Forschung* (Ed. H. J. Jusatz). No. 43 (1976): *Methoden und Modelle der geomedizinischen Forschung* (Ed. H. J. Jusatz). No. 51 (1979): *Geomedizin in Forschung und Lehre* (Ed. H. J. Jusatz). Steiner, Wiesbaden.

Hirsch, A. (1862–1864). *Handbuch der historisch-geographischen Pathologie*, 2nd edition. Stuttgart. (English edition 1883–1886, London.)

Hinz, E. (1983). *Afrika-Kartenwerk*, Series W. Monograph to sheet 14: Medical geography—West Africa. Bornträger, Berlin.

Jusatz, H. J. (1955). Das Tularämie-Vorkommen in Mainfranken 1949–1953, eine geomedizinische Analyse. *Arch. Hyg. u. Bakt.* (Berlin) **139**, 189–199.

Jusatz, H. J. (1958). Die Bedeutung der Landschaftsökologischen Analyse für die geographisch-medizinische Forschung. *Erdkunde* 12, 4, 284–289.

Jusatz, H. J. (1961). In *Welt-Seuchen-Atlas—World Atlas of Epidemic Diseases* (Eds E. Rodenwaldt and H. J. Jusatz), Vol. III, pp. 35–38b. Falk, Hamburg.

Jusatz, H. J. (1966). The importance of biometeorological and geomedical aspects in human ecology. *Int. J. Biometeorol.* 10, 3, 323–334.

Jusatz, H. J. (1974). Die Bedeutung der Geomedizin bei der Ökologischen Landschaftsforschungs. In *Deutscher Geographentag Kassel*, Vol. 39, pp. 418–439. Steiner Verlag, Wiesbaden.

Jusatz, H. J. and Wellmer, H. (1979). Landschaftsökologische Analyse der in Baden-Württemberg aufgetretenen Zecken-Encephalitis. *Beitr. naturkundl. Forschg. Südwest. Dtl.* 38, 155–160.

Learmonth, A. T. A. (1978). *Patterns of Disease and Hunger*. David and Charles, Newton Abbot.

Martini, E. (1955). *Wege der Seuchen*, 3rd edition. Enke, Stuttgart.

Paffen, KH. (1969). *Stellung und Bedeutung der physischen Anthropogeographie*. Wiss. Buchgem, Darmstadt.

Medizinische Länderkunde—Geomedical Monograph Series (1968–1980). Vol. I. *Libya* (H. Kanter). Vol. II. *Afghanistan* (L. Fischer). Vol. III. *Ethiopia* (K. F. Schaller and W. Kuls). Vol. IV. *Kuwait* (G. E. ffrench and A. G. Hill). Vol. V. *Kenya* (H. J. Diesfeld and H. K. Hecklau). Vol. VI. *Korea* (Ch. Th. Soh). Springer Verlag, Berlin, Heidelberg and New York.

Rodenwaldt, E. (1957). Die geomedizinische Bedeutung menschlicher Einwirkungen auf die Oberflächengestalt der Erd. *Z. Tropenmed. Parasit.* 8, 227–233.

Rodenwaldt, E. and Jusatz, H. J. (Eds) (1952–1961). *World Atlas of Epidemic Diseases—Welt-Seuchen-Atlas*, 3 Volumes. Falk, Hamburg.

Rodenwaldt, E. and Jusatz, H. J. (1966). *World Maps of Climatology—Weltkarten zur Klimakunde*, 3rd edition. Springer Verlag, Berlin, Heidelberg and New York.

Sitzungsberichte der Math.-naturwiss. Klasse der Heidelberger Akademie der Wissenschaften (1965–1982). Kauker, E. (1965). Milzbrand. *Jahrg.* 1965, 2 Abh., 171–215. Kauker, E. (1966). Tollwut. *Jahrg.* 1966, 4 Abh., 205–232. Rodenwaldt, E. (1968). Alberti. *Jahrg.* 1968, 4 Abh., 97–198. Jusatz, H. J. (Ed.) (1978). Zentraleurop. Zeckenencephalitis. *Jahrg.* 1978, 2 Abh., 105–166. Thimm, B. M. (1981). Brucellosis. *Jahrg.* 1982 (Suppl.). Wellmer, H. (1983). Dengue haemorrh. Fever. *Jahrg.* 1983. Springer Verlag, Berlin, Heidelberg and New York.

Thienemann, A. (1939). Grundzüge einer allgemeinen Ökologie. *Arch. f. Hydrobiol.* 35, 267–285.

Troll, C. (1953). Ein Markstein in der Entwicklung der Medizinischen Geographie. *Erdkunde* (Bonn) 7, 60–64.

Wellmer, H. and Jusatz, H. J. (1981). Geoecological analysis of the spread of tick-borne encephalitis in Central Europe. *Soc. Sci. Med.* 15D, 1, 159–162.

Zeiss, H. (1931). Geomedizin oder Medizinische Geographie? *Münch. Med. Wschr.* 78, 192–198.

Zeiss, H. (Ed.) (1942–1945). *Seuchen-Atlas*. Perthes, Gotha.

The geography of health in France and the Benelux countries

Yola Verhasselt

Geografisch Instituut, Vrije Universiteit
Brussel, Belgium

Some key studies

A common characteristic of the geography of health in France and the Benelux countries is its recent development. Indeed, strictly speaking, there are but few contributions by geographers to this subject in comparison with those in English-speaking countries. However, if we include studies by other scientists–epidemiologists, demographers, medical sociologists and others—the review broadens significantly. The problem then becomes one of making a choice in a very large field of research, where publications are dispersed over many scientific journals. We will try to include those contributions which start from a spatial and ecological point of view or with an emphasis upon geographical content and/or method. We distinguish between on the one hand, a geographical approach establishing links with physical and human environmental factors and, on the other hand, a spatial emphasis in a study. The bibliography comprises a comprehensive list of geographical contributions and only a selected list of publications written by non-geographers, but relevant to the scope of the geography of health. Only published material will be taken into account, and this review makes no claim to completeness.

In France pioneer work has to be mentioned. The most prominent geographer who made a substantial contribution to the progress of medical geography is Maximilien Sorre. In his extensive study on human geography he developed the essential notion of a pathogenic complex as an ecological way of thinking. This concept was first introduced in an article in 1933 (Sorre, 1933). Later, in his first volume on human geog-

GEOGRAPHICAL ASPECTS OF HEALTH
ISBN 0 12 483780 8

raphy (Sorre, 1943), Sorre devotes a first chapter to climate and man, studying the relationship between climatic elements and human organic functions. His second chapter describes the living environment and human nutrition, establishing the base of a geography of nutrition; the third, the human organism in struggle with the living environment. In this chapter on medical geography Sorre analyses pathogenic complexes as links between environment and transmission processes of tropical diseases, such as trypanosomiasis, malaria and yellow fever. He points out general problems of cartography which are still relevant even in the age of computer techniques. The distribution of diseases is treated as a zonal pathology with a distinction between Atlantic, Pacific and Asian areas. The work of Sorre is an ecological approach to human geography, in a sense of human ecology, long before this became a widespread scientific movement.

Two other interesting early contributions by French geographers are both related to malaria. Le Lannou (1936) studied the distribution of malaria and natural environment, historic examples of consequences of the spread of the disease, and links with human occupation. Gourou (1949) analysed the effect of malaria upon the geography of Brazil.

Very few publications on medical geography stemmed from the period 1945–1960. In the 1960s and especially the 1970s, an upward movement of interest and a recrudescence of activities can be recognized. This is confirmed not only by an increasing number of publications, but also by the founding in 1978 of a Working Group on Geography of Health by the National French Committee of Geography (Picheral, 1980). This may be compared with the IGU Commission on Medical Geography which had been established in 1948. The French Working Group functions under the direction of Professor Picheral, who has made substantial contributions to the geography of health. Annual meetings are organized at the *Journées Géographiques* and exchange of information is conducted through a newsletter. Close collaborative links have been established with Belgian and Canadian medical geographers. A Benelux Working Group on Mortality has also existed since 1979. Regular meetings are organized with participants from the disciplines of demography, sociology, medicine and geography.

In France, important books have been published during recent years. Picheral's (1976a) doctorate thesis *Espace et Santé: Géographie médicale du Midi de la France* is an outstanding regional study. Diseases and health care are analysed for nine departments situated between Pyrénées and Alpes Maritimes. This region is characterized by an excellent provision of medical care facilities and a high use of health services, by important mortality rates (with a considerable infant mortality even today) and by the continuation of several infectious diseases. Among the chronic diseases, special mention is made of diabetes mellitus in this area. Of course cardiovascular diseases and cancer are included in the study. Picheral defines the notion of sociopathogenic complex as the relationship between disease and environment including the effects of personal mechanisms, social behaviour and external elements. Health care infrastructure in the Midi is attributable to generally very high densities of physicians and good hospital equipment, but, within this overall scene, regional disparities and inequalities are demonstrated. The book is illustrated by cartographic material comparing the region with the whole of France.

Quite another field is covered by the excellent study of Labasse (1980), *L'hôpital et la ville. Géographie hospitalière*. From the standpoint of an urban geographer the author considers the hospital's image (*l'image hospitalière*) in the city. The book starts with a general overview of the hospital network in France with regional examples; the hospital itself as an organism is then analysed. The chapter related to centrality, localization and the impact of the hospital on its surroundings is the most interesting part. Finally, an analysis is made of the hospital's dynamics and its contribution to the whole urban and regional economy.

Two other books analyse specific major disease regions and are published in the same series. Each includes contributions by both geographers and non-geographers: one on tropical areas (Delvert, 1979) and one on temperate zones and developed societies (Picheral, 1981).

General features

In France as well as in the Benelux countries a great deal of research is related to the pathology of developed societies. Demographers have paid attention to a historical approach, in the sense of the spread of diseases and differences in mortality. Several articles published in the reviews *Population* and *Annales Economies, Sociétiés et Civilisations* evidence this trend among French scientists. Moreover contributions from the realm of medical sociology and demography have concerned correlations between mortality and socio-economic status (Febvay and Aubenque, 1957; Pressat, 1972; Leclerc, 1979).

In the Netherlands the effects of general demographic considerations upon mortality are widespread in many publications (Polman, 1951). Differences according to sex ratio (Van Brunschot, 1980), age (Polman, 1958), civil status (Van Poppel, 1976) and occupation (Van Raalte, 1979) in relation to cancer mortality are demonstrated. Spatial inequalities have been studied at different levels: provincial (Van Poppel, 1978), according to the degree of urbanization (Kruijsen, 1976), and within cities, e.g. Amsterdam (De Wolff and Meerdink, 1954; Habbema *et al.*, 1980; Van den Bos, 1981). An interesting research direction is apparent in studies of the relationship between dwelling and disease (Van Eijk, 1974; Giel *et al.*, 1975; Danz and Nieuwenhuijse, 1975).

In Belgium, numerous publications, mostly written by demographers and sociologists, concern changing trends in causes of death (mostly published in the journals *Population et Famille* and *Bevolking en Gezin*), and spatial distribution of mortality (Angelo, 1974; Van Houte-Minet and Wunsch, 1979; Grosclaude *et al.*, 1979). On this latter topic work has also been done by geographers (Saey, 1966; André, 1969, 1970; Verhasselt, 1971). In collaboration with a paediatrician, André (1971) wrote an interesting book upon infant mortality in Belgium. In spite of a serious decrease in the twentieth century, infant mortality is still higher in Belgium than in other West European countries. A regional analysis by *arrondissements* shows particularly high rates in the Hainaut province. Several studies (Girard *et al.*, 1960; Noel, 1974) involve the role of socio-economic and cultural factors as causes of spatial differentiation (Van der Auwera *et al.*, 1974). Infant mortality has been studied in several French regions (Brasseur, 1965; Picheral, 1971; Andrian, 1976) and is well accepted as a welfare-indicator. Beckers (1974) considers infant mortality as a parameter of health education and as an index of efficiency of sanitary infrastructure. Other health determinants are listed by Eylenbosch and Nuyens (1980) and Moens (1979), for example. Several publications are related to the definition of health status of the population (Klein-Beaupain and Lefevere, 1974; Clay, 1977; Damiani and Massé, 1978).

Heart disease

Among the chronic diseases, cancers and cardiovascular diseases have received most attention. If coronary heart disease is still the main cause of death in Western Europe, one can observe a decrease in the developed world (Picheral, 1981). Distribution patterns of heart (Derrienic *et al.*, 1977) and cerebrovascular diseases (Dubois and Dubois, 1978) have been studied in France, of cardiovascular disease in Belgium (Graffar, 1979), and of ischaemic heart disease in the Netherlands by size of municipality (de Haas, 1971). Climatic conditions of cardiovascular accidents have been analysed (Besancenot, 1981). Risk factors have been put forward (Rime, 1969; Kornitzer *et al.*, 1975). Detailed correlation studies, especially in connection with food intake habits, show for example in Belgium higher serum cholesterol levels and higher butter consumption in the southern part of the country, where higher mortality rates from heart disease also occur (Joossens *et al.*, 1977; Kornitzer *et al.*, 1979). An analysis of total male mortality in a soft-water region demonstrates that rates are not abnormally high (Sartot, 1979). Correlation between water hardness and cardiovascular mortality is discussed by Huel (1978).

Sites of cancer

The study of malignant neoplasms has generated numerous publications. Distribution patterns of cancer mortality have been a main topic of research from general analyses on a world scale (Van Molle and Verhasselt, 1974; Besancenot, 1975, 1979; Verhasselt, 1977, 1979) to the national situation with several cartographic approaches by Berlié (1979) for France, by De Laet (1975) and Verhasselt (1981) for Belgium, and by Diehl and Tromp (1958) for the Netherlands. Moreover a very valuable document for the Netherlands is the *Cancer Atlas* edited recently by the Central Bureau of Statistics (1980): maps for each site are shown for the country subdivided into 40 regions. Early contributions are related to cancer mortality in Paris (Montagnon, 1948) and to general patterns for France (Denoix, 1952; Specklin, 1955). The notion of "geocancerology" in the geographical sense of analysis of distribution patterns and correlation studies with environmental factors has been attempted in several publications (Verhasselt, 1976, 1977; Picheral, 1979). The urban situation has been studied particularly in connection with respiratory cancer by Firket (1958) and De Laet (1978, 1981) for Belgium, by Picheral (1978) for France, and with the evolution of cancer mortality and cardiovascular disease in Antwerp during the twentieth century (Vrijens, 1981, 1982).

Particular cancer sites received attention: for example, lung cancer (Denoix and Gelle, 1955; Firket, 1955; Verbeke, 1958), and bladder tumours (Berlié *et al.*, 1979). Cancer of the oesophagus has been studied thoroughly in France, where the incidence in Brittany is very high (Tuyns and Massé, 1973; Berlié, 1981); its correlation with alcohol intake has been demonstrated (Tuyns, 1970; Tuyns *et al.*, 1979). In Belgium, research related to gastric cancer (Maisin *et al.*, 1958; Ramioul and Tuyns, 1977; Verhasselt, 1981) deserves a particular mention because the north–south contrast is considerable (see Fig. 1). Links with food habits have been proposed; e.g. a higher fat intake in southern Belgium (Lederer, 1975; Joossens, 1978), or higher salt consumption (Joossens *et al.*, 1975). In the Netherlands, distribution of stomach cancer has been related to quality of drinking water (Tromp, 1954) and to soil composition, with higher rates on peat soils (Tromp and Diehl, 1955; Tromp, 1956). More generally

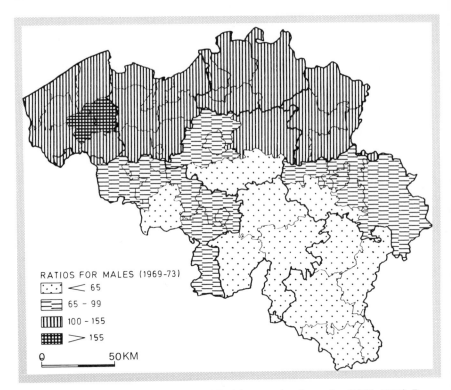

Figure 1. Stomach cancer—standardized incidence ratios for males (1969–1973). From *Geographia Medica* **II**, 107 (1981).

the same author has proposed links between geophysical factors and cancer distribution (Tromp, 1955, 1979). Other correlations with environmental elements have been indicated: such as nutrition and digestive cancers (Lederer, 1977; Massé, 1977; Meyer, 1977), alcohol intake (Lasserre *et al.*, 1967; Picheral, 1976), tobacco consumption (Damiani, 1966; Tuyns, 1979), occupational activities (Zielhuis, 1975; Lauwerys, 1979; Van den Oever *et al.*, 1981).

Other causes of mortality and morbidity have been examined spatially, such as deaths by accidents (Chesnais, 1974) and suicides (Mendelwicz *et al.*, 1970; Chesnais, 1978; Philippe, 1979; Bosman, 1980).

Infectious diseases

The occurrence of infectious diseases in developed societies (Bijkerk, 1974) has been analysed: for example, *fièvre de Malte* (Picheral, 1966), brucellosis (Picheral, 1969), malaria, (Jong, 1969), rabies (Bugyari *et al.*, 1979), leishmaniasis (Barabe *et al.*, 1981; Rioux *et al.*, 1981). Examples of historic studies concern the demographic consequences of plague in Brussels in 1667–1669 (Charlier, 1969) and a cholera outbreak in Leuven in 1849 (Van der Haegen and De Vos, 1980).

Urban studies

A very interesting topic from a geographical point of view is the spatial distribution of mortality and morbidity within a city. Besides the studies of cancer in urban settings already mentioned, distribution maps of causes of death have been published for Paris (Grisez, 1961). Other cities have been examined: Barcelona (Picheral, 1969), Amsterdam (De Wolff and Meerdink, 1952), Rotterdam (Schneider, 1980); Lyon and Marseille (Dubesset, 1971; Arnaud and Massini, 1973) as to the spread of tuberculosis. A general approach to urban mortality in France can be found in demographic and epidemiological work (Biraben, 1975; Bouvier *et al.*, 1980; McHarg, 1980). Urban mortality and morbidity deserve a greater emphasis as to distribution patterns and links with environmental factors and to comparisons between cities (Verhasselt, 1981).

Bioclimatology

There is a strong interest in human bioclimatology (*météoropathologie*) both in France and the Netherlands. Geographical contributions by Besancenot (1974) and Escourrou (1981) are representative of this field of research. Moreover, studies have been published from other disciplines (particularly in *Bioclimat* and *Presse Médicale*), establishing links between climatic factors and specific pathologic phenomena. For example, the meterological influence upon ischaemic heart disease appears mainly through sudden pressure changes (Coget, 1962). In the Netherlands the work of Tromp (1963) has led the way in the progress of biometeorology.

Nutrition

The geography of nutrition, although not specially oriented towards medical geography, contributes very useful elements to a most interesting field of social geography, where information is sparse. In France, Thouvenot and his team studied the relationship between environment and food intake, and the historic and socio-economic evolution of alimentary habits (Thouvenot, 1971, 1975, 1978). A general manual on the geography of nutrition has been published (Livet, 1969). Links between food habits (and alcohol intake) and disease or mortality have been established (Lennan and Meyer, 1977; Massart et al., 1980; de Lint, 1980). The study of trace-elements is promising (Bruaux and Lafontaine, 1978; Fouassin and Fondu, 1981).

Other research directions are worth mentioning, such as diseases of migrants (Lanier et al., 1979), health and tourism (Bailly, 1979; Reitel, 1975), impact of pollution (Rondia, 1973; Biersteker, 1966, 1975), haematology (a general spatial approach by Bernard and Ruffie, 1965, 1972) and geographical distribution of specific blood characteristics by Gourou (1961).

Tropical diseases

Tropical diseases deserve most attention. The continuing French tradition in tropical geography is also evident in the geography of health. Malaria (Borelly, 1975; Charmot et al., 1977; Rodhain and Roze, 1977), onchocerciasis (Picq and Albert, 1979), and schistosomiasis (Roze, 1978) are favourite topics of research in relation to environmental factors, and also infectious diseases like meningitis (Monnier, 1980) or syphilis (Maleville, 1976). Geographical and epidemiological contributions are included in a special issue of Cahiers d'Etudes Africaines (1981, No. 4) which is devoted to tropical Africa. Delvert's book (1979) already mentioned contains studies of important endemic diseases. A general introduction of tropical diseases (Gentilini et al., 1980) is illustrated with excellent maps and photographs and carried out by a team of physicians and a geographer. J.-M. Amat-Roze, who has made substantial contributions to the geography of tropical diseases.

Belgian epidemiologists have also done a great deal of work in connection with tropical illness. In the Annales de la Société belge de Médecine tropicale results of clinical and epidemiological research are published. Moreover thematic issues are devoted to one disease; for example Vol. 61, No. 2 (1981) to onchocerciasis and other human filariasis, Vol. 57, No. 4–5 (1977) to human trypanosomiasis. An ecological–geographical approach is employed upon the same disease in Zaire (Verhasselt, 1969–1970). Dutch contributions to the spread and ecology of tropical diseases can be found in Tropical and Geographical Medicine.

Health care

In the geography of health care regional disparities and inequality were demonstrated for France (Lebart *et al.*, 1974). Underprovision prevails in the north (Lasorne, 1968; Lottin, 1969), while a high density of physicians characterises the Paris area (Dekhli and Errahmani, 1979); spread of pharmacies has been studied in Vendée (Renard, 1981). Distributional studies of hospitals in Amsterdam (De Vries Reilingh, 1965) and socio-geographical aspects of hospital functions in the Belgian province of Luxemburg (Ek, 1976) were developed from a spatial point of view. Another geographical contribution considers the spread of physicians within Brussels (Vandermotten and Ots-Albitar, 1976). From the medical and governmental side, organizational problems in urgent medical assistance were spatially demonstrated for Belgium (Beckers, 1980). Examples of sociological approaches to general health care in Belgium are those by Foets and Nuyens (1980) and Nuyens (1980). As spatial planning is well organized in the Netherlands, a great deal of research is done with the aim of providing a well balanced health-care policy. A general statement on planning in health care (Stolte and Lapre, 1977) is one example of many publications related to this field. A special issue of *Tijdschrift voor sociale geneeskunde* (1980) is devoted to inequalities in health and health care. At the provincial level, interesting studies are those relating to the planning of hospitals in Friesland (*Provinciale Raad voor de volksgezondheid* in Friesland); among the factors taken into account is public opinion. A remarkable paper draws attention to the almost exceptional situation in borderlands regarding the use of medical services; a regulation of 1978 makes it possible for the inhabitants of the Dutch province of Zealand Flanders to go to Belgium for special treatment (Houtzager, 1978).

Problems of health care in the developing world are approached, for example, by Gentilini (1979) and by a special issue of *Annales de la Société belge de Médecine tropicale* (1979, Vol. 59).

Final thoughts

Thinking in medical geography in France has moved considerably from Sorre's original notion of a pathogenic complex linked with tropical and subtropical environments and transmission modes of endemic diseases, towards the concept of sets of socio-pathogenic complexes (Picheral, 1981) interfering with socio-economic factors and also towards the concept of techno-pathogenic complexes (George, 1981) involving technical progress and pollution. The future development of the geography of health in France will probably focus on these lines.

In comparison with publications in the anglophone world, geography of health in France and Benelux has been characterized by few methodological and theoretical contributions (De Lannoy, 1975; Verhasselt, 1977, 1981; Picheral, 1980), and few also in a historical perspective (Specklin, 1971; Comiti, 1980). Research should be stimulated in the field of health care. Interesting cartographic attempts have been made by Rimbert (1976) and Favier (1980). Collaboration between geography and other disciplines (especially epidemiology) has been realized in some fields (such as tropical diseases), but more teamwork approaches are still needed.

The geography of health is expanding now, particularly in France. The main problems are still related to the availability and reliability of statistical data.

Selected bibliography

André, R. (1969). La mortalité de la population de nationalité belge. Analyse régionale. *Rev. Inst. Sociol. ULB* **2**, 305–323.

André, R. (1970). Vieillissement et surmortalité en Hainaut. *Le Hainaut Franç. et Bel., A.E.D.E.* **2**, 107–163.

André, R. and Gyselings, A. (1971). La mortalité infantile en Belgique. Edit. Inst. Sociol. ULB, Bruxelles.

Andrian, J. (1976). La mortalité infantile dans le département de la Somme, 1959–1972. *Hom. et Ter. du Nord* **1**, 23–48.

Angelo da Silva, J. V. (1974). Surmortalité masculine aux âges actifs en Belgique. In *Deux études sur la mortalité en Belgique*, pp. 73–150. Centre d'Etude de la Population et de la Famille, Bruxelles.

Arnaud, J. L. and Masini, A.(1973). La population tuberculeuse dans l'agglomération marseillaise. Etude de géographie médicale urbaine. *Médit.* **1**, 3–28.

Bailly, P. (1979). Migration touristique et santé publique. *Rev. Santé publ.* **6**, 28–33.

Barabe, P. *et al.* (1981). Epidémiologie des leishmanioses en France. *Médit. méd.* **257**, 23–31.

Beckers, R. (1974). Les indices sanitaires. *Arch. belges Méd. soc. Hyg.* **32**, 9–10, 553–569.

Beckers, R. (1980). Problèmes d'organisation dans l'aide médicale urgente. *Arch. belges Méd. soc. Hyg.* **38**, 78–108.

Berlié, J. (1979). La répartition géographique de quelques cancers en France. *Prosp. et Santé* **10–11**, 111–131.

Berlié, J. (1981). La répartition géographique de la mortalité par cancer de l'oesophage en France. In *Etudes de géographie médicale, T II: Pays tempérés et sociétés développées* (Ed. H. Picheral), pp. 147–168. Com. Trav. hist. & scient., Bull. Sect. Géogr., LXXXIII, Paris, Bibl. Nat.

Berlié, J., Hanin, M. L., Hucher, M., Gest, J. and Brunet, M. (1979). Mortalité par cancer de la vessie en France de 1952–1976. Son évolution croissante et sa répartition géographique particulière dans le sud de la France. *Bull. Cancer* **66**, 3, 317–326.

Bernard, J. (1965). Esquisse d'une géographie des maladies du sang. *Ann. Géogr.* 403, LXXIV, 271–280.

Bernard, J. and Ruffie, J. (1972). *Hématologie géographique.* Masson and Cie, Paris.

Besancenot, J. P. (1974). Premières données sur les stress bioclimatiques moyens en France. *Ann. Géogr.* **459**, 497–530.

Besancenot, J. P. (1975). Regards sur la géographie du cancer. *Ann. Géogr.* **466**, LXXXIV, 665–698.

Besancenot, J. P. (1979). Le cancer primitif du foie à travers le monde. In *Etudes de géographie médicale, T I: Pays tropicaux* (Ed. J. Delvert), pp. 137–178. Com. Trav. hist. & scient., Bull. Sect. Géogr., LXXXIII, Paris, Bibl. Nat.

Besancenot, J. P. (1981). Le contexte climatique des accidents cardio-vasculaires sur la façade méditerranéenne de l'Europe. In *Etudes de géographie médicale, T II: Pays tempérés et sociétés développées* (Ed. H. Picheral), pp. 75–90. Com. Trav. hist. & scient., Bull. Sect. Géogr., LXXXIII, Paris, Bibl. Nat.

Biersteker, K. (1975). Health effects of specific industrial air pollutants in the Netherlands. *Tds. Soc. Gen.* **53**, 10, 299–305.

Bijkerk, H. (1974). Besmettelijke ziekten in Nederland. *Tds. Soc. Gen.* **53**, 10, 299–305.

Biraben, J. N. (1975). Quelques aspects de la mortalité en milieu urbain. *Popul.* **3**, 509–522.

Borelly, R. (1975). Le paludisme est un élément du sous-developpement. *Monde en dével.* **9**, 127–136.

Bosman, E. (1980). Een statistisch-sociologisch onderzoek inzake zelfmoord in België over het tijdvak 1930–1970. *Bev. en Gez.* **3**, 397–420.

Bouvier-Colle, M. H., Robine, J. R. and Favros, B. (1980). Surmortalité rurale ou sous-mortalité urbaine en France? *Rev. Epid. & Santé, Publ.* **28**, 1, 47–57.

Brasseur, A. (1965). La mortalité infantile dans la Région du Nord. *Hom. et Ter. du Nord* **1**, 7–31.

Bruaux, P. and Lafontaine, A. (1978). Exposition humaine aux éléments-traces. Effets possibles sur la santé. *Arch. belges Méd. soc. Hyg.* **36**, 401–426.

Bugyari, L. *et al.* (1979). La rage en Belgique. *Arch. belges Méd. soc. Hyg.* **8**, 465–480.

Central Bureau of Statistics (1980). *Atlas of Cancer Mortality in the Netherlands 1969–1978.* Staatsuitgeverij, The Hague.

Charlier, J. (1969). *La peste à Bruxelles de 1667–1669 et ses conséquences démographiques.* Pro Civitate, Bruxelles.

Charmot, G., Rodhain, F. and Roze, J. M. (1977). Relations entre le paludisme et le lymphome de Burkitt. *Bull. Soc. Path. exot.* **70**, 3, 274–281.

Chesnais, J. C. (1978). Le suicide par région. In *Les disparités démographiques régionales*, pp. 303–315. CNRS, Paris.

Clay, W. (1977). Meten van volksgezondheid. *Tds. Soc. Gen.* **55**, 26–31.

Coget, J. (1962). Les influences météorologiques et cosmiques dans l'infarctus du myocarde. *Presse méd.* **3**, 119–121.

Comiti, V. P. (1980). La géographie médicale de la Corse à la fin du XVIII siècle, Vol. 41. Librairie Droz, Genève.

Damiani, P. and Massé, H. (1978). Définition d'un indicateur du niveau de santé lié aux causes de décès. *J. Soc. Stat. Paris* **119**, 4, 357–366.

74   Yola Verhasselt

Danz, M. J. and Nieuwenhuijse, B. (1975). Mentale gezondheid en het wonen in hoogbouwflats; een methodologische beschouwing. *Tds. Soc. Gen.* **53**, 18, 566–576.

de Haas, J. H. (1971). Sterfte aan ischemische hartziekten naar gemeente-grootte. *Hart Bulletin* **2**, 67–75.

Dekhli, L. and Errahmani, E. (1979). Localités de l'Ile-de-France où sont installés plus de deux médecins libéraux pour mille habitants. *Cah Soc. Démogr. méd. France* **19**, 3, 64–68.

De Laet, H. (1975). Variations in the distribution of cancer mortality in Belgium. *Méd. Biol. Envir.* **3**, 2, 16–20.

De Laet, H. (1978). Lung cancer mortality in Belgian agglomerations. *Méd. Biol. Envir.* **6**, 2, 53–67.

De Laet, H. (1981). Studie van het verband luchtverontreiniging—longkanker in de Belgische agglomeraties. *De Aardr.* **1/2**, 185–192.

De Lannoy, W. (1975). Numerical grouping methods in medical geography. *Méd. Biol. Envir.* **3**, 2, 21–25.

de Lint. J. E. G. (1980). De invloed van het toenemende alcoholgebruik op het sterftepatroon. *Tds. Soc. Gen.* **14**, 547–551.

Delvert, J. (Ed.) (1979). *Etudes de géographie médicale, T I: Pays tropicaux.* Com. Trav. hist. & scient., Bull. Sect. Géogr., LXXXIII, Paris, Bibl. Nat.

Denoix, P. F. (1952). A propos d'une enquête géographique sur la morbidité par cancer en France. *Bull. Ass. fr. Cancer* **39**, 348–352.

Denoix, P. F. and Gelle, P. (1955). Estimation de l'importance comparée du cancer bronchopulmonaire en France et dans d'autres pays. *Bull Ass. fr. Cancer* **42**, 247–278.

Derrienic, F. *et al.* (1977). La mortalité cardiaque des Français actifs d'âge moyen selon leur catégorie socio-professionnelle et leur région de domicile. *Rev. Epid. & Santé, Publ.* **25**, 2, 131–146.

De Vries Reilingh, H. D. (1965). De ruimtelijke spreiding en vorm der Amsterdamse ziekenhuizen. *Geogr. Tds. KNAG* **2**, LXXXII, 4, 359–367.

De Wolff, P. and Meerdink, J. (1952). Le mortalité à Amsterdam selon les quartiers. *Popul.* **4**, 639–660.

De Wolff, P. and Meerdink, J. (1954). La mortalité à Amsterdam selon les groupes sociaux. *Popul.* **2**, 293–314.

Diehl, J. C. and Tromp, S. W. (1958). Geographical and geological distribution of cancer mortality. (A general analysis of basic assumptions and procedures.) *Acta Un. int. Cancr.* **14**, 580–590.

Dubesset, P. (1971). La population tuberculeuse dans l'agglomération lyonnaise. *Rev. Géogr. Lyon* **46**, 1, 91–120.

Dubois, A. F. and Dubois, H. (1978). Les disparités régionales de mortalité par maladies cérébro-vasculaires. In *Les disparités démographiques régionales*, pp. 333–344. CNRS, Paris.

Ek-Troisfontaines, A. (1976). Quelques aspects socio-géographiques de la fonction hospitalière dans la province de Luxembourg. *Bull. Soc. Géogr. Liège* **12**, 109–119.

Escourrou, G. (1981). Chaleur et mortalité. In *Etudes de geographie médicale, T II: Pays tempérés et sociétés développées*, pp. 59–73. Com. Trav. hist. & scient., Bull. Sect. Géogr., LXXXIII, Paris, Bibl. Nat.

Eylenbosch, W. and Nuyens, Y. (1974). Indikatoren voor een gezonde samenleving? *Tds. Soc. Gen.* **10**, 312–355.

Favier, A. and Thouvenot, C. (1980). Eléments de cartographie alimentaire. *Ann. Géogr.* **493**, LXXIX, 273–289.

Febvay, M. and Aubenque, M. (1957). La mortalité par catégorie socio-professionnelle. *Et. Stat. INSEE* **3**, 39–44.

Firket, J. (1955). Fréquence, facteurs étiologiques et repartition géographique des cancers du poumon. *Rev. méd. Gen.* **10**, 3–12.

Firket, J. (1958). The problems of cancer of the lung in the industrial area of Liège during recent years. *Proc. R. Soc. Med.*, **51**, 347–352.

Foets, M. and Nuyens, Y. (1980). Focus op de Belgische gezondheidszorg, Leuven, Sociol. *Studies en Documenten* **11**.

Fouassin, A. and Fondu, M. (1980). Evaluatie van het gemiddelde lood- en cadmiumgehalte in de dagelijkse voeding in België. *Belg. Arch. Soc. Gen. Hyg.* **1**, 1–14.

Gentilini, M. (1979). Aspects des problèmes sanitaires dans les pays en voie de développement. *Planif. Habit. Inf. Fr.* **95**, 13–19.

Gentilini, M., Brousse, G. and Amat-Roze, J. M. (1980). Risques infectieux et parasitaires intercontinentaux. Roche, Neuilly s. Seine.

George, P. (1978). Perspectives de recherche pour la géographie des maladies. *Ann. Géogr.* **484**, LXXXVII, 641–650.

Giel, R., Jessen, J. L. and Ormel, H. (1975). Flatbewoners en hun gezondheid. *Tds. Soc. Gen.* **53**, 10, 290–298.

Girard, A., Henry, L. and Nistri, R. (1960). Facteurs sociaux et culturels de la mortalité infantile. *Cah. I.N.E.D.* **36**.

Gourou, P. (1949). Paludisme et géographie au Brésil. In *Livre jubilaire offert à Maurice Zimmermann*, pp. 193–204. Imprimerie M. Audin, Lyon.

Gourou, P. (1971). Hématies en faucille et géographie humaine. *Homme* **1**, 90–94.

Graffar, M. (1979). Pathologie géographique des maladies cardiovasculaires en Belgique. *Rev. Epid. & Santé, Publ.* **28**, 5–6, 425–436.

Grisez, L. (1961). Les causes de décès à Paris depuis le début du siècle. *Inform. Géogr.* **1**, 1–10.

Grosclaude, A., Lux, B., Van Houte-Minet, M. and Wunsch, G. (1979). Mortalité régionale et comportements différentiels. Les déterminants de la mortalité masculine. *Popul. et Fam.* **3**, 1–43.

Habbema, J. D. F. *et al* (1980). Onderzoek naar verschillen in sterfte, ziekenhuisopname en langdurige arbeidsongeschiktheid tussen buurten in Amsterdam. *Tds. Soc. Gen.* **58**, 101–106.

Houtzager, A. O. (1978). Geneeskundige voorzieningen in het Nederlands-Belgisch grensgebied. *Benelux* **3**, 8–9.

Huel, G. *et al.* (1978). Dureté de l'eau et mortalité cardiovasculaire. Analyse critique des arguments de pathologie géographique. *Rev. Epid. & Santé Publ.* **26**, 349–359.

Jong, W. J. (1969). Malaria in Nederland. *Geogr. Tds. KNAG* **III**, 5, 458–459.

Joossens, J. V. (1969). Food pattern and mortality in Belgium. *Kon. Ac. Gen. B. Coll.* **31**, 133–161.

Joosens, J. V. *et al.* (1977). The pattern of food and mortality in Belgium. *Lancet* **8021**, 1069–1072; **8083**, 603.

Klein-Beaupain, Th. and Lefevere, G. (1974). Les indicateurs sociaux de santé. Une approche pour la Belgique. Edit. Univ. de Brux., Bruxelles.

Kornitzer, J., Kittel, F., Ruskin, R. M., Degre, V., Dramaix, M. and Thilly, C. (1975). Facteurs psychologiques et sociaux en relation avec les cardiopathies ischémiques. *Arch. Mal. Coeur et Vaiss.* **68** (suppl.), 35–44.

Kornitzer, M. G., De Vacker, M., Dramais, M. and Thilly, C. (1979). Regional differences in risk factor distribution, food habits and coronary heart disease mortality and morbidity in Belgium. *Int. J. Epid.* **1**, 23–31.

Kruijsen, A. (1976). Geografische verschillen in sterfte in Nederland. *Bull. NIDI* **18**, 1–3.

Labasse, J. (1980). *L'hôpital et la ville. Géographie hospitalière.* Hermann, Paris.

Lanier, P. *et al.* (1979). Expression de la pathologie des migrants. *Lyon-Médical* **242**, 16, 305–321.

Lasorne, C. (1968). L'équipement médical et hospitalier du Département de la Somme. *Hom. et Ter. du Nord* **1**, 79.

Lasserre, O., Flamant, R., Lelouch, J. and Schwartz, D. (1967). Alcool et cancer, Etude de pathologie géographique. *Bull. INSERM* **22**, 55–60.

Lauwerys, R. (1979). Pollution chimique professionnelle et cancer. *Arch. belges Méd. soc. Hyg.* **6**, 337–344.

Lebart, L., Sandier, S. and Tonnellier, F. (1974). Aspects géographiques du système des soins medicaux. Consommation. *Ann. CREDOC* **4**, 5–50.

Leclerc, A. (1979). Morbidité, mortalité et classe sociale. Revue bibliographique portant sur divers aspects de la pathologie, et discussion. *Rev. Epid. & Santé, Publ.* **27**, 4, 331–358.

Lederer, J. (1977a). Alimentation et cancer. *Nauwelaerts, Leuven*, **47**.

Lederer, J. (1977b). Facteurs nutrionnels induisant le cancer de l'estomac. *Acta Gastroent. Belg.* **38**, 329–346.

Le Lannou, M. (1936). Le rôle géographique de la malaria. *Ann Géogr.* **254**, XLV, 113–135.

Lennan Mac, R. and Meÿer, F. (1977). Food and mortality in France. *Lancet* **II**, 133.

Livet, R. (1969). *Géographie de l'alimentation.* Edit. ouvrières, Paris.

Lottin, J. J. (1969). Equipement sanitaire et hospitalier de la région Nord-Pas-de-Calais. *Hom. et Ter. du Nord* **1**, 75–82.

Maisin, J. H., Tuyns, A. and Goffin, R. (1958). Gastric cancer in Belgium. In *Proc. World Cong. Gastroent. Washington* **2**, 1119–1132.

Maleville, J. (1976). La syphilis et les tréponématoses endémiques. Distribution géographique et écologie. *Cah. Outre-Mer* **133**, 5–17.

Massart, L., Deelstra, H. and Hoogewijs, G. (1980). Vreemde stoffen in onze voeding. Nederlandsche Boekhandel, Amsterdam.

Massé, H. (1977). Mortalité par cancer: évolution de 1925 à 1974 et influence de l'environnement ainsi que de différents facteurs nutritionnels. *Méd. Biol. Envir.* **5**, 68–75.

McHarg, I. L. (1980). La ville: santé et maladie. *Cah. Inst. Aménagt. Urban, Rég. Ile de France* **58–59**, 154–158.

Mendelwicz, J., Wilmotte, J. and Defrise-Gussenhove, E. (1970). Les tentatives de Suicide. Résultats d'une enquête à Bruxelles. *Popul.* **25**, II, 797–809.

Meyer, F. (1977). Relations alimentation-cancer en France (estomac, colon, rectum, pancréas). *Gastroent. clin. biol.* **1**, 12, 971–982.

Moens, G. (1979). Gezondheidsekologisch onderzoek: mogelijkheden en beperkingen. Een literatuuroverzicht. *Arch. belges Méd. soc. Hyg.* **37**, 9–10, 562–588.

Monnier, Y. (1980). Méningite cérébro-spinale, harmattan et déforestation. *Cah. Outre-Mer* **130**, 103–122.

Montagnon, S. (1948). La mortalité par cancer à Paris. *Rec. Inst. nat. Hyg., Paris* **3**, 777–934.

Noel, F. (1974). Mortalité infantile: essai d'analyse socio-demographique. In

Deux études sur la mortalité en Belgique, pp. 3–68. Centre d'Etude de la Population et de la Famille, Bruxelles.

Nuyens, Y. (1980). *De eerste lijn is krom. Gezondheidszorg tussen onderzoek en beleid.* Van Loghum Siaterus, Deventer.

Philippe, A. (1979). Mortalité par suicide en France: Etude des disparités régionales. *Rev. Epid. & Santé, Publ.* **27**, 4–5, 479–482.

Picheral, H. (1966). Géographie de la Fièvre de Malte dans le Gard. *Bull. Soc. Langued. Géogr.* **4**, 631–660.

Picheral, H. (1969a). La bruxellose en France. Essai de Géographie médicale. *Ann. Géogr.* **426**, LXXVIII, 189–205. ·

Picheral, H. (1969b). Mortalité et Quartiers à Barcelone. *Bull. Soc. Langued. Géogr.* **92**, 3, 299–319.

Picheral, H. (1971). Le recul de la mortalité infantile en Corse (1950–1969). *Bull. Soc. Langued. Géogr.* **5**, 3, 301–318.

Picheral, H. (1976a). *Espace et Santé*. Paysan du Midi, Montpellier.

Picheral, H. (1976b). Alcoolisme et cancers de l'appareil digestif dans le Midi méditerranéen (France). *Méd. Biol. Envir.* **4**, 1, 26–36.

Picheral, H. (1978). Villes et cancers des voies respiratoires en France. *Bull. Assoc. Géogr. Fr. Paris* **451**, 125–137.

Picheral, H. (1979). Une géocancerologie urbaine en France: première approche. *Méd. Biol. Envir.* **7**, 2, 13–24.

Picheral, H. (1980a). L'essai récent des recherches françaises en géographie de la santé. In *Recherches géographiques en France* (Comité National Français de Géographie), pp. 151–153. Tokyo.

Picheral, H. (1980b). La géographie de la santé. In *La Recherche en Sciences Humaines, Sciences Soc.* D2, pp. 134–137. CNRS, Paris.

Picheral, H. (Ed.) (1981a). *Etudes de géographie médicale, T II: Pays tempérés et sociétés développées.* Com. Trav. hist. & scient., Bull. Sect. Géogr., LXXXIII, Paris, Bibl. Nat.

Picheral, H. (1981b). Santé et régions françaises: Etat de la recherche. In *Etudes de géographie médicale, T II: Pays tempérés et sociétés développées*, pp. 225–251. Com. Trav. hist. & scient., Bull. Sect. Géogr., LXXXIII, Paris, Bibl. Nat.

Picheral, H. (1981c). Le déclin récent de la mortalité par maladies coronariennes dans les pays développés. In *Etudes de géographie médicale, T II: Pays tempérés et sociétés développées*, pp. 91–107. Com. Trav. hist. & scient., Bull. Sect. Géogr., LXXXIII, Paris, Bibl. Nat.

Picq, J. J. and Albert, J. P. (1979). Onchocercose de savane et de forêt en Afrique de l'Ouest: un problème épidemiologique. *Rev. Epid. & Santé, Publ. Fr.* **27**, 5–6, 483–498.

Polman, A. (1951). *Ontwikkeling en huidige stand van de sterfte in Nederland en Belgie.* Ver. voor Demografie, 's Gravenhage.

Polman, A. (1958). Differentiële sterfte naar geslacht en leeftijd. In *Differentiële sterfte.* Vereniging voor Demografie, 's Gravenhage.

Pressat, R. (1972). La mortalité en France selon les catégories sociales. In *Sociologie médicale* (Ed. F. Steudler), pp. 145–156. A. Colin, Paris.

Prioux, F. and Vallin, J. (1978). Evolution des disparités de la mortalité infantile entre les départements français. In *Les disparités démographiques régionales*, pp. 391–399. CNRS, Paris.

Ramioul, L. and Tuyns, A. J. (1977). La distribution géographique des cancers du tube digestif en Belgique. *Acta Gastro-ent. bel.* 1977, 40, 129–147.

Renard, J. (1981). Répartition des pharmacies et géographie: Exemple de la Vendee. In *Etudes de géographie médicale, T II: Pays tempérés et sociétés développées* (Ed. H. Picheral), pp. 185–201. Com. trav. hist. & scient., Bull. Sect. Géogr., LXXXIII, Paris, Bibl. Nat.

Reitel, F. (1975). Le thermalisme en France: contribution à la géographie médicale et à l'aménagement du territoire. *Mosella* **5**, 1, 1–34.

Rimbert, S. (1976). Une expérience cartographique en géographie médicale: la répartition des décès par anomalies congénitales dans le Bas-Rhin. *Rech. Géogr. Strasbourg*, 229–241.

Rime, A. *et al.* (1979). L'épidémiologie de l'Atherosclerose des Coronaires en Belgique. *Acta Cardiol.* **24**, 5, 482–495.

Rioux, J. P. *et al.* (1981). Ecologie des leishmanioses dans le sud de la France. *Ann. Parasit.* **55**, 4, 445–453.

Rodhain, F. and Roze, J. M. (1977). Incidence géographique actuelle du paludisme. *Rev. Praticien* **27**, 37, 2347–2351.

Rodhain, F. (1979). La répartition géographique d'Aedes Aegypti et ses conséquences épidémiologiques. In *Etudes de géographie médicale, T I: Pays tropicaux* (Ed. J. Delvert), pp. 107–118. Com. Trav. hist. & scient., Bull. Sect. Géogr., LXXXIII, Paris, Bibl. Nat.

Rondia, D. (1973). Polluants et maladies de civilisation. *Liège, CEBEDOC* 41–60.

Roze, J. M. (1978). Les bilharzoses humaines à Madagascar. Etude de Géographie tropicale. *Bull. Assoc. Géogr. Fr.* **55**, 450–451.

Roze, J. M. and Charmot, G. (1979). L'onchocercose. In *Etudes de géographie médicale, T I: Pays tropicaux* (Ed. J. Delvert), pp. 119–136. Com. Trav. hist. & scient., Bull. Sect. Géogr., LXXXIII, Paris, Bibl. Nat.

Saey, P. (1966). De ruimtelijke differentiatie van de mortaliteit in Belgie. *Tds. Belg. Ver. Aard. Studies* T. XXXV, **1**, 67–78.

Sartor, F. (1979). Contribution de l'analyse démographique dans les enquêtes de toxicologie épidémiologique. Etude de la mortalité masculine "toutes causes" dans une région à eau douce. *Arch. Bel. Méd. soc. Hyg.* **37**, 537–560.

Schneider, J. H. (1980). Verschillen in de gezondheid van de Rotterdamse bevolking. *Tds. Soc. Gen.* **58** (suppl.), 107–114.

Sorre, M. (1933). Complexes pathogènes et géographie médicale. *Ann. Géogr.* **231**, XLII, 1–18.

Sorre, M. (1943). Les fondements biologiques de la géographie humaine. Essai d'une écologie de l'homme, A. Colin, Paris.

Specklin, R. (1955). La géographie du cancer en France. *Inf. Géogr.* **1**, 30.

Specklin, R. (1973). Géographie et médecine en Alsace (1920–1940) et progrès récents des recherches cartographiques. *Cah. Mulh. Géogr.* **4**, 164–175.

Thouvenot, C. (1971). La viande dans les campagnes lorraines. Evolution d'une habitude alimentaire. *Ann. Géogr.* **439**, LIII, 288–329.

Thouvenot, C. (1975). Consommations et habitudes alimentaires dans la France du Nord-Est. *Ann. Espace* **3**, 1–40.

Thouvenot, C. (1978). Studies in food geography in France. *Soc. Sci. & Med.* **12**, 1D, 43–54.

Tromp, S. W. (1955). Possible effects of geophysical and geochemical factors on development and geographic distribution of cancer. *Schweiz. Z. allg. Path.* **18**, 929–939.

Tromp, S. W. (1956). The geographical distribution of cancer of the stomach in the Netherlands (period 1946–1952). *Brit. J. Cancer*, **1**, 265–281.

Tromp, S. W. (1963). *Medical Biometeorology*. Elsevier, Amsterdam.

Tromp, S. W. (1979). Possible effects of geophysical factors on the geographical distribution of cancer. *Méd. Biol. Envir.* 7, 2, 52–57.

Tromp, S. W. and Diehl, J. C. (1954). A statistical study on the possible influence of soil and other geological conditions on cancer. *Experimentia, Basel* 10, 510–520.

Tromp, S. W. and Diehl, J. C. (1955). A statistical study of the possible relationship between cancer of the stomach and soil. *Brit. J. Cancer* 9, 349–357.

Tuyns, A. J. (1970). Cancer of the Oesophagus: Further evidence of the relation to drinking habits in France. *Int. J. Cancer* 5, 152–156.

Tuyns, J. (1979). Association tabac et alcool dans le cancer. *Bull. Acad. suisse et Sc. med.* 1–3, 151–161.

Tuyns, A. and Masse, Y. (1973). Mortality from cancer of the oesophagus in Britanny. *Int. J. Epid.* 2, 241–245.

Tuyns, A. J., Pequinot, G. and Abbatocci, J. S. (1979). Oesophageal cancer and alcohol consumption; importance of type of beverage. *Int. J. Cancer* 23, 443–447.

Van Brunschot, J. R. (1980). Sterfteverschillen tussen mannen en vrouwen. Een verkenning van verklaringen voor met name de Nederlandse situatie. *Tschr. v. Soc. Geneesk.* 58, 1, 14–18.

Van den Bos, P. (1981). Ongezondheid in de grote stad. *Medisch Contact* 1981, 12–20, 335–340, 13–27, 385–389.

Van den Oever, R., Vandendriessche, R. and A. Van den Berghe (1981). Kanker en beroep. *Tds. Soc. Gen.* 20, 37, 1197–1209.

Van der Auwera, J. C., Eylenbosch, W. J. and Meheus, A. Z. (1974). Sociaal-economische factoren in de mortinataliteit en de zuigelingensterfte van de stad Antwerpen in de periode 1962–1972. *Bev. en Gez.* 3, 455–472.

Van der Haegen, H. and De Vos, L. (1980). De Cholera-epidemie te Leuven in 1849. *Driem. Tds. Gemeentekrediet v. Belgie* 133, 197–210.

Vandermotten, C. and Ots-Albitar, M. (1976). Les médecins à Bruxelles. Différenciation sociale et philosophique de l'espace d'une grande ville. *Rev. belge Géogr.* 100, 2–3, 221–230.

Van Eijk, J. (1974). Wonen en ziek zijn. *Tds. Soc. Gen.* 7, 227–229.

Van Houte-Minet, M. and Wunsch, G. (1979). La mortalité masculine aux âges adultes. Un essai d'analyse régionale. *Popul. et Fam.* 43, 37–44, 19–48.

Van Molle, M. and Verhasselt, Y. (1974). Essai d'une géographie du cancer. Note préliminaire. *Méd. Biol. Envir.* 2, 3, 43–46.

Van Poppel, F. (1976). Burgerlijke staat en doodsoorzaak; een overzicht van de situatie in de 19e en het begin der 20e eeuw. *Bev. en Gez.* 1, 41–66.

Van Poppel, F. W. A. (1978). Provinciale sterfteverschillen in Nederland in de periode 1971–1975. *Geogr. Tds. KNAG* XII, 5, 406–412.

Van Raalte, H. G. J. (1979). Welk deel van de totale kankersterfte komt op rekening van het beroep? *Tds Soc. Gen.* 12, 398–401.

Verbeke, R. (1958). Longkanker als medisch-sociaal probleem. *Bel. Tds. Gen.* 14, 613–714.

Verhasselt, Y. (1969–70). The geographical environment and ecology of the tsetse-fly (*Glossina palpalis palpalis*) in Bas-Congo. *Geogr. Med.* 1, 7–20.

Verhasselt, Y. (1971). Contribution à la répartition spatiale des principales causes de mortalité en Belgique. *Geogr. Med.* 2, 23–32.

Verhasselt, Y. (1976a). Some Aspects of Geocancerology. *Méd. Biol. Envir.* 4, 1, 75–77.

Verhasselt, Y. (1976b). Quelques réflexions sur la géographie médicale. *Bull. Soc. Belge Etud. Géogr.* XLVI, **2**, 185–193.

Verhasselt, Y. (1977a). Quelques problèmes de géocancérologie. *Méd. Biol. Envir.* **5**, 122–123.

Verhasselt, Y. (1977b). Notes on Geography and Cancer. *Soc. Sci. Med.* **11**, 10, 745–748.

Verhasselt, Y. (1979). Approche d'une géographie du cancer. *Prosp. et Santé, Paris* **10–11**, 133–142.

Verhasselt, Y. (1981a). Geography of stomach cancer in Belgium. An approach. *Geogr. Med.* **11**, 104–115.

Verhasselt, Y. (1981b). Essai d'une géographie du cancer. In *Etudes de géographie médicale, T II: Pays tempérés et sociétés développées* (Ed. H. Picheral), pp. 129–146. Com. Trav. hist. & scient., Bull. Sect. Géogr., LXXXIII, Paris, Bibl. Nat.

Verhasselt, Y. (1981c). Geografie van de gezondheid en verstedelijking. *De Aardr.* **1/2**, 193–195.

Verhasselt, Y. (1981d). The Contribution and Future Development of Spatial Epidemiology. *Soc. Sci. Med.* **15A**, 333–335.

Vrijens, N. (1981). Evolutie van de mortaliteit en het doodsoorzakenpatroon in de gemeente Antwerpen 1900–1975. *Tds. Soc. Gen.* **59**, 6, 179–183.

Vrijens, N. (1982). Trends in mortality from diseases of the circulatory system and cancer by site in Antwerp, Belgium 1900–1975. *Soc. Sci. Med.* **16**, 293–302.

Zielhuis, R. L. (1975). Kankersterfte en chemische industrie. *Tds. Soc. Gen.* **53**, 776–797.

Three decades of medical geography in the United States

Gerald F. Pyle

Department of Geography and Earth Sciences,
University of North Carolina at Charlotte, North Carolina, USA

Early contributions

The *catalogue raisonnée* of the evolution of medical geography within the United States from the late 1940s to the early 1980s is intricately tied to concurrent expansions in international scientific knowledge and resultant technological applications. Conceptual approaches to the study of spatial aspects of human health problems within the United States have grown over the past several decades with scientific responses to expressed societal needs for changes, the proliferation of electronic computational capabilities, and a wide range of national health-related programmes resulting from policy decisions geared toward the general improvement of the well-being of the population. During this period, an ever-increasing body of knowledge about medical geography has been developed by drawing information and methodologies from a wide variety of scientific disciplines while at the same time taking advantage of the progress made within the parent discipline of geography. While some writers have referred to medical geography as either a "borderline discipline", a "foster child" or a "step child", the true strength of this general area of scientific endeavour has indeed become firmly established as an important ingredient of modern geography within the United States, and its best expression takes the form of contemporary spatial analysis. In addition, as with most areas of modern scientific undertaking, medical geography within the United States is a part of a larger international interest area. It is, in fact, impossible to trace the development of medical geography within the United States over the latter part of this century without taking into account the important impact of British, French and German scholars.

GEOGRAPHICAL ASPECTS OF HEALTH
ISBN 0 12 483780 8

As historical "chains of events" seem to impact upon the destiny of governments and science, a similar analogy can be drawn when viewing the conceptual developments which have taken place in American medical geography since the late 1940s. Consider this growth as chain-link inter-linkages of concepts. These linkages, best termed additive and incremental, have origins in both what had been broadly termed physical and human geography. While there are now greater degrees of sophistication and caution with regard to the utilization of such generalized labels, there is none the less still some residual conceptualization along these lines. These divisions were more clearly defined when Light released a trumpet call for a disease atlas in 1944. The post-war response of the American Geographical Society (AGS) had a lasting impact on American geography in general, and medical geography in particular: Jacques M. May, a French physician and geographer was contracted to accomplish a series of maps and studies that became the first major effort of an American geographical organization to produce a disease atlas (AGS, 1950–1955). May accomplished much more than was initially anticipated, and his somewhat dramatic exposition of medical geography *as disease ecology* within a natural environmental context strongly influenced at least two generations of American geographers and anthropologists (May, 1958). While May advised the study of sociocultural determinants of human health problems, initial interpretations of his contributions centred upon the identification of general environmental complexes wherein varying degrees of association could be found between "pathogens" and "geogens" (May, 1950). The earlier contributions of Max Sorre (1978), a French geographer more concerned with cultural complexes and disease ecology, were largely ignored by American geographers in their subsequent and various interpretations of May's statements.

A formative time: early emphasis on environmental complexes

During most of the 1950s, the branch of medical geography known to most professional geographers within the United States could actually best be described as an outgrowth of many decades of accumulated knowledge about disease risks to humans associated with the natural environment. While May's concepts substantially influenced such approaches, related works by American and German biomedical researchers had either already or simultaneously reinforced the importance of ecologically-oriented disease comparisons. The logic remains somewhat simplistic, but continues to have merit, especially when supported by realistic spatial-analytical testing. Certain environments do contain the necessary combinations of naturally-occurring phenomena that can cause a wide variety of human health problems, especially if control measures are not properly implemented.

The efforts of William Gorgas in developing control measures against yellow fever in Central America at the turn of this century contributed substantially to the completion of the Panama Canal (McCullough, 1977). The ecology of the disease associated with mosquitoes was beginning to be understood, and, with the support of Ronald Ross, who visited Panama in 1904, the recommendations of Gorgas gained international support. The Rockefeller Foundation supported many related searches for "ecological niches" during the early part of this century, and such common problems as hookworm and ringworm in the southern United States eventually were minimized.

On a broader scale, several atlas-like works of an international nature influenced the thinking of many American medical geographers during the 1950s and early 1960s. One such compendium used as a reference was an inventory of 80 "tropical" and 32 "temperate" disease risk regions identified by McKinley and his colleagues in 1935. During the period 1944–1954, Simmons *et al.* produced three similar descriptive volumes covering Africa, parts of Asia and the Pacific. These earlier contributions were clearly overshadowed by the three-volume *Welt-Seuchen-Atlas* produced by an international research group headed by the German medical geographers E. Rodenwaldt and H. J. Jusatz. Published from 1952 to 1961 with the support of the US Navy, the maps and textual materials within these volumes served as a comprehensive cartographic reference for many geographers concerned with the natural ecology of a variety of diseases. While any of the above works might be criticized for a variety of reasons in light of current medical knowledge, the single most important problem from a geographical perspective was the general lack of any spatial syntheses. May's methodological statements considered such associations, but two works by a British geographer, Sir Dudley Stamp, were both rapidly and widely accepted within the United States during the mid-1960s as important contributions in this general area (Stamp, 1964). Stamp, actually better known in the US for his works in "human" and regional geography, provided some useful insights to American medical geographers searching for methods of international regional synthesis.

The dual nature of approaches to medical geography as they emerged during this formative period was not dichotomous in any absolute sense; the emphasis on natural environmental complexes was simply more pronounced. In an early realization of the importance of culture and health conditions, Audy (1954) suggested that environmental change should not be ignored. Following this logic, in 1959, a US Senate Committee issued a report attempting to understand international health problems in relation to different cultural patterns. By the mid-1960s, Armstrong argued for more emphasis in medical geography on developing an understanding of culture and behaviour in relation to continually occurring disease hazards (Armstrong, 1965), and some of his subsequent research efforts in Malaysia have indeed broadened our horizons (Armstrong, 1980). An outstanding example of this approach is also seen in the efforts of Fonaroff (1968) to explain advances in agricultural activity in Trinidad in relation to intensified malaria control programmes. Environmental–cultural linkages associated with river blindness in Ghana were also carefully explained by Hunter (1966), and Meade's work a decade later on land development and human health in Malaysia added strength to our understanding of the linkages between these approaches (Meade, 1976).

It is important to stress particularly to students of medical geography that studies in the ecology of disease and the impact of changing environments continue to add to our knowledge of human health problems. In addition disease risks in relation to environmental change and the natural ecology are by no means restricted to tropical and/or exotic "foreign" places. Temperate climate examples include, but are by no means restricted to, arthropod-borne diseases that continue to present problems in the US. Such is the case of encephalitis viruses that are carried from forested valley areas in urbanized parts of Ohio by certain types of mosquitoes (Pyle and Cook, 1978). In addition, Rocky Mountain Spotted Fever continues to be a problem in the Piedmont area of the US south-east because this tick-borne disease seems to follow development in urbanizing fringe areas (Pyle, 1979). These associations in North America were initially identified through various forms of computer mapping, but regardless of the degrees of statistical sophistication that can be attained through use of modern technology, disease mapping *per se* has developed as an important linkage in medical geography in the US.

Improving disease mapping skills

As our skills in disease ecology were improved beyond the formative stages, so were our mapping abilities expanded by the computational advantages of computers. However, even before the widespread application of computer mapping programs to disease problems, an awareness

of the importance of data handling and general disease mapping procedures had emerged. One of the most important contributions of this
nature during the 1960s was made by Murray (1962, 1967) as he applied
mapping techniques initially introduced by Howe (1963) in Britain to
mortality rates in the United States. While other forms of disease mapping had clearly appeared before in American geographical journals,
Murray's contributions have been of lasting value due to his method of
presentation and the timeliness of publication with respect to emerging
trends, i.e. beyond traditional disease ecology. The era of computer-
assisted mapping followed the earlier contributions of Murray, and
during the mid-to-late 1960s Armstrong (1972) pioneered the use of
printer-oriented computer mapping in medical geography. The utilization of polynomial trend-surface computer mapping was introduced to
medical geography by Hopps (1968), and further applications of trend-
surface mapping to forecast disease patterns in the Chicago metropolitan
area were attempted during the late 1960s (Pyle, 1971). Computer-driven
pen plotters had also been used to map physician distributions during
this formative period (Shannon and Dever, 1974).

During the 1970s, "computer cartography" in health studies became
quite popular. Never exclusively within the defined parameters of medical geography at any given time (in fact, computer mapping in the US was
developed by "non-geographers"), computer-assisted mapping of health
data began to take the form of extensive collections of computer maps
produced by public agencies, often with little or no interpretation of
pattern. Some of the earlier attempts at such disease mapping were
crude, with no controls over numerical intervals (Burbank, 1971). Still,
some degrees of sophistication had been reached by the time the US
Government released national cancer atlases derived from computer
tapes and produced by mechanical plotters (Mason *et al.*, 1975). The
above publications do provide useful information to medical geographers studying problems in the US. During the 1970s, medical geographers in the US started to devote more attention to the resultant
patterns produced by computer maps than the actual technological
aspects of mapping. Also, given the widespread proliferation of micro-
computers during the late 1970s and early 1980s it is even more possible
for medical geographers to continue to perfect their disease mapping
skills (Achabal *et al.*, 1978). In fact, additional applications of McGlashan's
probability mapping techniques (McGlashan and Harington, 1976)
can now be accomplished rapidly through use of available micro-
computational systems. Improved disease mapping capabilities have
subsequently led to questions of associations with physical and human
geographical phenomena.

Expanding horizons

Biostatistical and public health researchers had perfected mathematical methods of testing hypothetical health–environmental associations in the US decades before the advent of computer-assisted associative analysis. In addition, while many geographers were still primarily concerned with finding explanations of spatial patterns through additional cartographic comparisons, sociologists had forged ahead in developing some understanding of socio-economic determinants of many urban and rural health problems (Theodorson, 1961). The "Quantitative Revolution" (Berry and Marble, 1968) within the discipline of geography in the US had a significant impact on medical geography because enhanced computerized capabilities led to the incorporation of many methodologies used by biostatisticians and sociologists into spatial research designs. In retrospect, three such thrusts during the late 1960s included socio-economic analysis of urban health conditions, location–allocation modelling of the use of health-care facilities and studies of disease diffusion.

A resurgence of social awareness in general during the 1960s led to a series of legislative "social-welfare" programmes primarily geared toward salvaging America's beleaguered cities. These changes were substantial, and they included Medicaid (health care for the poor) and Medicare (health care for the elderly). Inventories of health problems within sub-areas of cities were conducted by Social Welfare Councils (e.g. City of Chicago, 1967), municipal commissions, universities and a variety of concerned organizations. Many of these studies measured known poverty–ill-health associations. Increased use of continuously improving computer systems allowed for more thorough statistical testing and analysis, including more multivariate applications. At the same time, increased emphasis on utilizing these methods enabled geographers, centred primarily in Seattle and Chicago, to test prevailing theories on urban ecological structure (Rees, 1976).

Utilizing measures central to Social Area Analysis and more comprehensive "factorial ecology", i.e. socio-economic status, life-cycle shifts and minority segregation, medical geographers were able to develop a further understanding of spatial aspects of many urban health problems. In one of the earlier studies (Pyle, 1968), factor analysis was used as a descriptive mechanism isolating certain combinations of social and health indicators. Some of the combinations included a "poverty syndrome", with such diseases as gonorrhoea, measles and tuberculosis prevalent in lower-income areas of Chicago, and a "density syndrome" wherein such infectious diseases as whooping cough, chicken pox and scarlet fever clustered in the most densely populated parts of that city. Subsequent studies of this nature indicate that such associations persist in spite of the success of many of the revised health care programmes of the 1960s. Clearly, socio-economic studies of health conditions within cities are a part of the contemporary medical geographer's task; the results of such analysis must also be brought to public attention so that the effectiveness of health-care delivery mechanisms can be measured.

One of the most uniquely American trends in medical geography (at least during the late 1960s) consisted of detailed evaluations of how, and, to some extent, why, differing spatial patterns of the use of health-care facilities had developed over time within the United States. These approaches, now an integral part of medical geography, had their conceptual origins in the general area of locational analysis and allocation modelling. The earliest of such studies (Garrison et al., 1959) led to the more extensive five-year (1965–1970) Chicago Regional Hospital Study reports and publications (De Vise, 1973). Two of the researchers on that project, Morrill and Earickson, were able to identify some of the problems that can develop when the health-care system is allowed to function with little or no control within a free enterprise economy. For example:

(1) Hierarchies of hospitals can be identified, but locations have not been determined by principles of spatial equity with respect to access.
(2) There are specific cultural and behavioural determinants of health-care facilities selection and use within the United States.
(3) It is possible to utilize principles of locational analysis in planning the locations of new health-care delivery facilities, but policy decisions often overshadow "rational" solutions to location problems (Morrill and Earickson, 1968).

The ones already mentioned and additional studies of the same nature led many medical geographers of a more traditional bent to question whether such seemingly theoretical and quantitative approaches were not part of a divergent, indeed even dichotomous, spatial perspective on human health problems. Some geographers protested that such approaches were not in keeping with interpretations of medical geography according to May. Others suggested that knowledge of the ecology of diseases, from both natural and man-made environmental perspectives, can be incorporated into facilities' location models. Optimum recommendations utilizing such a combined model were issued for the Chicago Metropolitan Area in terms of treatment for heart disease, cancer and stroke in 1970; however, cost increases and policy shifts over the next decade indicated that while such procedures are theoretically desirable, they are not always "practical" in a profit-oriented health-care system (Pyle, 1968).

The incorporation of aspects of the geography of health-care delivery into American medical geography was actually a reflection of larger trends within the discipline—toward conceptual growth, modernization and a more broad-ranging understanding of the need for multidisciplinary efforts to combat spatial inequities in the delivery of services. This incorporation is best reflected in the 1974 work of Shannon and Dever that caused Learmonth (1978) to question whether there are "two medical geographies or one". Andrew's answer was one. Actually, social scientists from several disciplines, especially economics, had been concerned for nearly 20 years with many of the aspects of health services research addressed by Shannon and Dever:

(1) Distributional patterns of health care resources;
(2) manpower shortages;
(3) methods of payment;
(4) distances travelled to hospitals;
(5) different methods of planning for new facilities; and
(6) hierarchical arrangements of health-care delivery facilities.

The international comparison of hierarchical arrangements explained by Shannon and Dever was one of the most succinct of the time, and was partly an outgrowth of some of the earlier works of Shannon and Bashshur (1971). Later, when Shannon (1977) wrote, "Space, time, and illness behavior", he was attempting to explain to geographers where their health-related research might fit into a broader "medical care" context. According to Shannon, a gap between medical care geography and geographical epidemiology was still apparent in the research of many workers. Still more recently, Shannon and Crowley (1980) have devoted some attention to historical epidemiology with special emphasis on the diffusion of diseases within places.

Approaches to the spatial diffusion of diseases had been part of international medical geography since the nineteenth century. August Hirsch wrote about the spread of disease in the 1880s, and Rodenwaldt and Jusatz attempted some diffusion mapping in the *Welt-Seuchen-Atlas*. More recently, Hunter's work in northern Ghana explained the advance and retreat of river blindness (Hunter, 1966, 1981). By the late 1960s and early 1970s, studies of disease diffusion actually represented a third area of conceptual expansion for medical geographers working in the US. Partly initiated by historical and general accounts of cholera epidemics in the nineteenth century, three major epidemics within the US were reconstructed to determine if any contemporary principles of spatial analysis might help explain infectious disease diffusion patterns (Pyle, 1969). Both hierarchical city-size and distance-decay functions could be identified. Writing several years later in the *Annals* of the Association of American Geographers, Hunter and Young (1971) added to our knowledge of disease diffusion by comparing the spread of influenza in England and Wales in 1957 with population potential. In general these kinds of efforts demonstrated that US medical geography had grown substantially since the impact of May twenty years before. Still, many approaches were quite diffuse, and other claims persisted that American medical geographers of the mid-1970s were polarized with respect to their views on medical geography.

Crystallization or dichotomization?

Medical geographers were no more polarized during the 1970s than were geographers in general at that time; the use of innovative quantitative techniques had simply not diffused to sufficient universities. Other presumed conceptual dichotomies were posited by some scholars. For example, in 1972, during a meeting of the International Geographical Union Commission on Medical Geography in Guelph, Ontario, a group of British medical geographers (including Neil McGlashan, Andrew Learmonth, Melvyn Howe and Sheila Bain) met some of their American counterparts for the first time. (Alan Dever, Gary Shannon, Gerald Pyle and Joseph Schiel were among those present.) Initial impressions that formed during the paper presentation sessions were that most British medical geographers were primarily concerned with the ecology of human disease and most Americans were preoccupied with the geography of health-care systems. It eventually became apparent, and this is one of the purposes of such meetings, that there was a great deal of international exchange of ideas on the part of medical geographers from many countries. As a mechanism for the continuation of international communication, it was agreed that the IGU Medical Geography Newsletter would be edited by Gary Shannon and Alan Dever, and the newsletter was distributed from the US from 1972 to 1976.

Another organization for communication amongst medical geographers was established about a year after the Guelph meetings. In April, 1973, a group of American medical geographers met during the annual meeting of the Association of American Geographers and formed what still exists as the official special interest group on medical geography for that professional body. Included in that group were Richard Morrill, Robert Earickson, Gary Shannon, Alan Dever, John Hunter, Joseph Schiel and Gerald Pyle. After that meeting, a national communications network was established, mostly through the IGU Medical Geography Newsletter, and professional paper sessions during annual AAG meetings increased four-fold over the next nine years. This increasing interest in medical geography coincided with attempts to define the sub-area in a more comprehensive manner.

Meanwhile, the literature on medical geography was growing for several important reasons. Editors of professional journals were made aware of recent conceptual expansions of methodological approaches to medical geography. There were more students being trained in aspects of medical geography, and this trend led to more theses and dissertations. Symposia in addition to regularly scheduled AAG and IGU meetings were also held. One of the most noteworthy proved to be the First Carolina Geographical Symposium (on medical geography) held at Chapel Hill, North Carolina in 1973. That conference was a demonstration of the rising interest in medical geography at that time, and it resulted in a volume of methodological contributions (Hunter, 1974). Yet another volume was made available when Gerald Karaska, editor of *Economic Geography* suggested and supported a special issue of that journal devoted to medical geography (Pyle, 1976).

During the 1970s and 1980s, traditions in epidemiological geography were also growing in importance. Based in Hawaii, Armstrong directed teams of researchers in south-east Asia (Armstrong, 1973). In addition, Meade (1977) began publishing a series of contributions on the effects of development on human health conditions. These trends continued to add to the growing body of literature in the US, and the Second Carolina Symposium, organized at Chapel Hill, resulted in the publication of another collection of readings on medical geography (Meade, 1980).

In 1979, the first undergraduate text on medical geography was published in the United States (Pyle, 1979). The work was intended as a general introduction to the subject of medical geography to be used in conjunction with other materials. Major topics covered included disease mapping and measurement, elements of disease ecology, approaches to disease diffusion, methods of statistical association, the geography of health care and applications of computer-oriented geocoding systems in medical geography. The text has been adopted for existing and new courses in medical geography in the US and several other English-speaking countries.

International aspects of medical geography continue to be more important than the issue as to whether there is a special brand of the subject area that can be considered exclusively American. Even the highly specialized health-care delivery modelling techniques now seem to have more relevance when applied to developing nations than to an American health-care system so overwhelmingly caught up in cost and profit issues. There is little doubt that a truly international medical geography has emerged (Pyle, 1979).

The proliferation of ideas and techniques

As pursuits toward an international medical geography seemed to converge and become more holistic during the late 1970s and early 1980s, the same was true for studies that might be considered mostly American. The latter aspect is understandably difficult to label because Americans were continuing to develop analyses in "overseas" locations, many scholars originally from other countries (especially former Commonwealth areas) had clearly entered some sort of "mainstream" of US medical geography, and, perhaps of most importance, the journal that contained the majority of such "American" studies from 1977 to 1982 was published in Britain. In 1976, Pergamon Press of Oxford made the decision to divide *Social Science and Medicine* into several separate parts, with Peter J. M. McEwan, a sociologist, as Editor-in-Chief of four journals. Part D of the expanded series was devoted to medical geography, with Gerald Pyle and Gary Shannon as co-editors from November 1977 to November 1979, and Pyle as editor from December 1979 to December 1982. Again, the international focus of the journal was stressed, and as part of four issues per annum, special issues, including an extensive volume on Australia and New Zealand edited by Neil McGlashan (June, 1980) and an even larger one from the Tokyo Symposium on the Geography of Health-IGU edited by Andrew Learmonth (February, 1981), were produced. The international forum was created, and the result was a proliferation of ideas and techniques in medical geography.

Interests in medical geography initiated by May in the US 30 years ago seemed to multiply at an exponential rate with the publication of *Social Science and Medicine: Part D, Medical Geography* from 1977 to 1981.* Many scholars previously concerned with geographical methodologies made contributions to the growing literature in this fashion, and, of equal or greater importance, emerging researchers in medical geography found an outlet for their ideas. In addition to works by those who had been publishing in medical geography in a variety of general geography journals, physicians, public health workers and biostatisticians also made contributions. During this period, studies that could be considered

---

* *Social Science and Medicine* reverted in 1982 to being a single stream journal retaining the same groups of interest, and Pergamon added a new journal *Ecology of Disease* edited by G. M. Howe and published from Oxford.

mostly American in flavour continued to follow most of the general conceptual streams already mentioned. In fact, some directions were a direct result of an intellectual "critical mass" that had built up over the past dozen years.

Within the context of disease ecology, both traditional and innovative approaches were posited. For example, Meade (1978) offered further thoughts on the effects of development on health in peninsular Malaysia as she explained how voluntary agricultural resettlement increased some infectious and social disease hazards, while at the same time seemed to reduce population stress. Roundy (1978) also combined behaviour and disease ecology in another assessment of disease hazards in Ethiopia; he showed how diseases can be considered geographical hazard systems.* Haddock (1979) also produced an intensive review of the literature on Chagas' Disease hazards in Latin America during this period, with an examination of existing knowledge of the disease in different sub-regions. Innovative approaches to disease ecology included two different US examples. In one of these studies, Kovacik (1978) showed how malaria and other diseases influenced seasonal population movement patterns in colonial and antebellum South Carolina, and in the other Shafer (1979) explained the ecological history of health hazards produced by coal refuse bank fires in Scranton, Pennsylvania.

Cultural–ecological ingredients of medical geography also underwent some amplification during this period. Armstrong et al. (1978) produced a study explaining how nasopharyngeal carcinoma amongst Malaysian and Chinese populations in Selangor, Malaysia, could be differentiated on the basis of lower socio-economic status. In another community-based study of the Family Health Clinic in Calabar, Nigeria, Gesler (1979) examined both "traditional" and "modern" methods of seeking health care. The interface of such dual systems was explained in further detail by Good et al. (1979) when viewing health policy alternatives in Africa. Good and his co-workers showed how neither traditional nor modern health-care methods seem adequately to meet the needs of developing areas as they recommended policy decisions that would, in fact, be geared toward improving both methods of providing health care. The importance of culture change was also pointed out by Weil (1979) in an investigation of Bolivian peasants who migrated from marginal highland farmlands to newly opened tropical lowland areas. According to Weil, the immigrants have a better diet, but infant mortality rates appear to be higher in the lowlands than the highland areas. In a related analysis

---

* See also pp. 257–272.

based upon the premise that rural malnutrition forces migration to cities, Clark (1980) showed that in the Kingdom of Tonga, rural populations seemed to be generally more healthy than recent urban immigrants.

Studies using both traditional cartographic methods and more recent spatial analytical techniques were also produced in efforts to demonstrate the continuing importance of disease mapping. For example, Achabal *et al.* (1978) explained how interactive computer graphics can be used in designing and evaluating health-care delivery systems with Columbus, Ohio as an example. In more traditional mapping exercises, Hugg (1979) of the US Bureau of Census showed the relationship between poverty and work disability status, and Babin (1979) used stepwise discriminant analysis to regionalize US cancer mortality for the period 1950–1969. Further applications of spatial analytical techniques emerged in the works of Glick (1979) in unusual cartographic comparisons of cancer mortality using autocorrelation. Many of the more recent works have also demonstrated how cartographic-spatial analytical combinations in methodologies can help in our understanding of lower incidence diseases. In one such analysis, Shafer (1980) used computer graphics and contiguity-testing to identify statistically significant high and low probabilities of a rare disease (bone cancer) in Pennsylvania. A comparable analysis of Sudden Infant Death Syndrome in North Carolina was accomplished by Grimson *et al.* (1981). They used "adjacency" testing methods to isolate this problem in certain parts of the state. The contributions of biostatisticians and physicians to medical geography have increased substantially over the past five years in the US. Still, those with more specific training in geographical methods have explained more in the area of "associative" studies.

Within the context of what can now be clearly labelled "geographical epidemiology", US medical geographers have perfected many approaches to associative explanation. The series of such studies which have perhaps received the most attention are the seasonality in childhood lead-poisoning contributions of Hunter (1978). Hunter's findings indicate definite summer peaks in the incidence of this health problem. Other kinds of associations were identified by Robinson (1978) when he used the variable subset selection process for multiple regression modelling of heart disease mortality in north-eastern Ohio. He found that poor housing conditions and the percentage of the "foreign-born" population are good indicators of the disease in that area. In yet another application of regression, this time with path analysis, Bozzo *et al.* (1979) demonstrated how different demographic factors could be tested against air pollution problems. More naturally occurring variables were used by Miller (1979) in an epidemiological explanation of otitis media, while

Cleek (1979) and King (1979) raised several issues about the use of regression techniques and the selection of spatial units in associative modelling. Meade (1979) also used optimal regression techniques in exploring the cardiovascular mortality persistence in what has become known as the "Enigma Area" of the south-eastern US Atlantic coast.* Another sort of macro-regional problem was explained by Greenberg *et al.* (1980) in a massive data testing procedure for the infamous "Cancer Alley" of the US north-eastern Urban Corridor.[†] The use of urban ecological analysis also persists in the types of associative studies being produced in the US. Recently, Pierce (1981) completed such a study with special reference to the socio-economic status of women having abortions in Manhattan. He used factor analysis to show that poverty, work status and mobility are key indicators of the geography of this problem.

Known to be a controversial topic within the US, abortion also appears to demonstrate certain spatial regularities. Henry (1978) explained how acceptance of this procedure has diffused through different parts of the country. In general, she used regression techniques to show how the initial spread was contagious, followed by a more regular hierarchical pattern in accordance with city size. Given the magnitude of general disease diffusion problems, it is of interest that proportionately fewer studies than would be expected have emerged in the medical geography literature over the past five years. An interesting exception to this trend that is directly related to the planning of health-care facilities can be found in Baker (1979), who explains the diffusion of computerized tomography scanners in the US. Baker found that hospital size is a major determining factor in the rate of adoption; more so than urban hierarchical arrangements.

Generally, the relationship between emerging trends in medical geography and urban theory can best be understood when viewing works related to the planning of health-care facilities in the US. Many of the problems identified by Shannon and Dever in 1974, as well as the research directions set by Morrill and his colleagues during the Chicago Regional Hospital Studies of the late 1960s, can still be seen in the more recent literature. Given the nature of the health-care delivery system in the United States, a tendency toward real hardships due to incredibly spiralling costs and high degrees of bureaucratic ineptitude on the part of too many health-care planners, it is not surprising that the literature in this area is vast indeed. The more geographical components seem to be concentrated in four loosely-defined groups:

---

* See also pp. 175–196.
† See also pp. 157–174.

(1) studies concerned with hospital location and use;
(2) the location and use of Emergency Medical Services;
(3) physician distributions; and
(4) spatial aspects of the use of mental health facilities.

The last five years have, to some extent, been a frustrating time for those engaged in this research. The central problem does not rest with the lack of meaningful conclusions. Instead, it seems to be associated with the lack of communication of results to key policy-makers. Still, these trends must be encouraged in anticipation of more "spatial justice" with respect to the distribution and use of health-care facilities.

Recent examples of spatial studies of hospital location continue to shed some light on the magnitude of the problems. It is encouraging that over the last several years the American Hospital Association has employed several medical geographers in spatial data analysis efforts. Headed by Ross Mullner, this research team has completed studies (Mullner *et al.*, 1981) that have explained trends toward multi-hospital corporations and probabilities of hospital closure based on facility size. Efforts toward more established modelling techniques of the use of facilities also continue. Many of these methodologies are summarized by Roghmann and Zastowny (1979) in an effort to predict patient flow patterns in the Rochester, New York metropolitan area. Harner and Slater (1980) subsequently used hierarchical clustering to identify medical access regions in West Virginia, and Bennet (1981) used location-allocation modelling to determine the actual number of primary health-care facilities that would be needed to meet the needs of the 1990 population of Lansing, Michigan. Policy problems continue to haunt the geographer searching for optimal location models. For example, Kunitz and Sorensen (1979) explained just how difficult it can be to build a new hospital in a location where it really is needed.

It is of interest that research considered to be of assistance in planning for the allocation and reallocation of Emergency Medical Services (EMS) has generally been met with less opposition on the part of many US health-care planners. One reason for this circumstance is that major new hospital construction is not normally involved. Another reason is that many EMS programmes require degrees of local finance and other resources; also, locally elected officials are much more involved in the planning processes. While this might be a mixed blessing, at least there are clearly defined legal authorities within geographical areas. While the US Health Systems Agencies certainly have geographical areas, their authority is not local in nature. The local importance of spatial studies in EMS planning was pointed out by Mullner in his evaluation of the Illinois EMS system. At that time Mullner and Goldberg (1978) showed how patient outcomes are often overlooked by those seeking only distance minimization. The most important geographical aspect of such services seems to be how long it takes trained medics to reach patients. This finding was reinforced by Mayer (1979) in an analysis of Seattle's paramedic programme, and again by Williams and Shavlik (1979) in a related study of paramedic trips in San Bernadino. Given such findings, it is now possible to simulate EMS use for planning purposes, as was accomplished by Monro (1980) in Wisconsin.

The third interesting focus of health-care research is the location patterns of doctors' surgeries. Because the US has no National Health Service, physicians tend to locate in response to the market. This "market" is not always where population densities are greatest, as has been demonstrated by Rosenthal (1978). In a study of two Florida counties, Rosenthal came to the conclusion that physician practice locations shift in a direction toward more youthful, higher fertility age-group residences. Inequalities in physician locations were also identified by Gober and Gordon (1980) in a similar investigation of Phoenix, Arizona. They found that specialists are centralized in core areas and paediatricians are not necessarily located within proximity of their patients. Some have stated that many of these problems can be overcome with the increased use of family practice centres. In an attempt to fit an econometric model to such locations in metropolitan Northern Virginia, DiLisio (1981) found that the demand for primary-care physicians will soon outgrow the supply. In a similar study in West Virginia, Bosanac and Hall (1981) found that small area profile studies can be useful in modelling the provision of such primary-care resources.

The fourth domain of research endeavour in health-care studies in the US is the provision and use of mental health facilities. This is truly an emerging speciality within medical geography, and research directions have thus far been set by a limited number of scholars. One reason for the growth in concern for the geography of mental health has been a major shift in attitudes toward how the mentally ill have been treated. Traditionally, persons in need of mental health treatment were simply isolated from the general population, often with minimal custodial care for the remainder of their lives. Given the recent formation of Community Mental Health centres, much progress has been made. In addition to aspects of locating such centres, it is also useful to examine forms of adjustment. To some extent, as explained by Smith (1978), adjustment and chances of recidivism are directly related to environmental characteristics of neighbourhoods of former mental patients. National aspects of the general deinstitutionalization of the mentally ill presented by Smith and Hanham (1981) also indicate that certain time paths are associated, and aspects of modernization still require diffusion to some parts of the US.

Prospects for the 1980s and beyond

In summary, the research trends mentioned in this chapter are likely to continue over the next several decades. Advances in electronic micro-computational capabilities will enable future medical geographers to complete analyses at a much more rapid pace. As courses in the general area increase, there will be even more medical geographers to carry on with established methods and develop new techniques. The real future of medical geography in the United States is both multidisciplinary and international in scope. The International Geographical Union Working Group on the Geography of Health, for which Andrew Learmonth has spent so many years of effort, will continue to be the major focus for such cooperative endeavours.

References

Achabal, D. D., Moellering, H., Osleeb, J. P. and Swain, R. W. (1978). Designing and evaluating a health care delivery system through the use of interactive computer graphics. *Soc. Sci. Med.* **12D**, 1–6.

American Geographical Society (1950–1955). 17 sheets of the "Atlas of Disease" in *Geographical Review* **40**, 648–649; **41**, 272–273, 638–639; **42**, 98–101, 282–283, 628–630; **43**, 89–90, 253–255, 404; **44**, 133–136, 408–410, 583–584; **45**, 416, 572.

Armstrong, R. W. (1965). Medical geography: An emerging speciality? *International Pathology* **6**, 61–63.

Armstrong, R. W. (1972). Computers and mapping in medical geography. In *Medical Geography: Techniques and Field Studies* (Ed. N. D. McGlashan), pp. 69–85. Methuen, London.

Armstrong, R. W. (1973). Tracing exposure to specific environments in medical geography. *Geographical Analysis* **5**, 122–132.

Armstrong, R. W. (1980). Geographical aspects of cancer incidence in Southeast Asia. *Soc. Sci. Med.* **14D**, 299–306.

Armstrong, R. W., Kannankutty, M. and Armstrong, M. J. (1978). Self-specific environments associated with Nasopharyngeal Carcinoma in Selangor, Malaysia. *Soc. Sci. Med.* **12D**, 149–156.

Audy, J. R. (1954). A biological approach to medical geography. *British Medical Journal* **1**, 960–962.

Babin, E. (1979). United States cancer mortality regions: 1950–1969. *Soc. Sci. Med.* **13D**, 39–44.

Baker, S. R. (1979). The diffusion of high technology medical innovation: The computed tomography scanner example. *Soc. Sci. Med.* **13D**, 155–162.

Bennet, W. D. (1981). A location-allocation approach to health care facility location: A study of the undoctored population in Lansing, Michigan. *Soc. Sci. Med.* **15D**, 305–312.

Berry, B. J. L. and Marble, D. F. (1968). *Spatial Analysis: A Reader in Statistical Geography*, pp. 1–9. Prentice Hall, Englewood Cliffs.

Bosanac, E. M. and Hall, D. S. (1981). A small area profile system: Its use in primary care resource development. *Soc. Sci. Med.* **15D**, 313–319.

Bozzo, S. R., Novak, K. M., Galdos, F., Hakoopian, R. and Hamilton, L. D. (1979). Mortality, migration, income and air pollution: a comparative study. *Soc. Sci. Med.* **13D**, 95–110.

Brashshur, R. L., Shannon, G. L. and Metzner, C. A. (1971). Some ecological differentials in the use of medical services. *Health Services Research*, Spring 1971.

Burbank, F. (1971). *Patterns in Cancer Mortality in the U.S.: 1950–1967*. National Cancer Institute, Washington.

City of Chicago, Board of Health (1967). Preliminary Report on Patterns of Medical and Health Care in Poverty areas of Chicago and Proposed Health Programs for the Medically Indigent.

Clark, W. F. (1980). The rural to urban nutrition gradient: application and interpretation in a developing nation and urban situation. *Soc. Sci. Med.* **14D**, 31–36.

Cleek, R. L. (1979). Cancers and environment: the effect of scale. *Soc. Sci. Med.* **13D**, 241–248.

De Vise, P. (1973). "Misused and Misplaced Hospitals and Doctors: A Locational Analysis of the Urban Health Crisis". Association of American Geographers, Resource Paper No. 22.

DiLisio, J. E. (1981). Health manpower supply and demand: the case of a family practice residency program. *Soc. Sci. Med.* **15D**, 295–304.

Fonaroff, L. S. (1968). Man and malaria in Trinidad: ecological perspectives of a changing health hazard. *Annals Assoc. Amer. Geogr.* **58**, 526–556.

Garrison, W. L., Berry, B. J. L., Marble, D. F., Nystuen, J. D. and Morrill, R. L. (1959). *Studies of Highway Development and Geographic Change*. University of Washington Press, Seattle.

Gesler, W. M. (1979). Illness and health practitioner use in Calabar, Nigeria. *Soc. Sci. Med.* **13D**, 23–30.

Glick, B. (1979). The spatial autocorrelation of cancer mortality. *Soc. Sci. Med.* **13D**, 123–130.

Gober, P. and Gordon, R. J. (1980). Intraurban physician location: a case study of Phoenix. *Soc. Sci. Med.* **14D**, 407–418.

Good, C. M., Hunter, J. M., Katz, S. H. and Katz, S. S. (1979). The interface of dual systems of health care in the developing world: toward health policy initiatives in Africa. *Soc. Sci. Med.* **13D**, 141–154.

Greenberg, M. R., Preuss, P. W. and Anderson, R. (1980). Clues for case control studies of cancer in the northeast urban corridor. *Soc. Sci. Med.* **14D**, 37–44.

Grimson, R. C., Wang, K. C. and Johnson, P. W. C. (1981). Searching for hierarchical clusters of disease: spatial patterns of Sudden Infant Death Syndrome. *Soc. Sci. Med.* **15D**, 287–294.

Haddock, K. C. (1979). Disease and development in the tropics: a review of Chagas' Disease. *Soc. Sci. Med.* **13D**, 53–60.

Harner, E. J. and Slater, P. B. (1980). Identifying medical regions using hierarchical clustering. *Soc. Sci. Med.* **14D**, 3–10.

Henry, N. F. (1978). The diffusion of abortion facilities in the northeastern United States, 1970–1976. *Soc. Sci. Med.* **12D**, 7–16.

Hirsch, A. (1883–1886). *Handbook of Geographical and Historical Pathology* (Trans., C. Creighton, Jr.), 3 vols. New Sydenham Society, London.

Hopps, H. C. (1968). *Computerized Mapping of Disease and Environmental Data.* Department of Defense, Washington, D.C.

Howe, G. M. (1963). *National Atlas of Disease Mortality in the United Kingdom.* Nelson, London.

Hugg, L. (1979). A map comparison of work disability and poverty status in the United States. *Soc. Sci. Med.* **13D**, 237–240.

Hunter, J. M. (1966). River blindness in Nangodi, Northern Nigeria: a hypothesis of cyclical advance and retreat. *Geographical Review* **56**, 398–416.

Hunter, J. M. (Ed.) (1974). *The Geography of Health and Disease.* Studies in Geography No. 6, Department of Geography, University of North Carolina at Chapel Hill, Chapel Hill, N.C.

Hunter, J. M. (1978). The summer disease—some field evidence of seasonality in childhood lead poisoning. *Soc. Sci. Med.* **12D**, 85–94.

Hunter, J. M. (1981). Progress and concerns in the World Health Organization Onchocerciasis Control Program in West Africa. *Soc. Sci. Med.* **15D**, 261–276.

Hunter, J. M. and Young, J. C. (1971). Diffusion of influenza in England and Wales. *Annals Assoc. Amer. Geogr.* **61**, 637–653.

King, P. E. (1979). Problems of spatial analysis in geographical epidemiology. *Soc. Sci. Med.* **13D**, 249–252.

Kovacik, C. F. (1978). Health conditions and town growth in colonial and antebellum South Carolina. *Soc. Sci. Med.* **12D**, 131–136.

Kunitz, S. J. and Sorensen, A. A. (1979). The effects of regional planning on a rural hospital: a case study. *Soc. Sci. Med.* **13D**, 1–12.

Learmonth, A. (1978). *Patterns of Disease and Hunger.* David and Charles, Newton Abbot.

Light, R. U. (1944). The progress of medical geography. *Geographical Review* **34**, 36–41.

Mason, T. J., McKay, F. W., Hoover, R., Blot, W. J. and Fraumeni, J. F. (1975). *Atlas of Cancer Mortality for U.S. Counties: 1950–1969.* DREW Publication No. 75–780, Government Printing Office, Washington, D.C.

May, J. M. (1950). Medical geography: its methods and objectives. *Geographical Review* **51**, 9–41.

May, J. M. (1958). *The Ecology of Human Disease.* M.D. Publications, New York.

Mayer, J. D. (1979). Seattle's Paramedic Program: geographical distribution, response times, and mortality. *Soc. Sci. Med.* **13D**, 45–57.

McCullough, D. (1977). *The Path Between the Seas.* Simon and Schuster, New York.

McGlashan, N. D. and Harington, J. S. (1976). Some techniques for mapping mortality. *The South African Geographical Journal* **58**, 18–24.

McKinley, E. B. (1935). *A Geography of Disease.* George Washington University Press, Washington.

Meade, M. S. (1976). The impact of land development on human health in West Malaysia. *Annals Assoc. Amer. Geogr.* **66**, 428–439.

Meade, M. S. (1977). Medical geography as human ecology: the dimension of population movement. *Geographical Review* **67**, 379–393.

Meade, M. S. (1978). Community health and changing hazards in a voluntary agricultural resettlement. *Soc. Sci. Med.* **12D**, 95–102.

Meade, M. S. (1979). Cardiovascular mortality in the southeastern United States: the coastal plain enigma. *Soc. Sci. Med.* **13D**, 257–266.

Meade, M. S. (Ed.) (1980). *Conceptual and Methodological Issues in Medical Geography.* Studies in Geography No. 15, Department of Geography, University of North Carolina at Chapel Hill, Chapel Hill, N.C.

Miller, M. L. (1979). Epidemiology of Otitis Media: problem and research focus for geographers. *Soc. Sci. Med.* **13D**, 233–236.

Monroe, C. B. (1980). A simulation model for planning emergency response systems. *Soc. Sci. Med.* **14D**, 71–78.

Morrill, R. L. and Earickson, R. J. (1968). Variations in the use and character of Chicago Area Hospitals. *Health Services Research* **3**, 224–238.

Mullner, R. and Goldberg, J. (1978). Toward an outcome-oriented medical geography: an evaluation of the Illinois trauma/emergency medical services system. *Soc. Sci. Med.* **12D**, 103–110.

Mullner, R., Byre, C. S. and Kebal, J. D. (1981). Multihospital systems in the United States: a geographical overview. *Soc. Sci. Med.* **15D**, 353–360.

Murray, M. N. (1962 and 1967). The geography of death in the United States and the United Kingdom. *Ann. Assoc. Amer. Geogr.* **52**, 130 and **57**, 301.

Pierce, R. M. (1981). An ecological analysis of the socioeconomic status of women having abortions in Manhattan. *Soc. Sci. Med.* **15D**, 271–286.

Pyle, G. F. (1968). *Some Examples of Urban Medical Geography.* Unpublished Master's Thesis, University of Chicago.

Pyle, G. F. (1969). The diffusion of cholera in the United States in the nineteenth century. *Geographical Analysis* **1**, 59–75.

Pyle, G. F. (1971). *Heart Disease, Cancer and Stroke in Chicago.* Department of Geography Research Paper No. 134, University of Chicago.

Pyle, G. F. (Ed.) (1976). Human health problems: spatial perspectives. Special issue of *Economic Geography* **52**, April 1976.

Pyle, G. F. (1979). *Applied Medical Geography.* Winston, Washington.

Pyle, G. F. and Cook, R. M. (1978). Environmental risk factors of California encephalitis in man. *Geographical Review* **68**, 157–170.

Rees, P. H. (1976). Concepts of social space: toward an urban social geography. In *Geographic Perspectives on Urban Systems* (Eds B. J. L. Berry and F. E. Horten), pp. 306–394. Prentice-Hall, Englewood Cliffs.

Robinson, V. B. (1978). Modelling spatial variations in heart disease mortality: implications of the variable subset selection process. *Soc. Sci. Med.* **12D**, 165–172.

Rodenwaldt, E. and Jusatz, H. J. (1952–1961). *Welt-Seuchen-Atlas*, 3 vols. Falk, Hamburg.

Roghmann, K. J. and Zastowny, T. R. (1979). Proximity as a factor in the selection of health care providers: emergency room visits compared to obstetric admissions and abortions. *Soc. Sci. Med.* **13D**, 61–70.

Rosenthal, S. F. (1978). Target populations and physian populations: the effects of density and charge. *Soc. Sci. Med.* **12D**, 111–116.

Roundy, R. W. (1978). A model for combining human behavior and disease ecology to assess disease hazard in a community: rural Ethiopia as a model. *Soc. Sci. Med.* **12D**, 121–130.

Schafer, S. (1979). An ecological history of coal refuse bank fires in Scranton, Pennsylvania. *Soc. Sci. Med.* **13D**, 33–38.

Shafer, S. (1980). Mapping bone cancer death rates in Pennsylvania countries. *Soc. Sci. Med.* **14D**, 11–16.

Shannon, G. L. (1977). Space, time and illness behavior. *Soc. Sci. Med.* **11D**, 683–689.

Shannon, G. L. and Crowley, R. G. (1980). The Great Plague of London, 1665. *Urban Geography* **1**, 254–270.

Shannon, G. W. and Dever, G. E. A. (1974). *Health Care Delivery: Spatial Perspectives*. McGraw-Hill, New York.

Simmons, J. S., Whayne, T. F., Anderson, G. W. and Horack, H. W. (1944–1954). *Global Epidemiology: A Geography of Disease and Sanitation*, 3 vols. J. B. Lippencott Col, Philadelphia.

Smith, C. J. (1978). Recidivism and community adjustment amongst former mental patients. *Soc. Sci. Med.* **12D**, 17–28.

Smith, C. J. and Hanham, R. Q. (1981). Deinstitutionalization of the mentally ill: a time path analysis of the American States, 1955–1975. *Soc. Sci. Med.* **15D**, 361–378.

Sorre, M. (1978). Principes de cartographie appliquee a l'ecologie humaine. *Soc. Sci. Med.* **12D**, 238–250.

Stamp, L. D. (1964a). *Some Aspects of Medical Geography*. Oxford University Press, Oxford.

Stamp, L. D. (1964b). *The Geography of Life and Death*. Collins, London.

Theodorson, G. A. (Ed.) (1961). *Studies in Human Ecology*. Harper and Row, New York.

U.S. Senate Committee on Government Operations, United States Congress (1959). "Patterns of Incidence of Certain Diseases Throughout the World". Government Printing Office, Washington.

Weil, C. (1979). Morbidity, mortality and diet as indicators of physical and economic adaptation among Bolivian migrants. *Soc. Sci. Med.* **13D**, 215–222.

Williams, P. M. and Shavlik, G. (1979) Geographic patterns and demographic correlates of paramedic runs in San Bernadino, 1977. *Soc. Sci. Med.* **13D**, 273–280.

The evolution of medical geography in Canada

Jean-Pierre Thouez

*Department of Geography, University of Montreal,
Quebec, Canada*

Introduction

Research and teaching in medical geography is a relatively recent practice
in Canada. Until the 1970s, it was to some extent associated with
population geography and with social and cultural geography. When
compared with other social sciences, such as economics, sociology and
demography, medical geography has had a late start as a specific field of
research. It first came to the fore at a period when geography was
embarking on new and important methodological and conceptual trends
and at a time when young geographers were advocating, with greater
insistence, solutions to contemporary social and ecological problems. In
this respect, Anglo-Saxon, and in particular American geography exerted
great influence on its development.

Research development

Two information sources, which have been published since the early
1950s by the Association of Canadian Geographers, are indispensable for
an assessment of the evolution of medical geography in Canada: the
articles and comments published in the *Canadian Geographer*, and the
yearly *Newsletter* detailing research articles published by university
geographers (Barrett, 1980a).

There are several distinct categories which must be highlighted when
attempting to define the evolution of medical geography in Canada. They
are reports presented by Canadians to the annual conferences of Ameri-

GEOGRAPHICAL ASPECTS OF HEALTH
ISBN 0 12 483780 8

can and Canadian national associations or their regional divisions; research projects undertaken by Canadian university staff, such as those mentioned each year in the *Newsletter*; articles published by Canadians in national journals such as the *Canadian Geographer*, as well as regional reviews such as *Cahiers de géographie du Québec*, or foreign periodicals, in particular *The Geographical Review, The Journal of Tropical Geography* and *Social Science and Medicine (part D)*; and finally, master's and doctoral work in geography.

Before the 1970s, Canadian source materials in medical geography consisted of, for example, the reports of H. V. Warren, a geologist at the University of British Columbia, on the geography of disease (1964, 1965), and N. C. Field's work at the University of Toronto on *Land, Hunger and the Rural Depopulation Problem in the USSR* (1963). A number of articles were closely connected to population geography (Garry, 1964; Coulson, 1967). However, two writers may be considered to be exceptions to the rule and are worth mentioning in particular; they are John Girt and Roly Tinline.

British by birth, Girt studied at Leeds and was appointed by Memorial University in Newfoundland in 1968. His research concentrated on the analysis of health-care demand in the outlying communities of Newfoundland. Together with A. G. MacPherson and A. Hodd, Girt studied the historical demography of the province. In 1969, he joined Guelph University in Ontario. At the beginning of the 1970s, Girt was the most active medical geographer in Canada. His publications deal with the relations between chronic bronchitis and the ecological structure of Leeds, England (1972a), the role of distance of health-care use (1969, 1973), and non-vectored infectious diseases (1974).

In his study of the role of distance as a spatial factor of the interaction between disease and health facilities in a rural environment, Girt advanced the thesis that the probability of an individual consulting a physician for a given symptom is related to distance. Because the effects of illness and therapeutic behaviour cannot be measured independently, Girt decided to assess the effect of distance on attitude relating to certain cognitive processes thought to be involved in deciding whether to consult a physician or not. Approximately 1400 adults living in seven Newfoundland settlements at differing distances from their physician were interviewed and their attitudes towards certain aspects of the medical care process recorded. (It is to be noted that the cost of consultation in Canada is not a significant factor wherever such cost is defrayed by various government programmes.)

The individual dependence on the physician did tend to increase with the distance people lived from him. Readiness to consult with a physician was greater among those living in a settlement containing a cottage hospital than among those living 10–13 miles away, but it increased again for more distant settlements. This conclusion adds another dimension to the original finding that people appeared to be more sensitive towards ill-health with increasing distance from a doctor.

The locational effects of medical care facilities on levels of individual health appear to be significant and several conditional methods were used for linking disease and spatial behaviour: linear programming solutions to allocating health facilities, and multivariate models for assessing the ability of the hospital system to meet future demands. Girt's study indicates not only the need for considering the location of medical facilities from the point of view of providing opportunities accessible to all, but also the need for ascertaining the effect of location on revealed patterns of ill-health and as an agent influencing the success of measures aimed at raising the general health levels of populations.

Tinline is a Canadian whose first works dealt with the spread of epizootic foot and mouth disease (Tinline, 1970; Tinline and Hugh-Jones, 1976). His studies on disease diffusion can be consulted. Later, he took an interest in the relations between the ecology of foxes and rabies incidence in Ontario, as well as in data-gathering systems.

During this period, a number of master's theses were written on the organization of health services; for example, J. E. McMeiken (1971) on the study of the perception and attitudes of public health practitioners. Bottomley's (1970) thesis also studied, on a phenomenological plane, the location of doctors' surgeries in Vancouver.

The most complete study is the work of Michael Dear on health units for mental illnesses. English by birth, Dear's thesis dealt with the impact of health units for mental illnesses in a residential neighbourhood (Dear, 1974, 1975; Dear et al., 1975). Because of the decentralization policies in the United States with respect to health units for mental illnesses and their location in residential environments, public response was significantly negative (Dear, 1976). Dear et al. (1979) claim that three sets of factors are fundamental to the explanation of public response to community mental health facilities. These are the physical and social characteristics of the host neighbourhood, the attitudes of residents toward the mentally ill and the characteristics of the facility itself. Separating these three sets of factors does not imply that they exert a totally independent influence on public reaction to community mental health facilities. On the contrary, in any given situation, these factors work in combination to determine the fit between "form" and "context" (the facility and the neighbourhood) and therefore the acceptance or rejection of the facility by the host community. Empirical attentions are founded on the impact of community mental health facilities upon property values (Dear, 1977a,b), the relationships between attitudes toward the mentally ill and reactions to potential and existing facility locations (Dear, 1977c; Dear et *al.*, 1979, 1980b). Data used was collected in a questionnaire survey conducted in Toronto. The chief findings show that suburban divisions with a preponderance of owner-occupied single family housing are more vulnerable to the installation and implementation of community health facilities. In this case, the introduction of a facility is more likely to be visible and to be perceived as a threat to neighbourhood quality and to property values. This research shows the interest of the behavioural approach in locating and planning health units (Dear, 1978).

Dear *et al.* (1980a) show the need for a revised paradigm in terms of present-day analytical scenarios for community health care. He suggests that the field of medical geography, which has hitherto been dominated by a concern with spatial pattern to the almost complete exclusion of social process, should pay more regard to an historical approach.

The organization of emergency services is a relatively underdeveloped field of geographical research. David Ingram (1971, 1980; Ingram *et al.*, 1978) has recently studied the medical and social characteristics of patients using the emergency departments of two hospitals in Hamilton, Ontario. With a view to regionalizing emergency services, Ingram, using an elementary distance minimizing technique, underscores the impact in total travel distance that would result from the night-time closure of three locations. The results show that mutually exclusive catchment areas for hospitals can be defined using minimum travel distances, but that it must be recognized that potential patients do not possess perfect knowledge of hospital locations and therefore make journeys which are longer than necessary. The definition of catchment areas is a useful exercise for developing an assessment of the population which is most likely to use a particular hospital, for comparing the adequacy of facilities provided in different hospitals and for examining aspects of the problems of spatial variations in accessibility to hospitals.

Field's (1980) analysis of Canadian mortality over a 50 year period, at different scales, provides several fruitful and interesting observations. The author compares direct and indirect standardization methods for series of mortality data. He notes that the magnitude of the decline in the risk of dying, standardized for changes in the age–sex structure of the nation's population, can only be approximately specified by using these methods. These problems are shared with conceptually similar measures such as the Consumer Price Index and the Stock Exchange Index. At the root of the measurement problem in developing a standardized time series of mortality rates is the fact that changes in the age structure of the population have been accompanied by a substantial difference in the rate at which mortality probabilities have declined for the younger versus the older age groups. In general, mortality risks have undergone a much greater reduction in percentage terms for all age cohorts below 45 years than for those in the middle- to upper-age categories.

The most salient feature of the temporal trend of standardized mortality rates for the major geographical divisions of the nation has been a decline in the magnitude of the regional disparities over time, particularly in the pre-1960 period, as the high Quebec and low Western rates tended to move in the direction of the national average. Quebec's general mortality rating as a high risk area is mirrored in the rates for all of the major causal categories with the notable exception of diseases of the respiratory system, and revealed a tendency towards higher mortality rates in the more urbanized areas.

The broad overview of general mortality patterns across the nation that this study sought to provide brings to light many features that warrant more detailed investigation before socio-economic and environmental correlates of the mortality factor can be meaningfully evaluated. A still greater perspective would result if such studies were to transcend national boundaries and were to incorporate a comparison with the geographical patterns of the United States to the south. Measurements of risks at the level of individual urban centres and other units of a lower order than census divisions would be equally useful in studying the national geography of mortality associated with specific causes.

More directly related to the organization of services, the research of Bryan Massam (1975) is noteworthy. Between 1976 and 1978, Massam directed several master's theses on the distribution of mortality in Montreal in order to examine the spatial arrangement of selected causes of death by census tracts (Bouchard, 1976; Massam and Nisen, 1980). Statistical procedures were used to complement the production of maps by automated cartographic methods (Massam *et al.*, 1977; Massam and Bouchard, 1977). Massam's research on mortality or morbidity is directly related to the use of health services. There is scope for comparative behavioural surveys covering such factors as health attitudes and utilization of health services (Massam and Bouchard, 1976). Massam used data on the use of health services in Kuala Lumpur, Malaysia to illustrate this approach. First, he gave a classification of a set of health-care facilities based upon observed aggregate utilization patterns. Secondly, he endeavoured to explain the classification by analyses of the patient's travel patterns. By and large, familiar sources of health care continue to be used in spite of relocation. For example, rehoused squatters travel further and bypass more alternatives to get to facilities. Further work is needed to explain "attractiveness" but policy-making should clearly be based upon an understanding of the reasons why people choose a particular centre for a specific service.

Other Canadian geographers have conducted research in Third World countries. Frank Barrett (1975) has published a study of the geomedical aspects of goitre in the endemic regions of Africa. R. Aiken, Irish by birth, has been interested in the distribution of dengue haemorrhagic fever (DMF) in south-east Asia, and in particular, Malaysia and Singapore (Aiken and Leigh, 1978). His study recommends that future investigations should be based on local epidemiology conditions, vector ecology, origin of case detection, origin of infection and migratory movements in the area under investigation.

The role of seasons, as affecting favourable conditions for the development of illness and its transmission, has been surveyed not only in tropical countries but also in Canada. Simon Kevan has devoted time to the issue of the season of birth and season of death (Kevan and Chapman, 1980), especially with two of the more sensational causes of death: suicide and murder. The question is not so much the existence of seasonal variations of life and death, but rather explanation of causes. Regarding the season of birth, it seems that the winter-born appear to be at a slight disadvantage in terms of mental aptitude. Of far more concern to the medical profession has been the reconfirmation that people suffering from schizophrenia are born significantly more often during the late winter and early spring months than at any other time of the year (Kevan, 1978).

Research on seasonal variations of disease involves some difficulties (Kevan, 1980). First, the existence of a seasonal variation of some behavioural or pathological condition does not necessarily mean that meteorological factors are of any significant consequence—such distributions could be merely the effects of socio-economic conditions, coincident diet, or health factors or possibly even astro-physical forces. Another problem which is as serious, though it has been seldom mentioned, is that the use of monthly summarized meteorological data could mask the true importance of biometeorological relationships. Finally, there are also the more obvious problems associated with the use of regionally summarized data, especially when the regions are as large as a province or country. These problems, however, should be viewed as challenges for those interested in this field of medical geography.

French-speaking geographers have followed the same research patterns: spatial organization of health services particularly in the rural environment, and analyses of the variations in diseases and mortality. In the first case, the works of J.-P. Thouez, French by birth, may be cited. His principal research deals with the organization of hospital services and the problems of accessibility in rural areas (1978a,b, 1981). He has also been interested in geo-coded computer systems and has published a medical atlas of the eastern townships of Quebec (Thouez *et al.*, 1980b) and an atlas on the distribution of cancers in Quebec (Thouez *et al.*, 1980a).

Quebec is well suited to the analysis of components (physicians, paramedical personnel, beds, departments, and financial resources) which provide the basic elements for determining a classification of hospital units, because state payment for medical or hospital treatments provides the data necessary for study of the variations and delimitation of catchment areas and for determining the patient's diagnosis. However, the analysis of spatial behaviour in the patient must be supplemented by analysing attitudes and perception to health, sickness, and to medical personnel and resources (Thouez *et al.*, 1981b). The perception of the level of health by the respondents themselves is always the most important factor in explaining the number of medical visits. Alternative methods to express the state of health of the population of the eastern townships have been approached: the mapping and analysis of the spatial distribution of human blood components (Thouez *et al.*, 1980c) and the exploration of the contribution made by occupational status to leukocyte variability (Thouez *et al.*, 1981c).

A French-Canadian, Luc Loslier, has directed several research projects on the variation in mortality with respect to social areas of Montreal, on life-style and mortality in the Province of Quebec and on causes of mortality as associated with urban functions in Canada (Loslier, 1981a,b). For example, he finds that atmospheric pollution in downtown Montreal may explain the high mortality in areas where a well-off population lives. Similarly, mortality is inversely related to income levels for bronchitis, emphysema, asthma, cirrhosis of the liver in the 35–64 year age group and for motor vehicle accidents in the 1–14 year age group (Loslier, 1976).

For most causes of disease and especially for the young, mortality is higher among poorer than among richer inhabitants. Socio-economic inequalities reflect themselves in health conditions despite social and sanitary developments over the last decade. In order to improve the state of health, it may be more relevant to equalize income distribution, especially with regard to income security, rather than to increase health services. The individual sensitivity of each component of the socio-economic index (income, education, occupational status) would require examination to see which are susceptible to improvement.

Thus, the number of medical geographical scientists has increased, even though they are few in number in comparison with other geographical specialists. However, it is true to say that close cooperation and overlap exists between the specialized and the general fields of interest.

The teaching of medical geography in Canadian universities: influences and trends

At present, five departments of geography offer courses in medical geography at the university level. In 1975, Professor Thouez offered the first such course in Canada in this field for students at the master's level. The course was co-directed by Professor L. Munan, an epidemiologist with the Department of Community Health Sciences of the University of Sherbrooke. In 1980 this department offered a diploma course for geographers in this field of expertise. Since 1978, Professors Thouez and Foggin have offered, on an alternate basis, the same course for master's students and doctoral students at the University of Montreal. Since 1980, Professor Loslier has taught at higher degree level at the University of Quebec at Montreal. Beginning in 1977, English-speaking universities have also offered courses in medical geography for students at undergraduate level: Tinline at Queen's, Innes at Windsor, and Barrett at York University. All of these universities are located in Ontario.

Whether the courses are given at French or English-speaking universities, their content is similar. Diseases and mortality are emphasized as revealing factors for man–environment relations in time and space. It is acknowledged that disease must be globally defined and consequently, functions must not only be analysed specifically but also from the point of view of their interrelations. In other words, disease is viewed as a "paradigm" and it is necessary to study its sub-systems: the physical, biological, and socio-cultural environment influencing distribution. Other themes are also examined: regional disparities in health system organization, comparative analysis of health systems, etc. At York University and elsewhere, it has been realized that specific courses must be instituted to study health systems and nutritional geography (which in other departments are subjects incorporated into cultural geography).

Course expansion will allow more time to be devoted to the ecology of disease. On the other hand, any new course in the field of health services and nutritional sciences is usually subject to rejection by other departments or faculties of the same university if the possibility of academic conflict arises. This problem is negligible at York University because, in addition to the three courses mentioned above, the college has offered a medical geography seminar since 1980 and an interdisciplinary seminar on health, medicine and the social sciences.

The creation of medical geography courses, in particular at the master's and doctoral levels, has most definitely influenced the training of geographers interested in this specialization. These geography departments have several students who have written their theses within the scope of their own professor's research projects. In addition to the names given above, some 20 students have written master's theses in medical geography since 1970. Teaching, but above all, departments of community health and local community services centres, offer possible employment outlets for these specialized geographers.

Within the scope of these courses, several foreign professors have been invited to lecture in Canada. Professors G. M. Howe of Strathclyde and A. T. A. Learmonth of the Open University, in the United Kingdom, were invited to Windsor University by Professor Innes in 1977 and in 1980. They gave conferences in Quebec and in the United States. In 1977 and in 1980 Professor Thouez invited Professor Picheral of the University of Montpellier in France to the Universities of Sherbrooke and Montreal. Professor Picheral is the only French geographer to have written a doctoral thesis in medical geography.

The need for a more structured organization for medical geographers gave birth in 1976 to the creation of a Canadian medical geography work group. This group was first officially recognized in 1980 by the Association of Canadian Geographers and now publishes a news bulletin twice annually which is sent to some 50 members. Until 1980, the Medical Geography Commission of the IGU (which since 1976 has become the Working Group on the Geography of Health) had no Canadian members, although Girt had organized the 1972 Medical Geography Symposium at Guelph University. Since 1980, Professor Thouez has been appointed as the Canadian representative. This position will allow him to establish closer links with other national groups.

Since the 1970s, medical geography has undergone gradual but sustained growth. The challenge to geographers and other scientists posed by the high cost of medical services, the all too unequal geographical distribution of these services and the desire for improvements in the quality of life, all suggest to Canadian geographers the necessity for a more rapid development or, at least, for a more active participation in analysing these problems.

The future of medical geography in Canada

For the 1972–1976 period, the IGU's Medical Geography Commission projected four research trends: geography and nutrition; the creation of a composite community health index; the development of a syllabus for training medical geographers; and the relations between geography and pollution. In 1976, at Moscow, the Commission selected two themes: the distribution of several diseases and the demand for health care and the improvement of the environment. If one evaluates research and teaching activities in Canada against these fields of interest, both the weaknesses and the positive aspects of medical geography in Canada become clear.

Canadian scientists have devoted but slight attention to nutritional geography whether in the fields of medical or cultural geography. It is true that statistical information is hard to find and, where it exists, concerns local investigations by nutrition specialists. On the other hand, some studies on medication consumption have been conducted (Walker, 1977; Thouez, 1979). Three promising research trends, in our opinion, concern first the organization of health services, then the general ecology of diseases, and thirdly and in particular, the relations between pollution and disease.

In the first case, mental health and other health-care organization are under study by several scientists. Studies by Peter Foggin (1981) at the University of Montreal and Simpson-Housley (1980) at Calgary should be noted. The former study is based on data obtained from an investigation at 22 Metropolitan Montreal hospitals where Foggin examined 2242 patient files. Factorial component analysis of 42 variables disclosed seven factors used as independent variables in a multiple regression model. Attendance at psychiatric units could be linked to social aid workers, but for unemployed workers and the elderly there was no relation between psychiatric emergencies and spatial distribution of demand. Accordingly, the author suggests greater decentralization of emergency care. It is in this field that cooperation with other social scientists appears most promising for geographers because such cooperation utilizes their base training in spatial organization.

The distribution and spread of diseases and of mortality constitutes the second orientation in medical geography. Applications concern Canada and several developing areas: south-east Asia (Hyma and Ramesh, 1977), Africa (Stock, 1976) and Latin America. Among diseases most often analysed by Canadian geographers are foot and mouth disease, cancers and cardiovascular diseases. For example, Grant Sigsworth (1976, 1980) analysed the geographical dimensions of animal health in relation to the spread of foot and mouth disease in Mexico. The volume and precision of Mexican data do not permit a modelling of diffusion probabilities. However, the author shows that at the base level of the hierarchy the most prevalent type of transmission is between farms. Analysis of the geographical distribution of farms, production, marketing and transportation of animals allows the author to develop some strategies for an efficient eradication campaign.

The third potential for development concerns the way in which contaminated living conditions are, or may be, causatively related to man's health or man's diseases.

Frank Innes (1980) has analysed 28 variables such as the degree of urbanization, type of fuel used for home heating, employment patterns and ethnic origins in relation to a limited range of diseases at census tract level. Multiple regression was employed to try to establish these relationships but no conclusive findings resulted. He concluded that the unsatisfactory nature of the available information makes this approach one for further research. On the other hand, Thouez (1978c,d) in several publications on the relations between physical and chemical components of drinking water and cardiovascular diseases and cancers reached a number of interesting results. For example, there would seem to be a significant relation between soft water and cardiovascular incidence at the scale of municipalities in the eastern township region of Quebec. Similarly, significant relations for Quebec seem to exist between several components of drinking water such as copper, magnesium, lead, the softness and acidity of water, and certain cancers of the digestive tract, the rectum and the prostate (Thouez et al., 1980b). Robert Pampalon (1980, 1981) has provided further analyses of physical and human ecological relationships with health for the case of Quebec. It may seem surprising that medical geography has not extended its influence beyond Ontario and Quebec. There are some exceptions such as W. H. Allderdice of Memorial University in Newfoundland who studied the ecology of genetic diseases such as multiple sclerosis, and Gerda Bako, research associate at the Provincial Cancer Hospitals Board in Alberta. Her first works concerned the geographical distribution of mortalities from arteriosclerotic heart disease and fatal motor vehicle accidents (Bako 1973a,b, 1975, 1976a,b, 1977), and later her research has dealt with cancer incidence in Alberta. Since 1969 this province has collected significant data on demographic, socio-economic and life-style characteristics of patients attending hospitals in the main cities of this province. Using data for the 1969–1973 period, Bako et al. (1978, 1981) analysed the relations between these variables and chief cancer sites by the help of contingency tables. This research has a double interest: to evaluate the suitability of the collected information for statistical analysis by using a systematic epidemiological approach and to stimulate the research of associations between cancers and variables in order to clarify certain relationships which appeared during the analysis.

This commentary would not be complete without mentioning Barrett's (1980b) research on the conceptual foundations of medical geography during the eighteenth and nineteenth centuries, the works of A. Ray

(1975, 1976) on the spread of disease in relation to fur trade expansion in nineteenth-century Canada, and the research of Bordessa and Cameron (1980) on the history of the sanitary movement in Toronto. This shows an interest in integrating the historical dimension into medical geography proper.

During the last decade, important progress has been made in medical geography here in Canada. However, such a rapid expansion in use of new techniques and in breadth of study could not have been achieved without some error. It may be that the interest which geographers show in this specialization arises from a renewal in the discipline since the end of the 1960s, and consequently from the methodological anxiety which became widespread during that period. Thus, as Girt (1980) has aptly emphasized, before widening this field of research, it may be preferable to establish which geographical goals are most meaningful. Our potential contribution lies in social and environmental administration, particularly in its relation with diseases. We strive to benefit society. Many young people today demand that social sciences move from explaining and forecasting to establishing norms of action—norms which social scientists know how to implement, but still only too imperfectly.

References

Aiken, S. R. and Leigh, C. H. (1978). Dengue haemorrhagic fever in south-east Asia. *Trans. Inst. Br. Geogr.* **3**, 4, 476–497.

Bako, G. (1973a). *Alberta Medical Bulletin* **38**, 31–34.

Bako, G. (1973b). Mortality from Heart Disease in Alberta: Distribution and Environment. M.Sc. thesis, University of Alberta.

Bako, G. (1975). In *Report of the Task Force on Highway Accidents to the Minister of Social Services and Community Health*. Government of Alberta.

Bako, G., Mackenzie, W. C. and Smith, E. S. (1976a). Survey of impaired drivers, fatally injured or surviving, who caused fatal highway accidents in Alberta in 1970–72. *Can. med. Assoc. J.* **115**, 856–857.

Bako, G., Mackenzie, W. C. and Smith, E. S. (1976b). Effect of legislated lowering of the drinking age on fatal highway accidents among young drivers in Alberta, 1970–72. *Can J. publ. Hlth.* **67**, 161–163.

Bako, G. (1977). Recidivist Driver Involvement in Fatal Highway Accidents in Alberta, Canada, 1970–1972. Paper presented at the 7th International Conference on Alcohol, Drugs and Traffic Safety, Melbourne, 23–28 January.

Bako, G., Grace, M. and Smith, E. S. (1978). *Epidemiology of Cancer in Alberta, 1969–1973*. Provincial Cancer Hospitals Board and Government of Alberta.

Bako, G., Hill, G., Hannon, J. and Dewar, R. (1981). *Epidemiology of Cancer in Alberta, 1969–73. Specific Topic Supplement No. 3, Cancer of the Stomach.* Government of Alberta and Provincial Cancer Hospitals Board.

Barrett, F. A. (1975). Geomedical Aspects of Simple Endemic Goitre in Africa. Proceedings of the Canadian Association of African Studies, Toronto.

Barrett, F. A. (1980a). Medical geography as a foster child. In *Conceptual and Methodological Issues in Medical Geography* (Ed. M. S. Meade), pp. 1–15. Department of Geography, University of South Carolina at Chapel Hill.

Barrett, F. A. (Ed.) (1980b). The development and current status of medical geography in Canada. In *Canadian Studies in Medical Geography*, pp. 2–15. Geographical Monographs, York University.

Bordessa, R. and Cameron, J. M. (1980). Sanitation, water and health: two centuries of public health progress in Toronto. In *Canadian Studies in Medical Geography* (Ed. F. A. Barrett), pp. 121–146. Geographical Monographs, York University.

Bottomley, J. (1970). Physician Office Site Characteristics: A Cognitive–Behavioral Approach. Unpublished M.A. thesis, University of British Columbia.

Bouchard, D. C. (1976). Spatial autocorrelation and health care data: a preliminary study. *Cahier géo. Qué.* **20**, 51, 521–538.

Coulson, M. R. C. (1967). The distribution of population by age structure in Kansas City. *Annals Assoc. Amer. Geogr.* **58**, 155–167.

Dear, M. (1974). Locational Analysis for Public Mental Health Facilities. Ph.D. dissertation, Regional Science Department, University of Pennsylvania, Ann Arbor, Michigan.

Dear, M. (1975). The Neighborhood Impact of Mental Health Facility Setting. Discussion Paper Series No. 84. Regional Science Department, University of Pennsylvania, Ann Arbor, Michigan.

Dear, M. (1976). Spatial Externalities and Location Conflict. *London Papers in Regional Science* **7**, 152–167.

Dear, M. (1977a). Impact of mental health facilities upon property values. *Community Mental Health Journal* **13**, 2, 150–157.

Dear, M. (1977b). Locational factors in the demand for mental health care. *Econ. Geogr.* **53**, 3, 223–240.

Dear, M. (1977c). Psychiatric patients and the inner city. *Annals Assoc. Amer. Geogr.* **67**, 4, 588–594.

Dear, M. (1978). Planning for mental health care: A reconsideration of public facility location theory. *International Regional Science Review* **3**, 9, 23–112.

Dear, M., Wolpert, J. and Crawford, R. (1975). Satellite mental health facilities. *Annals Assoc. Amer. Geogr.* **65**, 1, 24–35.

Dear, M., Clark, G. and Clark, S. (1979). Economic cycles and mental health care policy. *Soc. Sci. Med.* **13C**, 43–53.

Dear, M., Taylor, S. M. and Hall, G. G. (1980a). Attitudes toward the mentally ill and reactions to mental health facilities. *Soc. Sci. Med.* **14D**, 281–290.

Dear, M., Isaak, S. and Taylor, M. (1980b). Community mental health facilities in residential neighbourhoods. In *Canadian Studies in Medical Geography* (Ed. F. A. Barrett), pp. 231–256. Geographical Monographs, York University.

Field, N. C. (1963). Land hunger and the rural depopulation problem in the USSR. *Annals Assoc. Amer. Geogr.* **53**, 4, 465–478.

Field, N. C. (1980). Temporal and spatial patterns of mortality in Canada. In *Canadian Studies in Medical Geography* (Ed. F. A. Barrett), pp. 32–58. Geographical Monographs, York University.

Foggin, P. (1981). Localisation des services d'urgence psychiatrique sur l'île de Montréal. *Santé mentale du Québec* **6**, 1, 10–15.

Garry, R. (1964). La loi de 1948 sur l'eugénisme national et l'évolution de la population Japonaise de 1949 à 1958. *Revue de geographie de Montreal* **1911**, 87–99.

Girt, J. L. (1969). Value orientations in seven Newfoundland communities. In *Newfoundland—Introductory Essays and Excursion Guides* (Ed. P. Crabb). Prepared for the Annual Meeting of the Canadian Association of Geographers at St John's, Newfoundland.

Girt, J. L. (1972a). Simple chronic bronchitis and urbal ecological structure in medical geography: techniques and field studies. In *Medical Geography: Techniques and Field Studies* (Ed. N. D. McGlashan), pp. 211–232. Methuen, London.

Girt, J. L. (1972b). The location of medical services and disease ecology: some conclusions on the effect of distance on medical consultations in a rural environment. *Geographia Medica* **2**, 43–62.

Girt, J. L. (1973). Distance to medical practice and its effects on ill health in a rural environment. *The Canadian Geographer* **17**, 2, 154–166.

Girt, J. L. (1974). The geography of non-vectored infectious diseases. In *The Geography of Health and Disease* (Ed. J. M. Hunter), pp. 81–100. Studies in Geography **6**. Department of Geography, University of North Carolina.

Girt, J. L. (1980). Some questions about the future of medical geography. In *Canadian Studies in Medical Geography* (Ed. F. A. Barrett), pp. 250–263. Geographical Monographs, York University.

Hyma, B. and Ramesh, A. (1977). *Cholera and Malaria Incidence in Tamilnadu, India. Case studies in Medical Geography*. Department of Geography Publication Series **9**, University of Waterloo.

Ingram, D. R. (1971). *Regional Studies* May, 33–36.

Ingram, D. R. (1980). Spatial aspects of emergency department use at two Hamilton hospitals. In *Canadian Studies in Medical Geography* (Ed. F. A. Barrett), pp. 211–230. Geographical Monographs, York University.

Ingram, D. R., Clarke, D. R. and Murdie, R. A. (1978). Distance and the decision to visit an emergency department. *Soc. Sci. Med.* **12D**, 55–62.

Innes, F. (1980). Medical geography: a preliminary investigation at two scales in Ontario. In *Canadian Studies in Medical Geography* (Ed. F. A. Barrett), pp. 95–119. Geographical Monographs, York University.

Kevan, S. (1978). The seasonal behaviour of Canadians' mental health. *Canadian Mental Health* **26**, 16–18.

Kevan, S. (1980). Season of life—season of death. *Soc. Sci. Med.* **13D**, 227–232.

Kevan, S. and Chapman, R. (1980). Variations in mortality rates in Canada. In *Canadian Studies in Medical Geography* (Ed. F. A. Barrett), pp. 65–77. Geographical Monographs, York University.

Loslier, L. (1976). La mortalité dans les aires sociales de la région métropolitaine de Montréal. Service des études épidémiologiques. Direction générale de la planification. Ministère des Affaires Sociales, Québec.

Loslier, L. (1981a). Les régions les plus éprouvées dans la province a la plus forte mortalité au Canada: le Québec. *Le médicin du Québec* **16**, 83–91.

Loslier, L. (1981b). Modes de vie, milieux de vie et disparités de santé au Québec. In *Comité des Travaux Historiques et Scientifiques* (Ed. H. Picheral), p. 133. Bulletin de la Section de Géographie, Paris.

Massam, B. H. (1975). *Location and Space in Social Administration*. Edward Arnold, London.

Massam, B. H. and Bouchard, D. (1977). Toward a framework for examining the utilization of a public facility: health care centres in Kuala Lumpur, Malaysia. *Geoforum* **8**, 113–119.

Massam, B. H. and Nisen, W. G. (1980). An analysis of mortality patterns in Montreal. In *Canadian Studies in Medical Geography* (Ed. F. A. Barrett), pp. 59–66. Geographical Monographs, York University.

Massam, B. H., Bouchard, D. and Nisen, W. G. (1977). Mortality patterns in Montreal. Report 4, Mimeo. Department of Geography, McGill University, Montreal.

McMeiken, J. E. (1971). Public Health Professionals and the Environment: A Study of Perceptions and Attitudes. Unpublished M.A. thesis, University of Victoria, B.C.

Ray, A. (1975). Smallpox: the epidemic of 1837–38. *The Beaver* Autumn, 8–13.

Ray, A. (1976). Diffusion of diseases in the western interior of Canada, 1830–1850. *Geo. Review* **66**, 2, 139–157.

Pampalon, R. (1980). Environment et santé au Québec. In *Canadian Studies in Medical Geography* (Ed. F. A. Barrett), pp. 16–30. Geographical Monographs, York University.

Simpson-Housley, P. and Hall, G. B. (1980). Paper presented at the 76th Meeting of the Association of American Geographers, Louisville, Kentucky.

Sigsworth, G. (1976). *Diss. Abstr. Int.* **XXXVI**, 9.

Sigsworth, G. (1980). Spatial structure of disease diffusion and control: foot and mouth disease in Mexico. In *Canadian Studies in Medical Geography* (Ed. F. A. Barrett), pp. 173–188. Geographical Monographs, York University.

Stock, R. (1976). Cholera in Africa: diffusion of the disease 1970–75 with particular emphasis on West Africa. Africa Environment Special Report 3, International African Institute, London.

Thouez, J. P. (1978a). L'utilisation de la cartographie automatisée dans un système régional d'information sanitaire. *Soc. Sci. Med.* **12D**, 192–203.

Thouez, J. P. (1978b). *Espace Régional et Santé*. Naaman, Sherbrooke.

Thouez, J. P. (1978c). Mortalité ischémique du coeur et la qualité de l'eau potable dans les Cantons de l'est. *The Canadian Geographer* **18**, 4, 308–321.

Thouez, J. P. (1978d). La dureté de l'eau potable et la mortalité cérébrale vasculaire dans les Cantons de l'est du Québec. *Bull. Assoc. Géogr. Franç.* **451**, 114–124.

Thouez, J. P. (1979). La consommation des médicaments à Sherbrooke, approche psycho-socio-démographique. Notes de recherche. Department of Geography, University of Montreal.

Thouez, J. P. (1981). La régionalisation des services hospitaliers: le cas des Cantons de l'est. In *Comité des Travaux Historiques et Scientifiques* (Ed. H. Picheral), 133, 203–244. Bulletin de la Section de Géographie, Paris.

Thouez, J. P. and Munan, L. (1981). Attitudes and opinions on health medical care. A case study of the rural population of the Eastern Townships, Quebec. *Geographia medica*.

Thouez, J. P., Beauchamp, Y. and Simard, A. (1980a). Atlas Oncologique de Québec, 1971–1976. Notes de Recherche, Département de Géographie, Université de Montréal, No. 80-02.

Thouez, J. P., Fortin, R. and Castonguay, J. (1980b). *Atlas Médical des Cantons de l'Est*. Naaman, Sherbrooke.

Thouez, J. P., Munan, L., Gagné, M. and Kelly, A. (1980c). The spatial distribution of leukocyte counts in a free-living population. In *Canadian Studies in Medical*

Geography (Ed. F. A. Barrett), pp. 147–172. Geographical Monographs, York University.

Thouez, J. P., Beauchamp, Y. and Simard, A. (1981a). Cancer incidence and the physico-chemical quality of drinking water in Quebec. *Soc. Sci. Med.* **15D**, 213–223.

Thouez, J. P., Munan, L. and Nabahi, I. (1981b). Factors associated with the utilization of health care services in rural areas. *Soc. Sci. Med.* **15D**, 379–387.

Thouez, J. P., Munan, L., Kelly, A., Gagné, M. and Labonte, D. (1981c). Relative leucopenia in the peripheral blood of asbestos miners: an epidemiologic analysis. *Scand. J. Hematology* **26**, 115–122.

Tinline, R. (1970). Lee wave hypotheses for the initial pattern of spread during the 1967–68 foot and mouth epizootic. *Nature* **227**, 860–862.

Tinline, R. and E. Hugh-Jones, M. E. (1976). Studies on the 1967–68 foot and mouth disease epidemic: incubation period and serial interval. *J. Hyg.* **77**, 141–153.

Walker, G. (1977). Report to the Non-medical Use of Drug Directorate. Health and Welfare, Ottowa.

Warren, H. V. (1964). Geology, trace elements and epidemiology. *Geogrl. J.* **130**, 525–528.

Warren, H. V. (1965). Medical geology and geography. *Science* **148**, 534–539.

Developments in medical geography in India

Attur Ramesh

Department of Geography, University of Madras, India

An historical perspective of medical geography in India

The earliest works in medical geography in India date back to the latter half of the nineteenth and the early twentieth centuries and were concerned with the distribution and study of diseases on a descriptive basis. Exemplars of this trend tended to concentrate on single particular themes in different regional contexts. For example, medical topography in the northern part of India was studied by McClelland (1859), McNamara (1880), Chevers (1886), Adams (1899) and Hamoston (1905). In similar descriptive vein were later works from southern India on public health at district scale (Hesterlow, 1930, 1931–1932; George and Webster, 1934; Ramachandra, 1937; Shivaramayya, 1938; Nityanandan Pillai, 1941). Hesterlow, one of the founding fathers of medical geography in India, worked at different regional levels, trying to correlate environmental factors with the incidence of various diseases (Hesterlow, 1929, 1931–1932).

The distribution and epidemiology of cholera and malaria have been the most widely researched topics, though it was not until the late 1920s that a cholera epidemic was first conceptualized within a framework which allowed such factors as the influx of pilgrims at different fairs and festivals to be examined in detail (Rogers, 1928, 1944). Subsequently, factors relating to the epidemiology of cholera (Russel and Sundarrajan, 1928; Banerjee, 1951) and its endemicity (Swaroop, 1951) were well established. Malaria incidence too was analysed at different regional levels (Rao, 1930; Russell and Ramachandra, 1940) and the influence of the work of geographers in developing an understanding of cholera and

GEOGRAPHICAL ASPECTS OF HEALTH
ISBN 0 12 483780 8

malaria deserve mention (Chakrabarti, 1954; Covell, 1955; Sen, 1957).

Work on cancer distributions also appeared in the early medical literature (Orr, 1933; Gault, 1955; Sarma, 1958). Studies such as that by Chopra *et al.* (1942) on the association of the incidence of crime with the local environment and two books on health and nutrition in the Indian sub-continent (Gangulee, 1938; Borker, 1957) illustrate the divergent paths taken by other disciplines prior to the formation of the IGU Commission on Medical Geography in 1948. This formal recognition and encouragement of the subject, noted in Indian journals in 1951 (Geddes, 1951; May and Walsh, 1951), as well as the earlier trends recorded above, stimulated a considerable broadening of interest in subsequent years.

The regional incidence of diseases

The most widely studied aspect of medical geography in India has certainly traditionally been the incidence and distribution of diseases. Perhaps this interest is a direct reflection of Professor Learmonth's many contributions. Earlier emphases on cholera and malaria incidence have persisted into recent time and this may be due to the far more reliable records now being maintained by public health departments. Geographers have also been influenced by the concern of other disciplines with such diseases as trachoma, goitre, cancer, guineaworm and infectious diseases.

During the 1960s medical geography in India appears to have become strongly established in the north in contrast to its dominance in southern India during the 1940s. For example, work on cancer (Indrapal, 1956, 1972), yellow water in parts of Uttar Pradesh (Indrapal, 1968) and on trachoma (Indrapal, 1970) have emerged from the north-western school centred at Jaipur in Rajasthan. In Bengal, work on cholera incidence gained greater importance (Sen, 1957; Basu, 1969) and goitre was widely studied in the Kumaon region and Maharashtra on a geomedical basis (Akthar, 1978b, 1979a; Krishnamachari, 1974). With regard to cholera in the latter part of the 1970s, yet another centre of medical geography was established at Madras, where, among other topics, cholera incidence at the state and city level was studied (Hyma and Ramesh, 1976, 1977; Kumaraswamy, 1981a,b).

Works on malaria are even more numerous, ranging in scale from national level studies (Learmonth, 1957) to state and micro-level studies (Nair and Samnotra, 1969). Colonization in new areas along the foothill zones of the *Terai* and at dam or reservoir sites and its impact on malaria incidence was highlighted by studies by medical geographers (Akthar,

1979b; Hyma and Ramesh, 1980). Subsequently malaria resurgence in many different parts of India became a matter of academic study (Learmonth and Akthar, 1979a; Hyma *et al.*, 1981), whilst state-level studies of the disease (Prasad, 1981) reinforced this growing concern.

In addition to malaria and cholera, geographers have also shown interest in the incidence of other diseases. Southern Asia as a whole was well surveyed by medical geographers with reference to the occurrence of dengue fever (Joshi and Despande, 1972; Jusatz, 1975). The geography of death from all causes at a state level was also defined by Ahmed (1973) using mortality statistics. Tuberculosis in different towns was surveyed by Bishit (1981) and Kumaraswamy (1981c) and smallpox was analysed with correlations on a regional basis (Singh and Dutta, 1981). Cancers at various sites were studied at a national level (Akthar, 1980).

A number of Ph.D. theses, written in different parts of the country, reflect a similar concern with the geography of diseases and their incidence in different states. For example, Singh and Singh's (1980) work on the Lower Chambal Valley, Pandurkar (1981) on Maharashtra, Mathur (1981) on Rajasthan and Rahman (1981) on the Brahmaputra Valley all deal with specific diseases and prove beyond doubt a growing interest in this field among Indian geographers.

Disease ecology

Most of the work published before 1950 on disease ecology concentrated especially on malaria and the work of non-geographers during the early period has influenced the work of geographers following on. In this category are Kendrick's (1919) study of malaria in relation to rice cultivation and Iyengar's (1930–1931) in relation to jungle. The influence of habitat upon the disease ecology of malaria has remained of interest to scholars (Russell and Ramachandra Rao, 1940) and malaria control and eradication have also been studied in great detail (Covell, 1955; Subramanyam, 1955; Alvarado, 1962; Bhatia *et al.*, 1957).

The year 1968 heralded large-scale entry into the field of disease ecology by geographers. The IGU met in New Delhi and was attended both by senior Indian academics and by large numbers of Indian research students who were exposed, many for the first time, to this field of study. One of the most important works to stem from that meeting was Indrapal and Mathur's (1970) research on trachoma and helminthic disease in Rajasthan and it deserves special mention because of its influence on later works. However, other geographers also started to examine the geo-ecology of a number of diseases in different regional contexts. In particular the geo-ecology of cholera (Jusatz, 1968; Banerjee and Hazra, 1974) together with its diffusion patterns (Dutta, 1973) were analysed in detail, as was the ecology of guineaworm disease (Tewari, 1968) and its biocoenesis (Mathur, 1970). Similarly, ecological factors influencing the patterns of different types of cancer in India had also been a subject of concern to medical scientists (Sharma, 1958; Wahi *et al.*, 1966) and they were followed by geographers (Jyssawalla, 1976; Akthar, 1980a, 1982c) with an interest in the epidemiology of cancer.

Developing the theme of Kendrick (1919), comprehensive analyses of climate, vegetation, tribal habitat and rice cultivation and their associa-tions with malaria were undertaken by Dutta, Akthar *et al.* (1980). Following Jacques May, Mukerjee (1980) examined the unique ecology of Chandigarh Dun where infectious diseases predominate and display a spatial association with pathogenic, geogenic and cultural factors.

In the field of disease ecology too, the Madras Symposium in 1981 revealed the diverse interests of Indian medical geographers. Spatial patterns of blood groups in southern India (Shanmuganandan), the ecology of tuberculosis (Singh and Singh), the establishment of new foci of schistosomiasis (Anantaraman), the spatial dynamics of disease (Dutta and Dutta) and the geogenic factors of eye disease (Indrapal and Mathur), were among the contributions. The Symposium also gave new impetus to interdisciplinary work between the fields of geography and health, which still tended to operate at a distance from each other. Geographers were brought face-to-face with medical viewpoints on changing modes of cholera control (Kapali), malaria ecology at new dam sites (Prasad) and the effects of insecticide spraying (Barai *et al.*). At several presentations, with vastly diverse topics, a many-sided interest was developed in the subsequent question and comment sessions.

Nutrition

Any review of the literature on the geography of nutrition in India reveals that a vast amount of work has come from a single institution, the Aligarh Muslim University in Uttar Pradesh, which has one of the oldest geog-raphy departments in the country. Research activity indicates a special concern with the study of agriculture and nutrition, leading on to research in such topics as food resources in relation to population, human geography on a regional scale and land utilization studies in different parts of northern India. These interests have resulted in at least 18 major theses, two of which directly relate to the fields of agricultural land use, nutrition and *deficiency diseases*. These are Akthar's (1978b) work on Kumaon and Alvi's (1974) work on Allahabad and Fatehpur districts.

The work from Aligarh can be divided into two groups. In the first are works on the deficiency diseases of different regions (Khan, 1968; Hussain, 1968; Siddiqi, 1972; Chouridule, 1973). An analysis of daily diets and deficiency diseases was also published for Ganga-Yamuna Doab (Farooqi and Khan, 1977), and for Agra and Mathura region (Qureshi, 1976, 1979–1980). The second group of work incorporates analyses of the calorific value of food in the villages of Uttar Pradesh (Siddiqi, 1966, 1968) and broader nutrition problems in relation to the food production of India (Shafi, 1967). This has led on to similar works at different regional scales (Khan, A. H., 1969; Khan, S. A., 1968; Hussain, 1969; Siddiqi, 1971–1972; Shafi, 1979).

From other parts of India has come the earliest recognized research into nutrition in India by Gangulee (1938), whilst subsequently Learmonth (1956) prepared a map of calorie and protein intake in the diets of poor Indians. Ayyar (1968), following the Aligarh tradition, has studied land use and nutrition, and aspects of protein malnutrition, whilst rural nutrition in Monsoon Asia was studied by Whyte (1968, 1974).

Work at the National Institute of Nutrition at Hyderabad has led to the production of the *Diet and Nutrition Atlas of India* (Gopalan, 1969) which, though interdisciplinary in nature, is a basic reference work. It lays down the standard caloric consumption of different sectors of the Indian population and quantifies the nutritive values of different grains and foodstuffs.

Most other geographical work on nutrition in India is influenced by Aligarh geographers. Caloric availability from foods by village blocks (Singh, 1968) and caloric levels against a framework of population pressure (Singh, 1971) are examples of this.

Environment and health

This aspect of medical geography has been studied either in relation to the incidence and distribution of diseases or as a part of ecological or nutritional studies. Work directly on the effects climate and atmospheric pollution and occupational health hazards, so common in the west, are unusual in India. However, among the few Indian studies, is one on human comfort zones at a limited number of stations in India representing a departure from the mainstream of Indian geographical work (Parthasarathy and Dhar, 1974). Similarly, southern India was classified according to human comfort zones (Subrahmanyam and Sarma, 1981) and the effects of climatic factors on the human body in India were studied by Subramanian and Seshami (1981). Although the well established effects of environmental pollution on human health have as a topic gained little attention from Indian geographers, there are a few notable exceptions; for example, Kumar (1980) on Kanpur; Singh (1981a) on Moradabad city and Kayastha *et al.* (1981) on health problems related to water supply in Varanasi district. A study of the occupational health hazards of leather- and shoe-workers in Agra (Singh, 1981b) provides a most interesting vignette, and another on the potential health risks from faecal bacteria in the highly polluted Cooum River of Madras city may well have wide relevance elsewhere in India (Azariah *et al.*, 1981).

Health-care delivery systems

Geographic study of health-care delivery systems in India has so far only a limited literature though there is tremendous scope for geographers to contribute to this aspect of medical geography. Most work has appeared only during the 1970s although rural health care was studied by a non-geographer, Dutta in 1955. Strassburger discussed the problems associated with health care in southern India in 1973 and other geographers have examined the spatial distribution and growth of health facilities in Rajasthan (Akthar, 1978a) and Maharashtra (Shinde, 1980).

The analysis of health facilities and efficiency is an important topic of current research. The spatial distribution of public health facilities in urban Tamilnadu (Ramesh, 1981), the efficient location of health facilities in Madras city (Kumaran and Jeyapal, 1981), problems of the redistribution of health services in Madras (Begum and Vembu, 1981) and health facilities in rural Upper Bhima basin (Job, 1981), are among the works in this field. Geographers have also assessed policy issues and their implications in the provision of rural health services (Mahadev and Thangamani, 1981) as well as examining the delivery of health care to backward tribal areas (Sukhdev, 1981). The role of traditional health-care systems in India has also been brought into the limelight. This system acts as a support to western medicine even in a metropolis like Madras (Hyma and Ramesh, 1981). The interaction of various systems of health care in India was also assessed by Banerjee (1981).

Certainly some of the papers at the Madras Symposium in 1981 indicated some changes in the interests of medical geographers in India and an increasing concern for health-care delivery systems. The role of health-care delivery in India as a whole was discussed (Akthar and Izhar) as well as a case study of primary health centres in the Poona District of

Maharashtra (Kamarkar and Pagnis). Various health programmes were also assessed in different regions (Bhatnagar) whilst an integrated child development scheme (Jayachandran), family welfare programmes (Kara), and the planning of maternity and child welfare centres are further examples. New arrangements for health facilities in Tamilnadu (Kapali) and Madhya Pradesh were also analysed (Choubey). The spatial distribution of specific centres such as leprosaria in Karnataka was also analysed (Karennavar). Even health resorts were assessed from an economic and climatic point of view (Subramaniam and Sambasiva Rao) and Marudachalam related economic levels with health status in his study of a rural region. Thus studies of planning for health facilities could be said to have emerged here for the first time as a major theme of research in medical geography in India. The studies stressed the need to take specific local aspects into consideration when planning health care in India. For example, Chauhan has illustrated the ecological approach to health problems in a desert environment. Finally, it can be pointed out that in recent years, the overall health-care system has become a major political concern of both Government and news media. This is evident from the wide coverage of the maldistribution of health services in India (*Indian Express*, 19 March 1982).

Community and social medicine

Cultural factors and social customs influence not only the occurrence of diseases, as indicated by studies of the incidence of deficiency diseases, but also the acceptance of innovations like family planning methods. These are the aspects of community and social medicine which Fonaroff and Fonaroff (1966) studied in the cultural environment of rural India. Their work, though carried out on a nationwide scale, has laid a most useful foundation for localized and rigorous follow-up. Also at a national level Learmonth and Akthar (1972) have examined the effects of cultural patterns on health and disease following this up with a further study in the same field just over a decade later, but stressing how the health risk element posed by cultural conditioning may be controlled (Learmonth and Akthar, 1982b). Anthropologists and sociologists have stressed the importance of the beliefs and attitudes of people towards disease and sickness. Two examples illustrate this. Beliefs among tribal populations in India about malaria were studied by cultural anthropologists (Dhillon and Kar, 1977) and the human factors in hookworm transmission were analysed in a limited rural context (Kochar, 1978). Such contributions from other disciplines certainly had a seminal influence on geographers, with the work of Mathur and John (1974) on the role of beliefs as a factor in smallpox and other infectious disease in southern India as a prime example.

Family planning is a part of the nationwide health campaign, and the spatial aspects of its diffusion in India were well analysed by Bladen and Karan (1975). The fact that there is a geographical pattern of acceptance of family planning methods in India was demonstrated by Bladen (1976). A study of family planning acceptance and its dynamic trends in two time periods was also a subject of interest to Gupta (1981).

That the public should be made aware of environmental health problems was stressed in a study of public awareness in the Calcutta Metropolitan area (Karan, 1980). Vaccination in south Asia, c. 1700–1865 (Greenough, 1980) and the immunization status of pre-school children in urban areas (Tyagi, 1981) represent work in this field. The need to involve the community in solving health problems is well recognized and has been discussed in a regional context (Agarwal and Tumasi, 1981).

Most of the studies by medical geographers in the area of community and social medicine have been done on a macro-scale. Much scope exists for micro-level studies which could be used for planning and for understanding how to offer the most efficient health-care system for a particular population recognizing their social habits and their awareness of health and sickness.

Sources of health-care data and mapping techniques

This is a neglected area of medical geography. New cartographic techniques and analytical methods would elevate the position of medical geography in India, though not much work has been done so far by geographers. However, what there is undoubtedly has been influenced by Learmonth's pioneering work on mapping. Good examples exist in the use of statistics for reviewing the incidence of cholera (Patnaik and Kapoor, 1967), for a mortality study in Rajasthan (Tewari, 1973) and in a description of mortality registration in Orissa followed by a note on mortality regions of this state (Ahmed, 1974). A Health Hazard Index for planning purposes using many variables, including infant mortality and distance from any health centre, was devised by Mukherjee (1976) for a small planning block.

Malaria has been well mapped and the various statistics on malaria have been used at different levels by geographers. Maps of malaria in India (Christopher and Sinton, 1978), ways in which a Malaria Parasite Index may be devised (Learmonth and Akthar, 1979b), and probabilities in the malaria cycle using a graphic approach (Learmonth and Hunt, 1980) exemplify the wide popularity of mapping the data of this disease. Ranking the intensity of the distribution of the disease in Tehri, Uttar Pradesh (Sharma, 1978), and the analysis of incidence of filariasis in Nagpur (Jain, 1980), represent some other works by geographers.

Most geographers in India (with a few exceptions) have used similar mapping techniques to show the incidence or mortality rates of a disease but have not devised any models or used sophisticated computer analyses. The major drawback is the non-availability, lack of standardization and unreliability of data. The work of Learmonth and Akthar in the use of mapping methods requires special mention. Learmonth (1958) and Learmonth and Pal (1959) have not only devised isopleth maps to show both variability and incidence, but also maps to illustrate both intensity and variability of the incidence of disease simultaneously. The use of health statistics in India and methodologies to cope with their weaknesses were also outlined by Akthar (1980b).

Conclusion and prospects

No geographer has contributed to Indian medical geography as much as Learmonth. From his early study of mortality and patterns of disease in the sub-continent (1952), he has moved to his present interest in malaria resurgence. The overall result has been that the position and importance of medical geography in south Asia can now be reflected at international level and has been recognized in Dutta's special publication "Contemporary Perspectives on Medical Geography of South and Southeast Asia" (1980). Two books by Akthar on the geography of health—one on nutrition and agriculture (1982a) and the other a bibliography of sources in the Geography of Health in India (1982b)—are also evidence of the international standing and importance of the field in India today.

During the last ten years interest in medical geography has been gradually developing and has spread its influence from one centre to another from the northern universities such as Jaipur, Baroda, Calcutta, Delhi and Kolhapur to the southern corner of India. Here Madras University at present offers a fully-fledged course in medical geography at the postgraduate level. Several other universities are planning to follow suit, such as Bombay, Hyderabad and Bangalore. The IGU meeting at Delhi in 1968 can be considered as the take-off point for a greatly increased level of involvement in work in medical geography in India. The National Association of Geographers in India (NAGI) subsequently gave support to this field of study by establishing its own Commission on the Geography of Health with participation at an encouragingly high level at the later meetings of NAGI in 1979, 1980 and 1981. Similarly, postgraduate studies in the field have increased, with several doctoral dissertations on medical geography recently completed in India.

The IGU Working Group on the Geography of Health met for the first time in India at Madras in 1981 and so helped the many potential young workers who were able to be present, to identify with the field. It initiated a useful dialogue between medical geographers and other disciplines and gave to overseas visitors a glimpse of the work of Indian medical geographers. It also provided an informal setting for Indian medical geographers to get to know their foreign counterparts. Professor Learmonth's valedictory address at this conference impressed on Indian geographers his personal views about the fields of development which he saw as most promising. Clearly there is vast scope for research in medical geography in India and those topics worthy of study include especially, infectious diseases, health-care systerms, disease mapping, nutrition and geographical aspects of traditional Indian medicine in both urban and rural India.

Acknowledgements

My thanks are due to Dr B. Hyma, Miss G. Sucharita and Dr R. Akthar for their kind help with this essay.

References

Adams, A. (1889). *The Western Rajputana States: A Medicotopographical and General Account of Marwar, Sirohi and Jaisalmer.* London.

Agarwal, and Tumasi, P. A. (1981). Community involvement in solving health problems. *Social Science and Medicine* **15A**.

Ahmed, Z. (1973). Geography of deaths in Orissa: some spatial patterns, trends and correlates of mortality. *Geographical Observer* **9**, 73–86.

Ahmed, Z. (1974). Mortality registration in Orissa. *Geographical Observer* **10**, 86–92.

Akthar, R. (1978a). Spatial distribution and growth of health facilities in Rajasthan. *Geographical Review of India* **40**, 3, 206–217.

Akthar, R. (1978b). Goitre zonation in the Kumaon region: A geo-medical study. *Social Science and Medicine* **12**, 157.

Akthar, R. (1979a). Environmental factors and health in India. *Philippine Geographical Journal* **23**, 3, 109–114.

Akthar, R. (1979b). Colonization and its impact on the incidence of Malaria in the Terai Region of Uttar Pradesh. Occasional Paper, 27. Centre for the Study of Regional Development, Jawaharlal Nehru University, New Delhi.

Akthar, R. (1980a). Geography of cancer in India. *Medecine-Biologie-Environment* (Belgium) **6.2**, 20–30.

Akthar, R. (1980b). Health Statistics in India: A methodological approach. Abstract of papers, National Association of Geographers—First Annual Conference, Chandigarh, Jan. 1980, **13**.

Akthar, R. (1982a). *Environment, Agriculture and Nutrition in Kumaon Region.* Marwar Publications, New Delhi.

Akthar, R. (1982b). *Bibliography of Sources in the Geography of Health in India.* Marwar Publications, New Delhi.

Akthar, R. (1982c). Geographical distribution of cancer in India with special reference to stomach cancer. *International Journal of Environmental Studies* (in press).

Akthar, R. and Izhar, N. (1981). Health Care Delivery in India. Proceedings of the IGU Working Group on the Geography of Health, Madras, 1–4 December.

Alvarado, C. A. (1962). Malaria eradication. *Health* **40**, 7, 164.

Alvi, Z. (1974). Agricultural Land Use and Nutritional Deficiency Diseases in Allahabad and Fatehpur Districts. Unpublished Ph.D. thesis.

Anantaraman, M. (1981). Is Bilharziasis likely to Establish itself in India? Proceedings of the IGU Working Group on the Geography of Health, Madras, 1–4 December.

Ayyar, N. P. (1968). Land Use and Nutrition in Bewas Basin, M.P., India. *Geographer* **15**.

Azariah, J., Sekhar, S. R. and Hilda, A. (1981). Potential Health Risks due to the High Incidence of Faecal Coliform Bacteria in the River Cooum, Madras. Proceedings of the IGU Working Group on the Geography of Health, Madras, 1–4 December.

Barai, D., Hyma, B. and Ramesh, A. (1981). The scope and limitations of insecticide spraying in rural vector control programmes in the states of Karnataka and Tamilnadu. Proceedings of the IGU Working Group on the Geography of Health, Madras, 1–4 December.

Banerjee, A. C. (1951). Note on cholera in the United Province. *Indian Journal of Medical Research* **39**.

Banerjee, B. and Hazra, J. (1974). *Geoecology of Cholera in West Bengal: A Study in Medical Geography.* Bagchi and Co., Calcutta.

Banerjee, D. (1981). The place of indigenous and Western systems of medicine in the health services of India. *Social Science and Medicine* **15A**.

Basu, R. (1969). Cholera in Calcutta—A case study in medical geography. *Geographical Review of India* **31**, 3, 1–12.

Begum, N. and Vembu, D. (1981). The Temporal and Spatial Incidence of Malaria in Madras City Neighbourhood. Proceedings of the IGU Working Group on the Geography of Health, Madras, 1–4 December.

Bhatia, M. L., Prakash, S. and Ramakrishnan, S. P. (1957). Malaria vectors and some epidemiological features of Rajasthan. *Bulletin of the National Society of India for Malaria and Mosquito-borne diseases* **5**, 2, 100–109.

Bhatnagar Sakuntala (1981). Integrated Child Development Scheme: A Coordinated Approach to Children's Health Care. Proceedings of the IGU Working Group on the Geography of Health, Madras, 1–4 December.

Bishit, L. S. (1981). Moradabad City—A Geographical Study in Tuberculosis Disease. NAGI 2nd Annual Conference, Tirupathi.

Bladen, W. A. (1976). Geographical patterns of acceptance of family planning methods in India. *The National Geographical Journal of India* **22**, 1 and 2, 25–42.

Bladen, W. A. and Karan, P. P. (1975). Spatial aspects of the diffusion of family planning methods in India. *The National Geographical Journal of India* **21**, 1, 1–5.

Borker, K. (1957). *Health in Independent India*. Ministry of Health, New Delhi.

Chakrabarti, N. (1954). Some factors influencing the mortality of cholera. *Calcutta Medical Journal* **51**.

Chauhan, B. S. (1981). Desert Medicine. Ecological Approach to Health Problems. Proceedings of the IGU Working Group on the Geography of Health, Madras, 1–4 December.

Chevers, N., McClelland, J. and MacNamara, F. N. (1886). *Diseases of India*. London.

Chopra, R. N., Chopra, G. S. and Chopra, I. C. (1942). Cannabis sativa in relation to mental diseases and crime in India. *Indian Journal of Medical Research* **30**, 155–171.

Choubey, K. (1981). Health care in Madhya Pradesh. Proceedings of the IGU Working Group on the Geography of Health, Madras, 1–4 December.

Chouridule (1973). Some aspects of nutrition and deficiency diseases in the Basin. *Journal of North East India Geog. Soc.* **5**, 57–65.

Christopher, S. P. and Sinton, J. A. A. (1978). A malaria map of India. *Indian Journal of Medical Research* **9**, 173.

Covell, G. (1955). Developments in malaria control methods during the past forty years. *Indian Journal of Malariology* **9**, 4, 305–312.

Dhillon, H. S. and Kar, S. B. (1977). Malaria eradication and investigation of cultural patterns and beliefs among tribal populations in India. *International Journal of Health Education* **8**, 5.

Dutta, A. D. (Ed.) (1980). Contemporary perspectives on the medical geography of South and Southeast Asia. *Social Science and Medicine* **14D**, 3.

Dutta, A. and Dutta, H. M. (1981). Disease Dynamics on South and Southeast Asia with Special Reference to India. Proceedings of the IGU Working Group on the Geography of Health, Madras, 1–4 December.

Dutta, A. D., Akthar, R. and Dutta, M. (1980). Malaria in India with particular reference to two east-central states. *Social Sciences and Medicine* (Ed. A. K. Dutta) **14D**, 317–330.

Dutta, M. K. (1973). The diffusion and ecology of cholera in India. *Geographical Review of India* **35**, 5, 248–269.

Dutta, P. C. (1955). *Rural Health and Medical Care in India*. Army Educational Press, Ambala.

Farooqi, M. Y. and Khan, Z. A. (1977). Daily diet and deficiency diseases in the villages of Ganga-Yamuna Doab. *The Geographer* **19**, 32–52.

Fonaroff, S. L. and Fonaroff, A. (1966). The cultural environment of medical geography in rural India. *Pacific Viewpoint* **7**, 1, 67–68.

Gangulee, N. (1938). *Health and Nutrition in India*. Faber and Faber, London.

Gault, E. W. (1955). Geographic distribution of carcinoma with special reference to South India. *Schwerz Ztschr. Allg. Path.* **18**, 732–749.

Geddes, A. (1951). Commission on medical geography. *Geographical Review of India* **13**, 1.

George, A. J. and Webster, W. J. (1934). Plague inquiry in the Cumbum Valley, South India. *Indian Journal of Medical Research* **22**, 77–104.

Gopalan, C. (Ed.) (1969). *Diet Atlas of India*. National Institute of Nutrition ICMR, Hyderabad, India.

Greenough, P. R. (1980). Variolation and vaccination in South Asia, c. 1700–1865: A preliminary note. *Social Science and Medicine* **14D**, 3, 345–347.

Gupta, N. L. (1981). A Changing Profile of Medical Termination of Pregnancy (M.T.P.) Acceptors—A Comparative Study of the Years 1977–78 and 1979–80. Third Indian Geography Congress, New Delhi.

Hamoston, I. (1905). *Some Aspects of the General and Medical Topography of Ajmeer.* Rajputana Printing Press, Jaipur.

Hesterlow, A. V. M. (1929). The geographical distribution of disease. *The Journal of the Madras Geographical Association* **4**, 3, 81–97.

Hesterlow, A. V. M. (1930). Public health in Coimbatore District. *Journal of Madras Geographical Association* **5**, 2 and 3, 134–149.

Hesterlow, A. V. M. (1931–32). Public health of Malabar. *Journal of Madras Geographical Association* **6**, 3 and 4, 179–184.

Hussain, S. S. (1968). Nutritional Deficiency Diseases in Budann and Shahjehanpur Districts, India. IGU Working Group on Medical Geography, New Delhi.

Hussain, S. S. (1969). Landuse and nutrition in Saharahpur District. *Geographical Review of India* **31**, 3, 26–37.

Hyma, B. and Ramesh, A. (1976). Geographic distribution and trends in cholera incidence. *Indian Geographical Journal* **51**, 1, 1–33.

Hyma, B. and Ramesh, A. (1977). Cholera and Malaria Incidence in Tamilnadu, India. *Department of Geography, Publication Series* **9**. University of Waterloo, Canada.

Hyma, B. and Ramesh, A. (1980). The reappearance of malaria in Sathanur Reservoir and environs: Tamilnadu. *Social Science and Medicine* **14D**, 337–344.

Hyma, B. and Ramesh, A. (1981). Traditional Indian medical systems as a field study for Indian medical geographers. *Geographica medica* **11**.

Hyma, B., Ramesh, A. and Barai, D. C. (1981). The Reappearance of Malaria in Tamilnadu and Karnataka: A Comparative Study. *National Association of Geographers India*, 2nd Annual Conference, Tirupathi, Jan. 1981.

Indian Express (1982). 19 March.

Indrapal (1956). Cancer in Home Corners. Mimeographed paper presented at International Geographic Conference, Aligarh Muslim University, Nainital.

Indrapal (1968). The Yellow Water Zone of Bijanore, Nainital and Moradabad District in Uttar Pradesh. IGU 1968, New Delhi.

Indrapal (1970). Geographical Distribution of Trachoma in Rajasthan, India. Abstract of papers given at the Twenty-First International Geographical Congress, Calcutta.

Indrapal (1972). Cancer in India and Abroad. Twenty-Second IGU Commission on Medical Geography, Guelph, Canada.

Indrapal and Mathur, H. S. (1970). Ecology of the Helminthic Disease in Rajasthan. Selected Papers, Twenty-First International Geographical Congress, Calcutta, pp. 400–403.

Indrapal and Mathur, H. S. (1981). Geogenic factors of Eye Disease in Rajasthan. Proceedings of the IGU Working Group on the Geography of Health, Madras, 1–4 December.

Iyengar, M. C. F. (1930–1931). Jungle in relation to malaria in Bengal. *Indian Journal of Medical Research* **18**, 259.

Jain, N. G. (1980). Mortality patterns and trends in filaria incidence in Nagpur City: A geographic analysis. *Transactions of Institute of Indian Geographers* **2**, 2, 101–108.

Jayachandran, S. T. (1981). Perspectives in the Planning of Health Care Facilities. A Study of Maternity and Child Welfare Centres in Dharmapuri District. Proceedings of the IGU Working Group on the Geography of Health, Madras, 1–4 December.

Job, A. S. (1981). Educational and Medical Facilities of Rural Settlements in Upper Bhima River Basin. Third Indian Geographical Congress, New Delhi.

Joshi, M. J. and Deshpande, C. D. (1972). Geographical distribution of some diseases common in southern Asia. *Geographica Medica* 3, 5–29.

Jusatz, H. J. (1968). Geo-Ecological Problems of Cholera. IGU, New Delhi.

Jusatz, H. J. (1975). The present distribution of dengue haemorrhagic fever in South Asia. *Applied Sciences and Development* 6, 119–126.

Jyssawalla, D. K. (1976). The problem of cancer in India: An epidemiological assessment from cancer in Asia. *Takashi Hirayama Research, Tokyo* 18, 265–173.

Kamarkar, P. R. and Pagnis, R. B. (1981). Health Care Systems in India. Case Study of Primary Health Centres of the Two Tahsils in Poona District (Maharashtra). Proceedings of the IGU Working Group on the Geography of Health, Madras, 1–4 December.

Kendrick, W. H. (1919). Malaria and rice cultivation. *Indian Journal of Medicine*. Proceedings of the Third All India Sanitary Conference, Lucknow, Calcutta.

Kapali, V. (1981). Changing Trends in Cholera Control in Tamilnadu with Special Reference to the Geographical Features. Proceedings of the IGU Working Group on the Geography of Health, Madras, 1–4 December.

Kara, P. K. (1981). Evaluation of Family Welfare Programmes. A Case Study of Themra P.H.C. of Sambalpur District of Orissa. Proceedings of the IGU Working Party on the Geography of Health, Madras, 1–4 December.

Karan, P. P. (1980). Public awareness of environmental problems in Calcutta metropolitan area. *National Geographical Journal of India* 26, 1 and 2, 29–34.

Karennavar, M. F. (1981). Leprosy Institutions in Karnataka State. Proceedings of the IGU Working Party on the Geography of Health, Madras, 1–4 December.

Kayastha, S. L. and Ram, B. (1981). The Importance of Water Supply to Rural Communities and Related Problems: An Environmental Assessment with Special Reference to Varanasi District. Third Indian Geography Congress. National Association of Geographers, New Delhi, India.

Khan, A. H. (1969). Food production and nutrition in Rohilkhand. *The Geographer* 16, 41–45.

Khan, S. A. (1968). Deficiency Diseases in Central Ganga-Yamuna Doab, India. IGU, New Delhi.

Kochar, V. (1978). Human factors in hookworm transmission in the rural West Bengal region. *Indian Journal of Preventive and Social Medicine* 9, 3, 97–124.

Krishnamachari, K. (1974). Endemic goitre in Maharashtra India. *Tropical and Geographical Medicine* 26, 147–151.

Kumar, V. L. (1980). Environmental pollution and human health: A geographical study of Kanpur City. *National Geographical Journal of India* 126, I and II, 60–69.

Kumaran, T. V. and Jeyapal, P. (1981). Health Facility Use and Locational Efficiency in a Madras Neighbourhood. Proceedings of the IGU Working Group on the Geography of Health, Madras, 1–4 December.

Kumaraswamy, K. (1981a). Cholera in Madras City—A Space Time Analysis. National Association of Geographers India. 2nd Annual Conference, Tirupathi.

Kumaraswamy, K. (1981b). Patterns of Cholera Incidence in Madras City. Proceedings of the IGU Working Group on the Geography of Health, Madras, 1–4 December.

Kumaraswamy, K. (1981c). Persistence of Tuberculosis in Madras City. Third Indian Geography Congress, National Association of Geographers, New Delhi, India.

Learmonth, A. T. A. (1952). Regional Differences in Natality and Mortality in India and Pakistan. Proceedings of the 8th General Assembly and 15th International Congress of the IGU, Washington.

Learmonth, A. T. A. (1956). A map of calories and proteins in poor Indian diet. *National Geographical Journal of India* **2**, 4.

Learmonth, A. T. A. (1957). Some contrasts in regional geography of malaria in India and Pakistan. *Transactions of Institute of British Geographers* **23**, 37–59.

Learmonth, A. T. A. (1958). Medical geography in Indo-Pakistan—A study of twenty years' data for the former British India. *The Indian Geographical Journal* **33**, 1–59.

Learmonth, A. T. A. and Akthar, R. (1972). Cultural patterns and health and disease in India. In *India: Cultural Patterns and Processes* (Eds A. G. Noble and A. L. Dutta), pp. 287–299. Westview Press, Boulder, Colorado.

Learmonth, A. T. A. and Akthar, R. (1979a). India's malaria resurgence, 1965–1978. *Geography* **64/3**, 221–223.

Learmonth, A. T. A. and Akthar, R. (1979b). Malaria Annual Parasite Index Maps of India by Malaria Control Unit Areas, 1965–1976. Faculty Research Paper No. 3, Open University, Milton Keynes.

Learmonth, A. T. A. and Hunt, J. (1980). Probabilities in the malaria cycle: A graphic presentation. *Geographica Medica* **3–11**.

Learmonth, A. T. A. and Pal, M. N. (1959). A method of plotting the variables such as mean incidence and variability from year to year on the same map, using isopleths. *Erdkunde* **13**, 145–150.

McClelland, J. (1859). *Sketch of Medical Topography and Climate on Soils of Bengal and North West Provinces*. London.

MacNamara, F. N. (1880). *Climate and Topography in Relation to Distribution of the Himalayan and Sub-Himalayan Districts of British India*. London.

Mahadev, P. D. and Thangamani, K. (1981). Policy Issues and Implications in Delivering the Rural Health Services. Third Indian Geography Congress, National Association of Geographers. New Delhi, India.

Marudachalam, V. M. (1981). Economic Development and Health Status in Rural Tamilnadu. The Case of Sriperumpudur Block. Proceedings of the IGU Working Group on the Geography of Health, Madras, 1–4 December.

Mathur, H. S. (1981). Spatial Distribution and the Possible Geogenic Causes of Blood Cancer in Rajasthan. Proceedings of the IGU Working Group on the Geography of Health, Madras, 1–4 December.

Mathur, R. K. and John, T. J. (1974). Population belief about smallpox and other common infectious diseases in South India. *Tropical Geography and Medicine* **25**, 190–196.

May, J. M. and Walsh, S. (1951). Medical geography: A programme of studies of the American Geographical Society. *Indian Geographical Journal* **26**, 6.

Mukerjee, A. B. (1980). The disease ecology of a small cul de sac: Chandigarh Dun. *Social Science and Medicine* **14D**, 3, 331–337.

Mukherjee, B. N. (1976). A simple method of containing health hazard index and its application in micro-regional health planning (India). *Regional Studies* **10**, 1, 105–123.

Nair, C. P. and Samnotra, K. A. (1969). A note on urban malaria in Broch Town, Gujarat State, India. *Tropical Diseases Bulletin* **56**, 5, 384.

Nityanandan Pillai, P. K. (1941). Public Health and its relation to environment. *Indian Geographical Journal* **10**, 16, 4.

Orr, I. M. (1933). Oral cancer in Betel-Nut-Chewers in Travancore. *Lancet* **ii**, 575–580.

Pandurkar, R. G. (1981). Spatial Distribution of some Diseases in Maharashtra—A Study in Medical Geography. Unpublished Ph.D. dissertation, Kolhapur.

Parthasarathy, B. and Dhar, O. N. (1974). A study of human comfort at a few stations in India. *The National Geographical Journal of India* **20**, 4, 216–222.

Patnaik, K. C. and Kapoor, P. N. (1967). Statistical Review of the Cholera Problem in India. Directorate General of Health Services, Ministry of Health and Family Planning, New Delhi.

Prasad, S. R. (1981). Spatial and Temporal Variables in the Incidence of Malaria in Orissa. National Association of Geographers India, 2nd Annual Conference, Tirupathi.

Qureshi, A. (1976). Food habits and deficiency diseases in the districts of Agra and Mathura. *The Geographer* **23**, 15–26.

Qureshi, A. (1979–80). Nutritional deficiency diseases in the districts of Agra and Mathura. *Geographical Outlook* **15**, 107–115.

Rahman, M. (1981). Patterns of Spatial Distribution of Certain Diseases in the Brahmaputra Valley: A Study in Medical Geography. Unpublished Ph.D. thesis. University of Gauhati.

Ramachandra, L. S. (1937). Public health of Kumbakonam. *Journal of Madras Geographical Association* **12**, 3 and 4, 146–149.

Ramesh, C. (1981). Spatial Organization of Health Facilities in Bulandshahar District of Uttar Pradesh. Abstract of papers NAGI: First Annual Conference, Chandigarh, 107–108.

Rao, T. R. (1930). Malaria in Madras Presidency. *Records of Malaria Survey of India* **1**, 4.

Rogers, L. (1928). The incidence and spread of cholera in India, forecasting and control of epidemics. *Indian Medical Research Memoirs* **9**.

Rogers, L. (1944). Cholera incidence in India in relation to rainfall, absolute humidity and pilgrimages: Innoculation of pilgrims as a preventive measure. *Transactions of the Royal Society of Tropical Medicine and Hygiene* **38**.

Russel, A. J. and Sundarrajan, E. R. (1928). The epidemiology of cholera in India. *Indian Medical Research Memoir* **12**.

Russell, P. F. and Ramachandra Rao, T. (1940). On habitat and association of species of Anophelina larvae in south-eastern Madras. *Journal of the Malaria Institute of India* **3**, 153–170.

Sarma, S. N. (1958). A study into the incidence and ecology of cancer of Laynix and adjacent parts in Assam. *Indian Journal of Medical Research* **46**, 525–533.

Sen, U. (1957). Distribution of cholera on the soil of West Bengal. *Geographical Review of India* **19**, 45–46.

Shafi, M. (1967). Food production efficiency and nutrition in India. *The Geographer* **14**, 23–27.

Shafi, M. (1979). Food consumption and nutritional requirements in the Islamic World. *The Geographer* **26**.

Shanmuganandan, S. (1981). The spatial patterns of distribution of ABO blood groups in India. Proceedings of the IGU Working Party on the Geography of Health, Madras, 1–4 December.

Sharma, J. P. (1978). Incidence, ranking and intensity of major diseases in District Tehri, Uttar Pradesh. *Geographical Review of India* **33**, 1, 37–49.

Shinde, S. D. (1980). A note on medical facilities in Maharashtra. In *Recent Trends and Concepts in Geography* (Eds R. B. Mandal and V. N. P. Sinha), pp. 313–319. Concepts Publishing Company, Delhi.

Shivaramayya, Y. (1938). Public health in Mangalore. *Journal of Madras Geographical Association* **XIII**, 3.

Siddiqi, M. F. (1966). Calorific value of food in rural Uttar Pradesh. *Man in India* **46**, 359–362.

Siddiqi, M. F. (1968). Studies on calorific consumption in the village of Kishanpur, Bundel Khand. *Man in India* **48**, 359–362.

Siddiqi, M. F. (1972). Deficiency disease combination in Uttar Pradesh. *Geographical Review of India* **34**, 4, 386–391.

Siddiqi, N. A. (1971–1972). Landuse and nutrition in the Central Ganga-Ghaghara Doab. *Geographical Outlook* **7**, 97–106.

Singh, A. and Singh, B. V. (1981). The Ecology of Tuberculosis Disease—A Study in Medical Geography. Proceedings of the IGU Working Party on the Geography of Health, Madras, 1–4 December.

Singh, B. B. (1968). The availability of calories for food in the village Baraut, District Meerut. *The Geographical Observer* **4**, 60.

Singh, B. V. and Singh, A. (1980). Environmental and Socio-economic Factors Influencing Spread of Cholera in the Lower Chambal Basin. Abstract of Papers, NAGI: First Annual Conference, Chandigarh, 103.

Singh, J. (1971). Optimum carrying capacity of land, caloric density and intensity of population pressure changes in Punjab, 1957–60. *National Geographical Journal of India* **17**, 31–49.

Singh, R. (1981a). Moradabad City—A Study of Environmental Pollution and Human Diseases. Third Indian Geography Conference, NAGI, New Delhi.

Singh, R. (1981b). Agra City—A Study of the Health of Shoeworkers. Third Indian Geography Congress, National Association of Geographers, India. New Delhi.

Singh, S. and Dutta, H. M. (1981). Smallpox patterns and its correlates. *GeoJournal* **5**, 1, 77–78.

Strassburger, E. (1973). Problems of health care in South Indian State. *International Development Review* **15**, 4, 22–26.

Subrahmanyan, V. P. and Sarma, A. A. L. (1981). A Climatic Study of Human Comfort Zones in South India. Proceedings of the IGU Working Group on the Geography of Health, Madras, 1–4 December.

Subramaniam, A. R. and Sambasiva Rao, A. (1981). Eco-Climatic Perspectives of Health Resorts in Maharashtra. Proceedings of the IGU Working Group on the Geography of Health, Madras, 1–4 December.

Subramanian, A. R. and Seshami, T. (1981). Effects of Some Climatic Aspects on the Human Body in India. Proceedings of the IGU Working Group on the Geography of Health, Madras, 1–4 December.

Subramanyam, H. (1955). Malaria control in Lower Bhavani Project Headwork, Coimbatore District, Madras State. *Indian Journal of Malariology* **9**, 131.

Sukhdev, S. C. (1981). Health Facilities in Kinnaur. A Study in Medical Geography (a case study of a tribal area). NAGI 2nd Annual Conference, Jan. 1981. Tirupathi.

Swaroop, S. (1951). Endemicity of cholera in India. *Indian Journal of Medical Research* **39**, 2 April, 185–196.

Tewari, A. K. (1968). Incidence and Ecology of Guineaworm Disease in Rajasthan, India. IGU, New Delhi.

Tewari, A. K. (1973). Geomedical methods and its applications in the study of medical geography of Rajasthan. *Rajasthan Medical Journal* **12**, 181–190.

Tyagi, R. C. (1981). An Enquiry into the Immunisation. Status of Pre-School Children in an Urban Environment—A Case Study of Hapur. NAGI: 3rd Indian Geography Congress, New Delhi.

Wahi, P. N., Lahiri, B. and Khar, U. (1966). Epidemiology of oral and oropharyngeal cancer: A study of regional factors in Uttar Pradesh. *Journal of Indian Medical Association* **46**, 171–181.

Whyte, R. O. (1968). Ecology of Protein Malnutrition in Monsoon Asia. IGU, New Delhi.

Whyte, R. O. (1974). *Rural Nutrition in Monsoon Asia*. Oxford University Press, Oxford.

Medical geography in Tropical Africa

R. Mansell Prothero

Department of Geography, University of Liverpool, England

Early contributions

It is difficult to identify with any degree of certainty the first contribution by a geographer to the study of medical geography in Tropical Africa. Certainly Gourou in *Les Pays Tropicaux*, first published in 1948, was concerned for the *insalubrité* of tropical lands, echoing in more general terms the specific attention which he had given to this in his works on the Tonkin delta (1936), Indochina (1940) and the Far East (1941). Gallais (1981) in a recent review of Gourou's work writes

> Un autre trait d'époque, dont il est bien regrettable qu'il ne soit pas encore de la nôtre, est l'interêt pour la géographie médicale et les conditions sanitaires. 12 pages sur le paludisme parmi les facteurs de la répartition de la population dans *L'Utilisation du sol.* . . . La réchèrche sur les grandes endemies tropicales prend son essor, à cette époque et ce souci se poursuivra dans les œuvres ultérieures de Pierre Gourou qui utilisera et interpretera avec soin et constance les progrés de la réchèrche médicale sous les Tropiques (pp. 131–132).

> [Another feature of that time, which unfortunately is not yet one of our own time, is the interest in medical geography and sanitary conditions. 12 pages on malaria as one of the factors in the distribution of the population in *The Utilisation of the Soil.* . . . Research into the great tropical endemic diseases advanced by leaps and bounds at this time and this preoccupation was continued in the later works of Pierre Gourou who carefully and steadfastly used and interpreted the progress made by medical research in the Tropics.]

Gourou's contributions were of a general nature and relatively deterministic in their interpretation of the association between geographical and medical factors. He was concerned more with the influence of the latter on the former—for example, the influence of malaria on the distribution of population—than with the way that many medical problems have important geographical perspectives to which geographers may effectively contribute.

GEOGRAPHICAL ASPECTS OF HEALTH
ISBN 0 12 483780 8

Though the work of Andrew Learmonth is associated particularly with the sub-continent of India, one of his earlier contributions is among the first of the forays made by geographers into medical problems in tropical Africa. In what is likely to be one of his least-known papers, in a volume of essays in memory of Professor A. G. Ogilvie of Edinburgh, Learmonth (1959) wrote on "Geography and health in the tropical forest zone". In this essay he was concerned to examine

> . . . some aspects of human health in communities in close contact either with the tropical rain forest proper or with other forest associations in the tropical zone.

It was based on the belief that

> Changing ecological patterns of health and disease developing because of these increased contacts between man and the forest are of geographical significance.

The paper reflects very clearly the ecological approach to medical geography which has characterized so much of Learmonth's work. It drew widely upon evidence for different diseases for different parts of the tropics, including trypanosomiasis in the Gambia and loiasis, a form of filariasis, in the south of the then British Cameroons. Sources of information for these two diseases were the research of medical workers, both doctors and medical entomologists. Commenting on one of these sources—on trypanosomiasis in the Gambia (Hutchinson, 1953)—in a later review of ecological medical geography, Learmonth (1975) comments that it

> . . . is really ecological human geography for it analyses the areal prevalence of trypanosomiasis in terms of man–tsetse contacts seen as daily or seasonal patterns of life and work. This includes male and female labour in particular sorts of fields, times and places of bathing and so on, while keeping in mind whether man and tsetse were, as it were, forced together for common needs for shade and water, or whether the fly can disperse widely in forest country and quite probably bite a jungle animal instead of infecting man with the trypanosome.

This approach differs from that of Gourou in being much more specific and more concerned with the influence of human activities on medical problems. It was an approach practised by a significant number of medical workers in Africa in the 1930s and 1940s, without doubt sound medical geography, though without any input from geographers and probably without much direct influence from geography. Geographers of any kind were then thin on the ground in tropical Africa and it is doubtful if there were any who were working in the field with the same degree of detail as were Hutchinson and others. This work of medical men is clearly needful of attention in this review of medical geography in tropical Africa.

Medical scientists and medical geography

From the early decades of this century a number of outstanding individuals, associated with the colonial medical services, were making
distinguished geographical contributions to the better understanding
and solution of problems with which they were confronted in Tropical
Africa. It is possible to do no more than sample from their work in an
unsystematic but reasonably representative fashion.

Among the many problems faced in attempting to improve and maintain health with limited resources, those associated with sleeping sickness received major attention. At the time of the consolidation of colonial
administrations, and the introduction of medical and other services, in
the last years of the nineteenth century and the early decades of the
twentieth century, the populations of great areas of tropical Africa were
swept by epidemics of sleeping sickness. The causes of these epidemics
have been investigated by Ford, a noted worker on sleeping sickness, in
The Role of the Trypanosomiases in African Ecology (Ford, 1971). They were
the result of major changes in ecological relationships consequent on
political, social and economic factors associated with European penetra-
tion and control of Africa (e.g. Deshler, 1960).

The epidemics were manifested in clearly apparent morbidity and
mortality and to these there was a ready response. The campaigns which
were launched to reduce sleeping sickness involved deliberate changes
being made in ecological conditions to reduce habitats favourable to the
breeding of the tsetse-fly vectors, with planned resettlement of population to remove people from tsetse-infested environments and the
creation of conditions in which tsetse-free environments could be maintained. This work was carried out by colonial medical and entomological
personnel such as Morris in the Gold Coast (Morris, 1951–1952) and later
in East Africa (Morris, 1960), Hutchinson in West Africa (Hutchinson,
1953, 1954), Duggan (1962) and Nash (1944, 1948) in Nigeria, and Ford and
Swynnerton in east and south-central Africa (e.g. Swynnerton, 1936;
Ford, 1960, 1969). The approach of Hutchinson has already been indicated; the work of any of the above might be used to illustrate their
appreciation of the holistic nature of the problems with which they were
confronted. That of Nash in northern Nigeria exemplifies this appreciation and is selected for its intrinsic value and because of its influence on
the author of this paper.

In the late 1930s and early 1940s Nash, a medical entomologist, played
a major part in establishing the Anchau "Corridor" in Zaria Province in
northern Nigeria. Sleeping sickness surveys in this area in the 1930s had
shown incidence rates of between 30 and 50 per cent in a population
living largely dispersed in small villages and hamlets. The Anchau

scheme was an integrated project relating health improvement to wider ranging rural development, ". . . the first large scale attempt at rural development to be made in British West Africa" (Nash, 1948). It involved the creation of a tsetse-free environment, necessitating the concentration of the previously dispersed population, with the movement into new settlements of about 10,000 people in such a way that they would be provided with adequate and suitable farmland and with supplies of water and of wood. The essence of the Anchau scheme was that it left little to chance. It was premised on the belief that satisfactory change would be effected only on the basis of planning from what was known and proceeding from this to determine what was needed.

> The scheme has been treated throughout as a scientific experiment. The preliminary investigations necessitated an ecological study of the local Hausa peasant in relation to his environment. Europeans are far too prone to consider that their own methods are best and therefore must be intro-duced. When one studies native methods—the inherited wisdom of gener-ations—one finds how sound they are in many things, and how wrong are our preconceived ideas, based subconsciously on our European experience. (Nash, 1948)

The project team undertook a thorough survey of the existing con-ditions—ecological, demographic, social, economic and administrative. Population structure and characteristics were evaluated, land-use sur-veys were undertaken to calculate land needs, land capability for agricul-tural production was determined on the basis of vegetation indicators which were used by the Hausa people of the area. Water and fuel consumption were measured over a 12-month period so that allowance could be made for seasonal variations in needs. The result of all these investigations was a geographical survey *par excellence*. There have been few projects for development at any scale in tropical Africa before or since which have been based on such comprehensive knowledge. Nash's report was certainly an inspiration to a geographer beginning work in Nigeria in 1950.

Though the Anchau "Corridor" did not remain tsetse-free, and though subsequent anthropological work demonstrated that not all things essen-tial to its success had been taken into account, what is both remarkable and depressing is that similar comprehensive and integrated approaches were not adopted in respect of other medical problems in Tropical Africa in the 1950s and 1960s. None the less, it was in these two decades that geographers first became fully involved in studies of medical problems there. It followed the establishment of geography departments in univer-sity institutions which were set up in Tropical Africa after the Second World War.

Geographers as consultants in medical geography

In the 1950s, Tropical Africa shared with other malarious parts of the world, the euphoria associated with prospects for the global eradication of malaria within a limited time period (Macdonald, 1957). The required scientific and technical knowledge were available in the form of drugs and insecticides to be used in a concerted action against the malaria parasites and the anopheles mosquito vectors. The means were available for dealing with two of the three factors in the malaria complex as set out by May (1950) in his classic statements on medical geography. However, pilot projects and more extensive programmes for eradication soon revealed that these means could be successfully operated only if the third factor (rather a set of factors) could be dealt with satisfactorily. For the most part in tropical Africa this proved to be impossible. A great range of "human factors" militated against the successful use of the available drugs and insecticides. These factors were operational, logistic, administrative, political, social and economic; some of them could not have been foreseen, some although recognized were given insufficient attention, while others need not have presented major problems if they had been given sufficient forethought.

Despite recognition of their importance human factors in malaria in Tropical Africa were not accorded the attention that was given to parasites and vectors. In malaria eradication programmes parasites and vectors were studied by trained and experienced personnel, while human factors were left to be dealt with by personnel who were insufficiently equipped or had insufficient time (usually both) to cope with them adequately.

Through the initiative of Bruce-Chwatt* the author of this chapter worked as the first geographer consultant to the World Health Organization in 1960, to be followed by further consultancies in 1962 and 1970. Each of these was concerned particularly with problems arising from population movements which contributed to malaria transmission and prejudiced programmes planned for the control and eradication of the disease. They were also concerned with the influence of human factors in general. They were undertaken at progressively more detailed scales of consideration—for tropical Africa in 1960 (Prothero, 1961, 1962), for Morocco in 1962 (Prothero, 1964), and for a malaria eradication experimental project at Garki in Kano State, Nigeria in 1970 (Molineaux and

---

* Then Director of Research and Technical Intelligence for the Division of Maleria Eradication, WHO; formerly Senior Malariologist in Nigeria and subsequently Director of the Ross Institute, London School of Hygiene and Tropical Medicine.

Gramiccia, 1980). Each consultancy highlighted the problems associated with mobility and other human factors and the need to provide more adequately for dealing with them (e.g. Prothero, 1965, 1977). For the most part these are factors which cannot be eliminated for they are part of the essentials of human life. They therefore need to be better understood so that provision can be made for them in programme planning, through cross-sectional studies, though preferably through longer-term longitudinal investigation.

While these consultancies influenced the thinking of those involved in anti-malarial work and provided for greater geographical inputs in planning for this work, there is no doubt that the human factors in the malaria complex continue to be treated in a relatively Cinderella-like fashion. Indeed an offer made to provide an independent geographical input for the Garki project in Kano State in 1970 was declined on the grounds that it would be administratively difficult to accommodate!

Global malaria eradication has been shown to be impossible, and for many reasons progress in Tropical Africa has been more limited than in any other part of the world. These include resistance by parasites and vectors to drugs and insecticides respectively, technical and logistical difficulties, and political, social and economic problems. Over the years the reports of the WHO Expert Committee on Malaria have continued to acknowledge the significance of human factors, but this has been little more than lip-service to the need to tackle them. For example, at the end of 1972 when a WHO inter-regional conference discussed *Malaria Control in Countries where Time-limited Eradication is Impracticable at Present* (WHO, 1974), it recognized the socio-economic problems of anti-malaria programmes in Africa and suggested that feasibility, planning and operation activities should be undertaken by

> a team of specialised personnel comprising a medical officer (malariologist), an entomologist, an operations technical officer (sanitary engineer or a senior sanitarian) . . . and possibly assisted by a statistician.

The statistician seems to have been included almost as an afterthought and, with due respect, might be someone not competent to evaluate the socio-economic problems. The old story continues of expert experience available to deal with the parasite and vector aspects of a programme, but with the human host remaining largely unprovided for. In view of their unpredictability human factors should be given at least as much, if not more, attention as parasite and vector factors. Environmental influences (such as natural hazards), over which there is limited control, if any, may also operate in less developed parts of the world where major malaria hazards still remain.

The experience of working with the WHO in respect of malaria has been salutary, and not altogether disillusioning. Some useful input has been made. Furthermore, the experience of other geographers has demonstrated that the value of their contribution to the understanding of problems relating to other diseases has been appreciated. As a consultant in the planning of a major WHO/World Bank Onchocerciasis Control Programme, Hunter (1972) has extended his original work on the advance and retreat of settlement in north-east Ghana consequent on population pressure and on onchocerciasis (river blindness) respectively (Hunter, 1966, 1980). This very costly programme aims to eradicate the disease from the river valleys of northern Ghana, Upper Volta and the Ivory Coast. It is still in progress and involves not only the reduction of the disease through the elimination of the vector (the black fly, *simulium damnosum*), but also the planned resettlement and agricultural development of the valleys with supporting economic and social infrastructure (roads, wells, schools, health facilities).

The geographical work on onchocerciasis initiated by Hunter in north-east Ghana was extended by Bradley and developed in greater detail in the Hawal valley in north-east Nigeria. His study of the interrelationships between settlement, economy and onchocerciasis demonstrated the decline of settlement through depopulation and consequent loss of economic viability (Bradley, 1975, 1976). Bradley's work, like that of Hunter, provides a means for predicting future developments as well as providing explanatory analysis of what has happened, and was taken up and used by the World Health Organization.

All of this consultative work in medical geography emphasizes the importance of maintaining close links between geographers and medical colleagues, *to mutual advantage*. Without such close links it is possible for each to be naïve about matters in which the others have the necessary expertise. There is ample evidence that medical workers often operate at levels of generalization in matters geographical which they would abhor in matters medical, and no doubt the reverse is true. For example, Learmonth (1975) has drawn attention to the investigation of Burkitt's lymphoma (Burkitt, 1962) which suggested the possibility that this condition was associated with a mosquito-borne virus; this was subsequently shown by McGlashan (1969) and others to be an oversimplification, and was later refined in collaborative work by Burkitt and Cook, a geographer (Burkitt and Cook, 1970).

McGlashan worked for some time with the South African Institute for Medical Research and produced in the 1960s and 1970s a range of significant studies in medical geography relating to south-central Africa (e.g. McGlashan, 1968a, 1969, 1972a). These studies exemplify

McGlashan's views of the tasks and contributions of medical geography (McGlashan, 1966); they are integrative in their approach and have made methodological and technical contributions.

General studies in medical geography

The contributions so far considered have all involved direct contact in various ways between geographers and medical workers. For the most part they also represent the precursors of work in medical geography by geographers, which has developed on a much wider scale in Tropical Africa since 1970. It is not possible to detail all of this work and the examples given are representative. It may be categorized on the basis of the variety of scales at which it has been practised.

There have been a number of studies which range over the whole or the greater part of Tropical Africa. By far the most important and the most quoted in geographical, medical and other literature on development is the masterly overview by Hunter and an anthropologist colleague of the all-too-often neglected relationships between disease and development (Hughes and Hunter, 1970). Knight (1971) and Kloos and Thompson (1979), in article-length studies, have considered trypanosomiasis (both human and animal) and schistosomiasis respectively, utilizing a wide range of medical and other literature to draw out in the light of their own experience the major geographical factors and issues involved in these diseases, the ways in which they have been coped with and the prospects for dealing with them in the future.

Stock (1976) has brought together historical and contemporary material relevant to the study of the diffusion of cholera in Africa. The main thrust in this work is directed to the diffusion of cholera El Tor in the period 1970–1975 when it appeared in Africa for the first time for nearly a century. Using data from the *Weekly Epidemiological Report* of the World Health Organization, Stock investigated the diffusion of cholera in time and in space, with particular detail for West Africa to establish major systems of diffusion—coastal, riverine, urban, hierarchical and radial. While casting light on the processes of diffusion in greater detail than ever previously attempted (and to much greater effect than the study of cholera diffusion in West Africa by Kwofie (1976)) Stock also develops a predictive model which may be used for forecasting spread in future epidemic conditions.

There are a variety of works at the national scale. These include the *Atlas of Disease Distribution in Uganda* (Hall and Langlands, 1975), the only work of its kind in Africa and one of the few examples in the world. Two

Medizinische Landerkunde (Geomedical Monograph Series) sponsored by the Heidelberg Academy of Sciences, have appeared for countries in tropical Africa. The volume on Ethiopia (Schaller and Kuls, 1972), one of the earliest in the series, brings together a great deal of valuable information on the geography of health and disease, though in a largely encyclopaedic fashion. In contrast, one of the most recent volumes on Kenya (Diesfeld and Hecklau, 1978) provides a much more penetrating analysis and achieves a much greater integration of the medical and geographical data presented. It is without doubt the most successful of the monographs published. A further volume on Nigeria is in preparation but at present there is no foreseeable date for publication (Prothero, 1976).

At more detailed scales the studies undertaken range very widely. Some are essentially descriptive analyses, though not in any respect less important for this reason. An outstanding example is work of Roundy (1976) on the significance of altitudinal mobility for disease transmission and health status in Ethiopia, where there are such striking contrasts between the plateau at an average altitude of 2000 m above sea-level, the deeply-gouged river valleys which are cut into it and the lowlands which surround it. There is a variety of studies based on available data from health authorities and even more based on data generated by their authors. Examples of such work have been published in a recent issue of *GeoJournal* devoted to medical geography in Africa (Prothero, 1981) and in a special issue of *Rural Africana* (Roundy, 1981).

The study of local mobility and measles in a rural area of Kenya by Ferguson and Leuwenberg (1981) which appears in each of the above collections is a further example of a joint geographical/medical effort. At a smaller scale of consideration, Turner (1981) at the community level in Botswana and Rossington (1981) for individual children in Ibadan, Nigeria, have examined socio-economic factors affecting standards of nutrition. The latter extends work on seasonal variation in nutrition status pioneered by Hunter (1967) in northern Ghana; furthermore this study gained much from being set in a long-term longitudinal survey of children being carried out by the Institute of Child Health, University Hospital, Ibadan.

Almost all the studies so far considered have been undertaken by expatriates working in Africa. It is important, particularly for the future, to draw attention to the increasing volume of work in medical geography which is now beginning to come from African geographers. As yet the number is small and not all those working are identified here. In seeking contributions for the recent issue of *GeoJournal* there was no response from university geography departments in anglophone territories in East and south-central Africa, and only isolated and unpublished pieces of work have been undertaken in the University of Ghana (Disu, 1976; Iyun, 1978). The greatest output has come from Nigeria (e.g. Ajaegbu and Mann, 1975; Adesina, 1981), and particularly in recent years from geographers at the University of Calabar (e.g. Olu Sule, 1981; Uyanga, 1979, 1981). Research on population mobility and the diffusion of water-related diseases is planned for the immediate future, to involve the cooperative efforts of a Nigerian parasitolologist and an expatriate geographer, both working at the University of Ilorin in Kwara State (Edungbola and Watts, 1981). The latter is especially welcome in providing an example of close interdisciplinary links between medicine and geography, something which as yet has not been readily apparent in the work of African geographers.

Geographers and health care

The work discussed so far all falls under the broad heading of ecological medical geography. It includes the major contributions which have been made in this field in Tropical Africa by geographers and by medical scientists working with geographical perspectives. Concern for health-care provision and utilization has existed from the introduction of western-style services by the colonial authorities. Throughout, efforts have been directed to greater or lesser extent towards trying to match scarce resources with demands which are generally greater than the means to satisfy them. There is much evidence of the involvement of medical workers in determining ways and means of allocating scarce resources (King, 1972; Fendall, 1963), though the methodology they have employed has for the most part been of a relatively general and simplistic nature. For example, the determination of the catchment areas of health facilities has been based on crude linear distances to be travelled by potential users, with limited attention paid to constraints relating to seasonal accessibility, the availability and cost of transport, the inevitable incapacity of those seeking facilities, and the perceptions of facilities by potential users.

On the whole the larger urban places in Tropical Africa are better provided with health facilities to the detriment of rural areas. For example, Kano State, Nigeria, with a total population of over 6 million, was served in 1970 by 25 qualified doctors, of whom 21 were located in the metropolitan area of Kano city with a population of one million. Various measures have been introduced to redress such gross imbalance, of which the most important is the selection and training of paramedical personnel to serve the basic needs of the majority of the population who live in the rural areas (Newell, 1975). A major example of change in this direction has come with the reorganization of rural medical services in Tanzania, associated with the concentration of population through "villageization", thus making for the better provision of health and other social facilities (Van Etten, 1976).

Particular groups of people present special problems in making adequate social provisions available to them. Such problems are especially acute among nomadic pastoralists, whose continual mobility makes fixed health facilities of limited efficacy. The provision of mobile facilities to meet their needs has been considered in general terms for north-east Africa (Prothero, 1972). Mobile health facilities (Medical Field Units) serving sedentary as well as mobile populations were operated in northern Ghana several decades ago (Waddy, 1956). Such units can provide basic services only, though these are sufficient to serve everyday needs. Some measure of specialized attention for mobile people and for those living in inaccessible areas can be provided by a flying doctor service, such as that in Zambia which has been the subject of a geographical analysis (Jackman, 1972).

Studies by geographers of the availability and use of health services have, like studies in ecological medical geography, been carried out at a variety of scales. There have been country-wide analyses of hospital facilities in Zambia and in Malawi (McGlashan, 1968b, 1972b), the applications of techniques of locational analysis to achieve the optimal, least-travel cost location of facilities (Okafor, 1981), and in-depth field studies in limited areas over time (Stock, 1980).

Stock's work on health-care behaviour in Hadejia District, in the north-east of Kano State, Nigeria, is worthy of note for two reasons. It provides detailed analysis of field data recording the utilization of several categories of health facility (e.g. rural dispensary, rural health centre, district hospital) and examines the range of factors which influence their use. It also relates the use of these western-style health services to the availability and use of traditional health-care services which are available in a variety of forms (Good, 1977; Good et al, 1979; Stock, 1981). This integrated approach accords with contemporary thinking on the provision of medical services in developing countries in general and in tropical Africa in particular, to achieve a maximum satisfaction of need from limited available resources.

Future prospects

There is nothing to be gained from engaging in lengthy discussion as to whether the geography of health care is more important than ecological medical geography, or vice-versa. To this author this has always seemed to be fruitless and unnecessary in any part of the world. In tropical Africa to be so engaged would be wasteful of time and effort, since in each of these areas of concern there is so much to be done that all energy should be directed to tackling the many problems awaiting investigation.

Africa provides unbounded scope for the practice of medical geography whatever definitions are employed to denote its nature and purpose. Man and environment are closely linked in complex relationships which frequently present conditions of disequilibrium in which diseases flourish and health is impaired. These conditions are to be found not only in the rural areas where the majority of the population are at risk but also in the urban areas into which increasing numbers of people are being drawn.

The range of diseases encountered in Africa is particularly wide. It includes the classic diseases of the tropics and the sub-tropics—malaria, sleeping sickness, schistosomiasis, trachoma and yaws—involving not only the factors of the physical environment which favour them, but also the socio-economic factors which are of considerable influence. In addition there is now evidence in Africa for an increasing prevalence of diseases which previously seemed to figure largely in the more economically developed parts of the world—cancers, degenerative diseases of the circulatory system, tuberculosis and psychiatric disorders. Directly and indirectly associated with both the above groups of diseases are chronic and acute malnutrition which affect a very high proportion of people in Africa. Furthermore, it has been shown strikingly in the last decade in various parts of the continent that food shortages causing severe undernutrition may still occur.

All the above problems of disease and health have important geographical aspects, which are at least recognized, even if not always sufficiently, by members of the medical profession as well as by geographers. The work of geographers on geomedical problems in Tropical Africa has been inevitably limited to date by the relatively small numbers who have been involved. However, the varied nature of this involvement has been examined and exemplified in this chapter. All approaches by medical geographers to medical problems have important elements of description, in each there is analysis and interpretation; in all there is some degree of prescription, in some there are elements of prediction. They all make important contributions to the problems which they confront; these are contributions additional to what might be expected from the expertise and experience of those in the medical profession.

To this author it seems possible to be an effective medical geographer only with close reference to and relationship with medical colleagues. These do not diminish the function of the former, they simply emphasize the maximum return which can be achieved in an inter-disciplinary field through integrated effort, through the mutual exchange of skills based on recognition of the contributions that each discipline may make. Many medical geographers working in Africa have enjoyed these close relationships with medical colleagues. Every effort should be made to foster them in the future. We shall hope for more direct involvement like that of Bradley, whose research on river blindness has been cited. Subsequently he has worked as a medical geographer in an inter-disciplinary public health project in northern Nigeria carried out jointly by the Department of Community Health, Ahmadu Bello University and the Liverpool School of Tropical Medicine (see e.g. Bradley et al., 1977). He is now a member of the Medical Research Council Laboratory, Fajara, Gambia, which has been involved for more than 25 years in cross-sectional and longitudinal studies of health problems. Undoubtedly there are roles for medical geographers in the design and promotion of programmes for evaluating disease problems and for promoting public health. In broad context these contributions relate to the UNDP/World Bank/WHO Special Programme for Research and Training in Tropical Diseases which was set up in the last decade and in which there is a Working Group on Socio-Economic Research with geographical representation.

It may seem trite to say that all human diseases and all activities to promote the health of human beings involve seemingly disparate factors which are related to the physical and human environment in which they are set and of which they are part, but this is so (e.g. Prothero, 1968). It may seem even more trite to state that all these factors need to be given full attention, but it is a fact that such attention is frequently not given. Medical geography has contributed and may further contribute to what is lacking and what is needed in these respects. It is a field of study of long-standing, which has now come of age in Africa and elsewhere. We are as yet seeing only fragments of its potential contribution to the understanding and solution of contemporary problems and hopefully to the limitation and prevention of problems in the future. Medical geographers in tropical Africa as elsewhere, in what they have done and in the directions they may go, have inevitably been inspired and guided in their work to a varying extent by the example of Andrew Learmonth.

References

Adesina, H. O. (1981). A statistical analysis of cholera diffusion characteristics in Ibadan city 1971. *Social Science and Medicine* **15D**, 121–132.

Ajaegbu, H. I. and Mann, C. E. (1975). Human population and the disease factor in development in Nigeria. In *The Population Factor in African Studies* (Eds R. P. Moss and R. J. A. R. Rathbone), pp. 123–138. U.L.P., London.

Bradley, A. K. (1975). The effects of disease on rural economy, social structure and settlement: a case study of onchocerciasis in the Hawal Valley, Nigeria. Unpublished Ph.D. thesis, University of Liverpool.

Bradley, A. K. (1976). Effects of onchocerciasis on settlements in the Middle Hawal Valley, Nigeria. *Transactions Royal Society of Tropical Medicine and Hygiene* **70**, 225–229.

Bradley, A. K. (1981). Local perceptions of onchocerciasis in the Hawal Valley, Nigeria. In "Studies in medical geography in Africa" (Ed. R. M. Prothero), *GeoJournal* **5**, 357–362.

Bradley, A. K., Gilles, H. M. and Shehu, U. (1977). Malumfashi Endemic Disease Project, 1. Some ecological and demographic considerations. *Annals of Tropical Medicine and Parasitology* **71**, 443–449.

Burkitt, D. P. (1962). A children's cancer dependent on climatic factors. *Nature* **194**, 232–234; Can tumours be transmitted by insects? *Nature* **194**, 222–226.

Burkitt, D. P. and Cook, P. (1970). An epidemiological study of seven malignant tumours in East Africa. Mimeographed report, Medical Research Council, London.

Deshler, W. (1960). Livestock, trypanosomiasis and human settlement in north-eastern Uganda. *Geographical Review* **50**, 541–554.

Diesfeld, H. J. and Hecklau, H. K. (1978). *Kenya*. Geomedical Monograph Series 5. Heidelberg Academy of Sciences. Springer-Verlag, Berlin.

Disu, D. (1976). The spread of schistosoma haematobium (bilharzia) along the Afram and Pawmpawmaya areas of the Volta lake. Unpublished M.A. thesis, University of Ghana, Legon.

Duggan, A. J. (1962). A survey of sleeping sickness in northern Nigeria from the earliest times to the present day. *Transactions Royal Society Tropical Medicine and Hygiene* **56**, 439.

Edungbola, L. D. and Watts, S. (1981). Population mobility and the diffusion of water-related diseases in Kwara State, Nigeria. Unpublished research proposal, University of Ilorin, Nigeria.

Fendall, N. R. E. (1963). Health centres: a basis for a rural health service. *Journal Tropical Medicine and Hygiene* **66**, 219.

Ferguson, A. and Leuwenberg, J. (1981). Local mobility and the spatial dynamics of measles in a rural area of Kenya. In "Studies in medical geography in Africa" (Ed. R. M. Prothero). *GeoJournal* **5**, 315–332.

Ford, J. (1960). The advance of *Glossina morsitans* and *Glossina pallidipes* into the Sabi and Lundi River basins, Southern Rhodesia. Proceedings 8th Meeting International Scientific Commission on Trypanosomiasis. C.C.T.A. Publication No. 62, 219.

Ford, J. (1969). The control of the African trypanosomiases with special reference to land use. *Bulletin World Health Organization* **40**, 879.

Ford, J. (1971). *The Role of the Trypanosomiases in African Ecology*. Clarendon Press, Oxford.

Gallais, J. (1981). L'evolution de la pensée géographique de Pierre Gourou. *Annales de Géographie* **90**, 1290–150.

Good, C. M. (1977). Traditional medicine: an agenda for medical geography. *Social Science and Medicine* **11**, 705–713.

Good, C. M. et al. (1979). The interface of dual systems of health care in the developing world: toward health policy initiatives in Africa. Social Science and Medicine 13D, 141–154.

Gourou, P. (1936). Les Paysans du delta tonkinois. Editions d'Art et d'Histoire, Paris.

Gourou, P. (1940). L'utilisation du sol en Indochine française. Centre d'Etudes de Politique Etranger, Paris.

Gourou, P. (1941). La terre et l'homme en Extreme-Orient. Colin, Paris.

Gourou, P. (1948). Les pays tropicaux. Presses Universitaires de France, Paris.

Hall, S. A. and Langlands, B. W. (1975). Atlas of Disease Distribution in Uganda. East Africa Publishing House, Nairobi.

Hughes, C. C. and Hunter, J. M. (1970). Disease and development in Africa: the continuing need for an ecological appraisal. Social Science and Medicine 3, 443–493.

Hunter, J. M. (1966). River blindness in Nangodi, northern Ghana: a cyclical hypothesis of advance and retreat. Geographical Review 56, 398–416.

Hunter, J. M. (1967). Seasonal hunger in a part of the West African Savanna: a survey of bodyweights in Nangodi, north-east Ghana. Transactions Institute of British Geographers 41, 167–185.

Hunter, J. M. (1972). Geographical aspects of onchocerciasis control in northern Ghana. Report of a mission, June/August 1972. World Health Organization unpublished document. PAG Mission RAF/71/188-AFRO-2202.

Hunter, J. M. (1980). Strategies for the control of river blindness. In Conceptual and Methodological Issues in Medical Geography (Ed. M. S. Meade). Studies in Geography 15. Department of Geography, University of North Carolina at Chapel Hill.

Hunter, J. M. (1981). Progress and concerns in the World Health Organization onchocerciasis control programme in West Africa. Social Science and Medicine 15D, 261–275.

Hutchinson, M. P. (1953). The epidemiology of human trypanosomiasis in British West Africa. Annals Tropical Medicine and Parasitology 48, 75.

Iyun, B. F. (1978). Spatial analysis of health care delivery in Ibadan city. Unpublished Ph.D. thesis. University of Ghana, Legon.

Jackman, M. E. (1972). Flying doctor services in Zambia. In Medical Geography: Techniques and Field Studies (Ed. N. D. McGlashan), pp. 97–103. Methuen, London.

King, M. (1972). Medical Care in Developing Countries. OUP, Nairobi and Oxford.

Kloos, H. and Thompson, J. (1979). Schistosomiasis in Africa: an ecological perspective. Journal of Tropical Geography 48, 31–46.

Knight, C. G. (1971). The ecology of sleeping sickness in Africa. Annals Association of American Geographers 61, 23–44.

Kwofie, K. M. (1976). A spatio-temporal analysis of cholera diffusion in western Africa. Economic Geography 52, 127–135.

Learmonth, A. T. A. (1959). Geography and health in the tropical forest zone. In Geographical Essays in Memory of A. E. Ogilvie (Eds R. Miller and J. W. Watson), pp. 195–220. Nelson, London.

Learmonth, A. T. A. (1975). Ecological medical geography. Progress in Geography 7, 203–226.

Macdonald, G. (1957). Epidemiology and Control of Malaria. OUP, Oxford.

May, J. (1950). Medical geography: its methods and objectives. *Geographical Review* **40**, 9–41.

McGlashan, N. D. (1966). The medical geographer's work. *International Pathology* **7**, 81–83.

McGlashan, N. D. (1968a). The distribution of certain diseases in central Africa: an approach to medical geography in an underdeveloped country. Unpublished Ph.D. thesis, University of London.

McGlashan, N. D. (1968b). The distribution of population and medical facilities in Zambia. *Medical Journal of Zambia* **2**, 17–25.

McGlashan, N. D. (1969). The African lymphoma in Central Africa. *International Journal of Cancer* **4**, 113–120.

McGlashan, N. D. (Ed.) (1972a). *Medical Geography: Techniques and Field Studies.* Methuen, London.

McGlashan, N. D. (1972b). The distribution of population and medical facilities in Malawi. In *Medical Geography: Techniques and Field Studies* (Ed. N. D. McGlashan), pp. 89–95. Methuen, London.

Molineaux, L. and Gramiccia, G. (1980). *The Garki Project: Research on the Epidemiology and Control of Malaria in the Sudan Savanna of West Africa.* WHO, Geneva.

Morris, K. R. S. (1951–1952). The ecology of epidemic sleeping sickness. *Bulletin Entomological Research* **42**, 427–443.

Morris, K. R. S. (1960). The epidemiology of sleeping sickness in East Africa. *Transactions Royal Society Tropical Medicine and Hygiene* **54**, 71 and 212.

Nash, T. A. M. (1944). A low density of tsetse flies associated with a high incidence of sleeping sickness. *Bulletin Entomological Research* **35**, 51.

Nash, T. A. M. (1948). *The Anchau Rural Development and Settlement Scheme.* HMSO for the Colonial Office, London.

Newell, K. M. (Ed.) (1975). *Health by the People.* WHO, Geneva.

Okafor, S. I. (1981). Expanding a network of public facilities with some fixed supply points. In "Studies in medical geography in Africa" (Ed. R. M. Prothero). *GeoJournal* **5**, 385–390.

Olu Sule, R. A. (1981). Spatial patterns of urban mental health: Calabar (Cross River State), Nigeria. In "Studies in medical geography in Africa" (Ed. R. M. Prothero), *GeoJournal* **5**, 33–330.

Prothero, R. M. (1961). Population movements and problems of malaria eradication in Africa. *Bulletin World Health Organization* **24**, 405–425.

Prothero, R. M. (1962). Population mobility and trypanosomiasis in Africa. *Bulletin World Health Organization* **28**, 615–626.

Prothero, R. M. (1964). Geographical factors and malaria eradication: the case of Morocco. *Pacific Viewpoint* **5**, 182–204.

Prothero, R. M. (1965). *Migrants and Malaria.* Longman, London.

Prothero, R. M. (1968). Pastoralism, politics and public health in the Horn of Africa. Sixth Melville J. Herskovits Memorial Lecture. Northwestern U.P., Evanston.

Prothero, R. M. (1972). Problems of public health among pastoralists: a case study from Africa. In *Medical Geography* (Ed. N. D. McGlashan), pp. 105–118. Methuen, London.

Prothero, R. M. (1976). Towards a geomedical monograph of Nigeria. In *Methoden und modelle der geomedizinischen forschung* (Ed. H. J. Jusatz), pp. 90–97. Steiner Verlag, Wiesbaden.

Prothero, R. M. (1977). Disease and human mobility: a neglected factor in epidemiology. *International Journal of Epidemiology* **6**, 259–267.

Prothero, R. M. (Ed.) (1981). Studies in medical geography in Africa. *GeoJournal* **5**, 298–390.

Rossington, C. E. (1981). Environmental aspects of child growth and nutrition: a case study from Ibadan, Nigeria. In "Studies in medical geography in Africa" (Ed. R. M. Prothero). *GeoJournal* **5**, 347–356.

Roundy, R. W. (1976). Altitudinal mobility and disease hazards for Ethiopian populations. *Economic Geography* **52**, 103–115.

Roundy, R. W. (Ed.) (1981). Rural health problems in Africa. *Rural Africana* **8/9**. Michigan State University, East Lansing.

Schaller, K. F. and Kuls, W. (1972). *Ethiopia*. Geomedical Monograph Series 3. Heidelberg Academy of Sciences. Springer-Verlag, Berlin.

Stock, R. (1976). *Cholera in Africa*. African Environment Report No. 3. International African Institute, London.

Stock, R. (1980). Health and health care in Hausaland. In *Canadian Studies in Medical Geography*. (Ed. F. A. Barrett), pp. 199–210. York University Geographical Monographs, Ontario.

Stock, R. (1981). Traditional healers in Hausaland. In "Studies in medical geography in Africa" (Ed. R. M. Prothero). *GeoJournal* **5**, 363–368.

Swynnerton, C. F. M. (1936). The tsetse flies of East Africa. *Transactions Royal Entomological Society London*, **84**, 579.

Turner, N. (1981). A nutritional survey in moshaneng, Ngwaketse Botswana: preliminary findings and observations. In "Studies in medical geography in Africa" (Ed. R. M. Prothero). *GeoJournal* **5**, 339–346.

Uyanga, J. (1979). Food habits and nutritional status in southeastern Nigeria. *Journal of Tropical Geography* **49**, 88–91.

Uyanga, J. (1981). The regional correlates of child nutrition in rural southeastern Nigeria. In "Studies in medical geography in Africa" (Ed. R. M. Prothero). *GeoJournal* **5**, 331–338.

Van Etten, G. M. (1976). *Rural Health Development in Tanzania*. Van Gorcum, Assen, Amsterdam.

Waddy, B. B. (1956). Organisation and work in the Gold Coast Medical Field Units. *Transactions Royal Society of Tropical Medicine and Hygiene* **50**, 313–343.

WHO (1974). *Malaria Control in Countries where Time-limited Eradication is Impracticable at Present*. WHO Technical Report Series. No. 537. Geneva.

Part Two

Environmental toxicology in the United States

Michael Greenberg

School of Urban and Regional Policy, Rutgers University,
New Brunswick, New Jersey, USA

Introduction

Geographers are typical social and physical scientists in so far as they
have not played a major role in the relatively new field of environmental
toxicology. The limited role does not represent a lack of interest. The field
of environmental toxicology has rushed out at us in a bewilderingly short
period of time. There is so much going on that accurate perception is
difficult to achieve. With this *caveat* in mind, this chapter is divided into
an initial, small background section for those readers who are unclear
about the scope of the field. A review of major research needs and roles
for geographers constitutes the much longer second section. In the
absence of a substantial geographical literature, the author has drawn
upon the geography, environmental toxicology and epidemiology literatures and has used the State of New Jersey in the United States as a case
study to illustrate specific types of research conducted by geographers.
Since the combined literatures are massive, citations are selective largely
to direct the reader to additional literature, especially those journals and
publishers which print most of the literature.

Background

The term toxic is derived from the Greek word referring to poisons in
which arrows were dipped. Civilizations including Egyptian, Greek,
African, Arab and early European were aware of and used some of these

GEOGRAPHICAL ASPECTS OF HEALTH
ISBN 0 12 483780 8

substances. While it is appropriate to begin an academic paper with the note that toxicology began more than 30 centuries ago, considerable public interest dates only from the late nineteenth century when occupational exposure in an increasingly industrial society began to threaten a noticeable segment of the working population.

The public has become all too aware of the field of toxicology during the last three decades. At first, it was viewed in a positive light. Economic (drugs, additives, pest and vegetation control) and forensic (medical, legal) toxicology were presented as positive products of science. Within the last 15 years, however, environmental toxicology, the science of studying the harmful effects of toxins has claimed the headlines.

Sources of toxins

Exposure to toxic substances occurs in the home, workplace and other indoor and outdoor environments. The home environment is a major source of chronic exposures. Toxins are found in and produced by the use of cigarettes, food and food additives, alcohol, drugs, cosmetics and other household and consumer products. It will be the rare reader who does not have cigarette smoke, stove emissions, insecticides, assorted cleaning agents and paint remover and other potentially toxic products in their home.

The workplace environment contains two ingredients for serious acute and chronic exposures: the use of compounds, the properties of many of which are not known; and stress due to heat, humidity, improper ventilation, noise and shifts in circadian biorhythms due to changing work shifts. The fact that many workers manifest acute symptoms of workplace exposures is widely acknowledged.

The role of work in producing chronic effects has been hotly debated, especially during the last half decade. At present cancer is at the centre of the occupational exposure controversy. Until recently, it was rare to find a researcher who was willing to attribute more than five per cent of male cancers to occupation. Within the last few years, the relatively low share has been challenged by health researchers who argue that the estimate should be raised to at least 20, possibly 40 per cent.

An unknown amount of human exposure and contamination of the natural environment occurs because of water and air emissions and discharges onto the land. Spraying, seepage from dump sites and accidents are some of the more notorious emissions because they can produce acute as well as chronic effects.

Effects of toxins

Depending upon the source, toxic substances enter the body through inhalation, ingestion or absorption through the skin. If not blocked by the skin, or eliminated by cilia, mucous, phagocytes or in faeces, the immediate chemical, biological and physical effects of toxins can include irritation, interference with the immunological system, sensitization, narcosis and damage, alteration and destruction. Symptoms are both acute and chronic. Acute effects include behavioural changes such as depression and irritability, eye irritation and loss of eyesight, skin rashes and burns, kidney and liver damage and mild to fatal poisoning. Chronic exposures can lead to lung and heart disease, sterility, birth defects, nervous system damage, mutation, cancer and death.

A substance may have different effects depending upon the dose and route of exposure. The pre-existing condition of the individual can be important. For example, asbestos workers who also smoke have a much higher incidence of respiratory disease than those who engage in only one of those activities. Some chemicals enhance the toxic effects of others (e.g. cadmium and zinc on fish), while others produce a less toxic effect (e.g. lead and calcium).

Toxic substances have had negative impacts on the natural environment. The most obvious examples are fish kills. Other more subtle but serious impacts include interference with reproductive cycles of birds, fish and other wildlife, elimination of beneficial predators, stunted or eliminated ecosystems, and local and perhaps global climatic changes.

A research agenda that includes geographers

The following agenda has three broad, sequential foci which begin with identifying and end with controlling toxic substances.

Identifying the toxicity of substances

The most pressing need is to determine which substances are toxic under particular conditions. This task is astounding in scope. It is estimated that 70,000 chemicals are in general use and that 1000–2000 new chemicals enter the environment every year (Interagency Task Force, 1978). The initial list of potentially toxic substances produced by the US Environmental Protection Agency (EPA, 1977) is three volumes thick and contains over 40,000 entries.

Carcinogenicity is receiving priority. Yet only ten per cent of the chemicals in commerce have been tested for carcinogenicity. Of those tested, 10–15 per cent have proved to be carcinogenic in animal tests. Because suspected substances have been included in the testing, the actual amount of carcinogenic substances is probably between five and ten per cent.

Scientists will develop, test and implement protocols which determine toxicity, especially mutagenicity. Because of economic pressures, short-term, inexpensive tests like the Ames test have and are likely to receive priority. A related set of tasks is to calculate dose-response relationships primarily from animal data and determine how such relationships may be extrapolated to humans.

Geographers are unlikely to play much of a role in these endeavours, but will have to become informed in order to keep abreast of research priorities.

Toxins in the outdoor, personal and occupational environments

The most optimistic person among us cannot foresee the end of toxins in the environment. Monitoring toxins in the environment and human population studies of exposure are therefore important. The following presentation is in two parts: (i) outdoor, and (ii) personal and occupational. The organization and space devoted to these two parts reflects the author's belief that outdoor studies, while not necessarily more important than the other two, are and will continue to be more feasible. Personal and occupational studies have been and will continue to be difficult to execute because of a lack of information made available to the public.

Toxins in the outdoor environment

The fate and implications of toxins in the air, water and land environments have been hotly debated for decades. Atmospheric pollution as a source of exposure, especially to carcinogens, is typical. Briefly, many studies have shown an excess of cancer in urban compared to rural areas (Pike et al., 1975). Air pollution is suggested as a contributing agent to urban–rural differences. Opponents of an air pollution factor contend that cigarette smoking, occupational exposures and data deficiencies explain the difference (Greenberg, 1983).

Debates about toxins in water and on the land are by comparison to air more recent, but are probably even hotter than those about air contamination. A recent set of studies suggests that drinking water may play a role in gastrointestinal cancer (Russell, 1978). The evidence, like the evidence for the air–respiratory cancer link, is easily attacked. Almost all of the approximately two dozen studies followed the same design. County-scale cancer mortality rates were correlated with county-scale indicators of water supply (surface *vs* ground, chlorinated *vs* unchlorinated) while controlling for urbanization, industrialization, ethnicity, socio-economic status and other confounding factors. Only a few studies (e.g. Wilkins and Comstock, 1981) were confined to a population in which the ecological fallacy and confounding variable problems could be tightly controlled.

Contamination of the land and soil arrived on the front page only recently. Disposal of toxic wastes on the land has become the biggest environmental issue of the 1980s in the United States and an important problem in countries like West Germany and the Netherlands.

Whether air, water and land contamination are producing acute and chronic effects will no doubt be debated for many years because of legal, political and economic implications. While charges are exchanged and laws are considered, some answers will be obtained through monitoring of the environment.

With respect to air significant monitoring began during the early 1960s (Sawicki and Westphal, 1961). Hydrocarbons, especially polycyclic aromatic hydrocarbons (PAH), and asbestos have received most of the attention because of their toxicity and ubiquity (Pike *et al.*, 1975). PAH and asbestos and their interactions remain at the top of the research list. However, the fate of many other substances is now being studied ranging in geographical scale from the impacts of local industrial emissions from a pesticide factory (Matanoski *et al.*, 1980) to long-distance transport of secondary pollutants (Cleveland and Graedel, 1979). Special attention seems to be focused on acid rainfall, diesel exhaust, lead, vinyl chloride, benzene and other ubiquitous substances which are also toxic. Acute effects produced during air pollution episodes and exposure to high risk groups of children and persons with pre-existing health problems are also receiving high priority (Seskin, 1977; Calabrese, 1978a, 1978b).

Substantial data gathering about toxins in the water and land environments began later than that for the air. Initial data (Office of Toxic Substances, 1975) precipitated immediate concern about contamination of groundwater and chlorination of water supplies. Other recent studies have focused on a broad spectrum of concerns including responses of different bodies of water (e.g. oligotrophic *vs* eutrophic lakes) to toxic substances because of different chemical and biological properties, the effects of acid mine drainage, of depositing sludge and uranium mill tailings on land and especially of placing or even storing hazardous waste in landfills and on land.

Geographers have become increasingly interested in environmental pollution. The research of Bach (1972), Shafer (1979), Bland (1976), Greenland (1980), Ling (1981) and Muschett (1981) covers air quality topics including smog, particulates, and populations at risk. Geographers have contributed, for example, to the study of atmospheric lead. In a series of papers, Hunter (1976, 1977, 1978) analysed the presence of lead in the childhood environment. Caprio *et al.* (1975) examined the relationship between childhood blood levels of lead and distance from major roads. The work of Carey *et al.* (1972), Greenberg (1976, 1979), Smith (1978) and Mrowka (1978) illustrates a wide spectrum of interest in water and land contamination ranging from literature synthesis to siting of landfills, water quality monitoring and modelling.

New Jersey is an excellent place for those who wish to study the geographical distribution of toxins in the atmosphere because New Jersey has both the highest population density, probably the highest automobile traffic density, and by far the greatest density of chemical production in the United States as well as large rural areas. To date, only limited sampling has occurred primarily for the purpose of establishing a baseline. The initial data has not only provided a baseline, but also a sense of the extent of concentrations of toxins in different environments and initial clues about associations between land use and air quality.

The data gathered during the first year were 100 samples of six metals and about 300 samples of 11 organic chemicals. The data from the second set focused on an expanded set of 20 volatile organic substances at six sites. Samples were taken for 24 hours at six-day intervals in one rural and several urban and suburban sites.

With respect to the first data set, among the 11 organics only benzene with a modal value of 1·4 parts per billion (p.p.b.) had a modal value above the minimum detectable level. The high value of benzene, a proven leukaemogen and ubiquitous substance, was expected because it has been found at about the same or even higher concentrations in most urban areas. The mode for three of the 11 substances was the minimum detectable value and was non-detectable for the remaining seven organic substances. Only in ten per cent of samples did the values of most of the chemicals exceed 1·5 p.p.b. The metals occur naturally in the environment. Therefore, they were expected and were found more often. Their concentrations, like those of the organics, were, with very rare exception, several orders of magnitude below threshold values considered to be hazardous to workers.

Multivariate statistical analyses identified some common chemical and spatial patterns related to probable source. With respect to the 11 organic substances, five tended to be consistently found in urban sites: benzene, trichloroethylene, tetrachloroethylene, 1,2-dichloroethane, and 1,1,1-trichloroethane. Emitted by industry and by automobiles, several of these substances are so ubiquitous in the urban environments that chemists doubt samples which do not show them to be present.

Two other much less prevalent groups of chemicals were found in industrial areas probably because they are manufactured together. p- and o-dichlorobenzene and nitrobenzene were found in one industrial area, while carbon tetrachloride and chloroform were found in another.

With respect to metals, the major finding was relatively high lead readings near major highways. This observation is in agreement with the work of others.

Working with over 1000 samples of about 50 substances, analyses similar to those for the air studies have also been made for water-borne toxins (Greenberg et al., 1981a; Page, 1981). Briefly, like the air data, in 90–95 per cent of the samples contaminants are non-detectable or have the minimum detectable values. Secondly, toxins were found more often in surface than in ground waters probably because of greater dispersion in surface water. For the same reason, however, the highest concentrations of toxins were found in ground not in surface waters. Statistical analyses have shown strong tendencies for gross contamination of pesticides to occur in agricultural neighbourhoods and gross contamination of light chlorinated hydrocarbons to occur in industrial–commercial areas. No geographical tendency was found for metals (Greenberg et al., 1982).

In the state with the greatest concentration of chemical plants it is not surprising that research on chemical spills and abandoned dump sites is continuing. In a pilot study, Greenberg et al. (1981b) found that a significant proportion of oil and chemical spills occur on important ground water aquifers, amidst population concentrations and near wildlife habitats. Analyses of abandoned hazardous dump sites in New Jersey and selected places in the United States are continuing with the goal of finding economic, social and political correlates of dump sites.

Overall, studying the spatial distribution of toxic substances in the outdoor environment is an avenue of great potential for geographers with an environmental science orientation. Policy makers will want to know the relationships between the distributions of toxic substances in the outdoor environment and the sources of toxins such as landfills, industries, electricity generating stations and highways. They will find it necessary to take into account short-term meteorological conditions such as temperature and wind speed, direction and duration in transporting toxic substances. Likely variations by season and time of day will also be sought. Decision makers will have to know more about the chemical and biological properties of surface and underground water bodies, and, in the case of the latter, a better idea of the direction and flow properties of water. Finally, efforts have been and will continue to be made to tie together sources of toxic substances with atmospheric and water transport and, in turn, with public exposure.

Toxins in the personal and occupational environments

John Higginson, the founding Director of the World Health Organization's International Agency for Cancer Research (1979) attributes between 65 and 75 per cent of cancers to personal and life-style factors and another 2–6 per cent to workplace exposures. Thus, tracing the fate of toxins in the personal and occupational environments are important tasks and should be promising research areas for geographers. Based on the track record, however, the promise is unlikely to be fulfilled.

There is no shortage of literature and hypotheses. A massive literature about smoking, nutrition, drugs, anthropogenic and natural radiation, viruses, genetics and occupational exposure exists. The literature, however, is based almost exclusively on small sample studies and on national surveys. Comparisons between nations are possible. For example, Kagawa (1978) reviews the impact of western nutritional habits on Japanese disease profiles. At the other extreme, laboratory tests have shown that the copying process used to copy this paper contains toxic substances.

What is lacking is reliable, sub-national aetiological data. The only geography of smoking* that can be constructed in the United States is of cigarette sales by state gathered annually by the Tobacco Tax Council (1980) for 1950–1980. Cigarette sales cannot be equated with cigarette consumption because of bootlegging, tourists and commuter sales. Upon eliminating states that have many tourists, bootlegging of cigarettes or incomplete data, one finds a tendency toward a spatial convergence of cigarette smoking evenly across the United States. Only sample surveys have been taken at finer geographical scales. Similar data problems hinder research on the geography of alcohol consumption. There are state sales data and some states have county data; however, few states have the same data for the same time periods.

---

* See also pp. 241–255.

Most occupational exposure data have been gathered in response to complaints rather than with a systematic design in mind. While some workers (e.g. asbestos, nickel workers) are known to be at high risk, not all industries have been studied with equal vigour. Thus, it was surprising to learn that industrial and scientific instruments (solder, asbestos, thallium) exposed more workers to toxic chemicals than the chemical industry which would have been expected to rank first in exposing workers (National Institute for Occupational Safety and Health, 1977). Olson (1979) has shown how geographers can use workplace data. However, there is a dearth of data about occupational exposures at the usual scales geographers study. Until specific chemicals are linked to specific workers, and data about the location of these workers are made public, it will be difficult to do anything but speculate about occupational exposures from ecological correlation studies (e.g. Blot et al., 1977, 1979).

Geographical studies of diet, drug use, exposure to anthropogenic sources of ionizing radiation and pesticide and insecticide use are not possible to construct because of a lack of data. Ethnicity, race, socio-economic status, family status and other typical census variables are available. As the author and many others have found, at best these data provide initial clues, and, at worst, false leads about where to look for aetiological factors. For example, our New Jersey–New York–Philadelphia region studies found strong correlations between stomach cancer mortality rates and the presence of Polish-born Americans and between childhood and 'teenage leukaemia, Hodgkin's Disease and non-Hodgkin's lymphoma cancer mortality rates and the presence of persons born in the USSR (Greenberg et al., 1980). We suspect that Polish in the first association is a surrogate for diet and that the USSR in the second is a surrogate for Russian-born, Jewish-born Americans. In both cases, the best that we could accomplish was to suggest specific places to study these diseases and control factors to the New Jersey Departments of Health and Environmental Protection. We may have provided them with valuable clues, but maybe we have diverted their attention away from something potentially more productive.

In an effort to overcome some of these deficiencies, the United States Environmental Protection Agency (USEPA) recently began testing personal monitors (Mage and Wallace, 1979). If the monitors prove to be reliable, data could become available for those who are interested in studying the relationship of daily and weekly activity patterns to exposure to toxic substances. Among geographers, the work of Armstrong (1976; Armstrong et al., 1978) demonstrates the potential of such an approach. Indoor air pollution may become a second, new, important source of data on indoor exposure to toxic substances.

In conclusion, in the absence of a strong political swing in favour of gathering and disclosing detailed personal and occupational data, it will be at best difficult to trace toxic substances in these environments.

Controlling toxic substances

The control of toxic substances will only be an important priority during a period of economic stress if it receives widespread public support. Since the late 1970s, the support has been focused squarely on toxic waste disposal, and it is likely that this focus will continue in the near future. Abandoned dump sites near Niagara Falls (Love Canal), and Elizabeth, New Jersey (Chemical Control Corporation) have drawn and held public attention. The geographers Ebert (1980) and Cutter and associates (1980) have reported these cases with particular insight about historical, institutional and public perception concerns.

But how long will support continue? Sewell (1980) provides an astute analysis of the fluctuations of support for environmental programmes. Undoubtedly, there will be further opportunities for geographers to perform analyses of public reaction to a hazardous waste menace.

The potential international repercussions of producing, selling and disposing of toxic products in the developing nations are paring away the credibility of the western nations. The United States exemplifies the dilemma. As American laws have become more stringent, primary production stages have moved elsewhere. Italy is one of the places which has realized the employment benefits as well as the environmental impacts, including the widely publicized atmospheric release at Seveso of dioxin. This highly toxic substance has caused political problems in other settings. Irrespective of its impact on health, the legacy of the herbicide "Agent Orange", which contains dioxin, is being felt in Vietnam, Australia and the United States among returned servicemen.

Dioxin is not the only toxic substance which may regenerate the spectre of the "ugly American". With cigarette sales levelling off in North America and Europe, the African market has been successfully pursued with the support of government foreign aid funds. In a similar manner, African and Latin American nations have been approached by American industry as possible disposal sites for toxic wastes. The complex implications of exporting hazardous substances to developing nations were reported by the geographer, Goldman (1980).

Overall, there should be ample opportunities for political geographers. Comparisons can be made within nations of laws regulating the transportation and disposal of toxic materials. Siting regulations seem particularly worthy of investigation. At the international scale, researchers should focus on the political implications of the flow of toxic substances and wastes and international efforts to control them.

Controlling toxic substances requires not only public support, but also technical studies beyond those previously noted; these may be divided into engineering, data management and data analysis. Engineering will be necessary to provide the least expensive control technologies ranging from monitoring equipment to incinerator ships. Geographers will probably not play much of a role in this engineering research. They can, however, play important roles in data management and analysis. Monitoring toxic substances has undergone a major revolution during the last five years. Sophisticated chemical equipment that can identify substances at concentrations of parts per trillion has been developed and is being deployed. The data presented in the outdoor environment section (above) were gathered during some of the earliest attempts to use this equipment for detailed geographical surveys.

The explosion of data management equipment parallels that of the data monitoring equipment. Micro-computers, special software packages and hardware configurations have made it possible to conduct analyses that were not previously feasible. For example, the author has used an interactive, centralized computer system, UPGRADE, for rapid statistical and graphical analyses of mortality and aetiological factor data sets.

Another relatively new system, RAMIS, has been used for the New Jersey industrial carcinogen survey (Greenberg et al., 1981a). The data set for this survey consists of the use, production, inventory and emissions of 155 chemicals by thousands of manufacturing facilities. Tables varying from plant-by-plant reports to county, river basin and state summaries can be generated within the package. Confidential data can be protected. UPGRADE and RAMIS are only two of the data management methods that geographers interested in environmental toxicology will increasingly encounter.

Unfortunately, improved monitoring and data management methods cannot overcome data deficiency problems and gaps in statistical methods. Many of these are all too familiar to geographers: serial and spatial autocorrelation; ecological fallacy; outlier detection; multicollinearity; weighted versus unweighted correlation methods; mixing point with area-based data; and the reliability of aerial photography for locating abandoned dump sites and catching midnight dumpers.

The author has had to grapple with all of the above deficiencies during the last five years while working with the State of New Jersey. We have often had to make *ad hoc* extrapolations. For example, as an alternative to health-based water quality standards for ground water, the State of New Jersey asked us to try to develop an approach for non-degradation standards. Outlier detection methods were tested. Because these methods had not previously been applied to that end *ad hoc* estimating methods had to be rapidly developed and tested (Page and Greenberg, 1983). Therefore, geographers with a quantitative interest are urged to consider applying their creative skills to the data sets produced in the field of environmental toxicology.

Even if public support continues and technical problems are reduced, controlling toxic substances will be difficult. The painfully slow processes of testing substances, of studying their fate in the environment and especially of controlling substances stand in sharp contrast to public demands for quick and decisive action embodied in legislation.

American agencies have tried to take decisive action but with relatively little success. For example, the Occupational Safety and Health Administration and the Consumer Product Safety Commission have tried to regulate groups of chemicals by a generic approach. The EPA proposed carbon filtration of organic substances for public water agencies whose sources are surface waters and which serve more than 75,000 customers. None of these quick and decisive approaches has been very successful.

At the root of the arguments of opponents of these proposals is the theme that the benefits of chemicals outweigh their alleged costs, especially because the case against most chemicals is supposedly weak while the benefits of chemicals seem obvious. Variations of the theme include the following: chemicals are crucial to our standard of living and our health; even the most hazardous substances (e.g. dioxin—Smith, 1978) have been found to occur naturally in the environment, and we have been exposed to them, so a bit more does not matter; regulation of chemicals feeds inflation; a little risk from chemicals is acceptable because we implicitly accept risk every day, for example, when we drive our cars; and proponents of regulation are fanatics seeking to regulate everything that we "eat, drink and breathe" (Tucker, 1978). Opponents of strict controls argue that if chemicals must be regulated, then cost-benefit methods must be applied to the regulatory process.

Proponents of regulation counter that, if anything, the risk is understated and the agencies are not moving fast enough. They argue that the human system has slowly evolved over the millenia and is incapable of warding off masses of interacting chemicals, most of which have been in substantial use for less than two decades. Furthermore, they contend that there is a population of particularly high risk people who must be protected. Those who doubt cost-benefit methods argue that there are no magic numbers for acceptable exposure and therefore, regulation on the basis of extraordinarily imprecise cost-benefit numbers is misguided and short-sighted.

Added to the difficulties of contending with many thousands of chemicals and the attack on the regulatory process both by opponents and proponents, is the difficulty of co-ordinating the agencies involved. In the United States the USEPA, the Occupational Safety and Health Administration, the Food and Drug Administration, and the Consumer Product Safety Commission are the major agencies, but other agencies such as the Department of Transportation are involved. The author's review of specific parts of 20 federal laws addressing the control of toxic substances revealed that they differ considerably in who or what they seek to protect, the degree of protection sought, the type of control (emission, ambient), assignment of the burden of proof, weighting of costs and even definition of a dangerous substance. An inter-agency regulatory liaison and a toxic substances strategy committee have been formed to try to rationalize these and other differences. They face a difficult job and are working under great pressure.

Siting of, and living with, hazardous waste processing, storage and disposal facilities will probably be the most hotly debated environmental issue of the early 1980s and the single issue that can most benefit from the participation of geographers. The issue is EPA's "highest priority" (Blum, 1979) because the air and water legislation has increasingly closed out those media as disposal options. In addition, the record of toxic waste disposal in the United States is frightening.

The intent of the EPA is to reprocess for use, destroy or bury in secure facilities waste that is hazardous. Before this major land programme can be accomplished, the government will have to overcome public fear which has made it "almost impossible to locate new hazardous waste facilities" (Temple, 1979).

Whether their particular interest is urban or rural, physical or human, whatever their orientation may be, geographers bring a perspective of viewing things holistically in a spatial context to the study of controlling toxic substances. They have made contributions ranging from evaluation of evacuations (Barnes *et al.*, 1979; Ziegler *et al.*, 1981) to the evaluation of the failure of integrative pest management strategies (Manners, 1979), to the weighing of risk (Whyte and Burton, 1980; Greenberg and Page, 1981). The 1981 national meetings of the Association of American Geographers offered a session on hazardous waste management facilities and another on the economic impact of air emission controls. Geographers should be in a good position to participate in other important projects including the evaluation of methods of protecting water supplies and retrospective studies of the geographical dimensions of alternative regulatory approaches.

With respect to selecting the sites for hazardous waste management, three issues stand out as having important spatial dimensions. One is deciding whether to centralize or disperse hazardous waste facilities. A second is how much compensation, if any, should communities receive that allow a facility to be located inside or near their borders. Thirdly, and beyond these two broad elements, is the tedious process of selecting, weighing and mapping geological, hydrological, topographical, climatological, demographic, economic and political criteria that influence siting. In New Jersey, Anderson and Greenberg (1981) developed and tested approaches for screening sites for facilities. The pilot study included almost 100 criteria in 272 cells each of which is about 1·5 square miles. Interest groups provided assistance on the importance of the water, other physical, demographic and economic criteria. Then, using statistical and mapping methods, the least disadvantageous cells were identified. To determine if any of these initial, least disadvantageous, cells are feasible sites they should be studied using finer data gathered during site visits.

Discussion

Designing studies to evaluate and control toxic substances may be the single most difficult environmental problem that the United States has ever faced. Uncertainty is rampant. We are not sure what substances are toxic, where the important sources of toxins are to be found, who will be affected and when the effects will occur. To call for control in the face of so much uncertainty is troublesome because the implications of control may be drastic changes in the ways we live, work and recreate. Such changes will be made, if at all, with great reluctance and some anger. Not to call for controls ultimately may be judged to have been a catastrophic mistake. Geographers who contribute to the field of environmental toxicology will be making a badly needed and worthy commitment.

Acknowledgements

The author would like to thank Robert Roundy for his helpful comments on the initial draft of this chapter.

References

Anderson, R. and Greenberg, M. (1981). A macro screening process for siting hazardous waste management facilities: A case study on the Lower Raritan/Middlesex County 208 Area, New Brunswick, New Jersey. Report prepared for the NJDEP. (See also (1982). Hazardous waste facility siting; A role for planners. *Journal of American Institute of Planners* **48**, 204–218.)

Armstrong, R. (1976). The geography of specific environments of patients and non-patients in cancer studies with a Malaysian example. *Economic Geography* **52**, 161–170.

Armstrong, R., Kutty, M. and Armstrong, M. (1978). Self-specific environments associated with nasopharyngeal carcinoma in Selangor Malaysia. *Social Science and Medicine* **12D**, 149–156.

Bach, W. (1972). *Atmospheric Pollution*. McGraw-Hill, New York.

Barnes, K., Brosius, J., Cutter, S. and Mitchell, J. (1979). Response of impacted populations to the Three Mile Island nuclear reactor accident: An initial assessment. Discussion Paper No. 13, Department of Geography, Rutgers University, New Brunswick, N.J.

Bland, W. (1976). Smog control in Los Angeles County: A critical analysis of emission control programs. *Professional Geographer* **28**, 283–289.

Blot, W., Mason, T., Hoover, R. and Fraumeni, J. (1977). Cancer by county: etiologic implications. In *Proceedings of the Cold Spring Harbor Conferences on Cell Proliferation, Origins of Human Cancer* (Eds H. Hiatt, J. Watson and J. Winsten), pp. 21–32. Cold Spring Harbor, New York.

Blot, W., Stone, B., Fraumeni, J. and Morris, L. (1979). Cancer mortality in U.S. counties with shipyard industries during World War II. *Environmental Research* **18**, 281–290.

Blum, B. (1979). ES&T Currents. *Environmental Science and Technology* **13**, 1025.

Calabrese, E. (1978a). *Pollutants and High-risk Groups*. Wiley-Interscience, New York.

Calabrese, E. (1978b). *Methodological Approaches to Deriving Environmental and Occupational Health Standards*. Wiley-Interscience, New York.

Caprio, R., Margulis, H. and Joselow, M. (1975). Residential location, ambient air lead pollution and lead absorption in children. *Professional Geographer* **27**, 37–42.

Carey, G., Zobler, L., Greenberg, M. and Hordon, R. (1972). *Urbanization, Water Pollution and Public Policy*. Centre for Urban Policy Research, Rutgers, New Brunswick, N.J.

Cleveland, W. and Graedel, T. (1979). Photochemical air pollution in the northeast United States. *Science* **24**, 1273–1278.

Cutter, S., Decter, S., Brosius, J. and Kelly, C. (1980). Institutional and individual responses to toxic chemical fires: The Chemical Control Corporation Fire, April 21, 1980, Elizabeth, N.J. Discussion Paper, Department of Geography, Rutgers University, New Brunswick, N.J.

Ebert, C. (1980). Love Canal: An environmental disaster. *Transition* **10**, 3–11.

Goldman, A. (1980). The export of hazardous industries to developing countries. *Antipode* **12**, 40–46.

Greenberg, M. (1976). *Solid Waste Planning in Metropolitan Regions*. Centre for Urban Policy Research, Rutgers, New Brunswick, N.J.

Greenberg, M. (1979). *A Primer on Industrial Environmental Impact*. Centre for Urban Policy Research, Rutgers, New Brunswick, N.J.

Greenberg, M. (1983). *Urbanization and Cancer Mortality*. Oxford University Press, Oxford.

Greenberg, M. and Page, G. (1981). Planning with great uncertainty: A review and case study of the safe drinking water controversy. *Socio-Economic Planning Sciences* **15**, 65–74.

Greenberg, M., Preuss, P. and Anderson, R. (1980). Clues for case control studies of cancer in the Northeast Urban Corridor. *Social Science and Medicine* **14D**, 37–43.

Michael Greenberg

Greenberg, M., Burke, T., Caruana, J., Page, G. and Ohlson, K. (1981a). Approaches and initial findings of a State-sponsored research programme on population exposure to toxic substances. *Environmentalist* **1**, 53–63.

Greenberg, M., Frumkin, M. and Lyons, E. (1981b). The potential implications of the geographical distribution of chemical and oil spills on public health and the environment: A case study. Unpublished paper.

Greenberg, M., Anderson, R., Keene, J., Kennedy, A., Page, G. and Schowgurow, S. (1982). An empirical test of the association between gross contamination of wells with toxic substances and surrounding land use. *Environmental Science and Technology* **16**, 14–19.

Greenland, D. (1980). Atmospheric dispersion in a mountain valley. *Annals of the Association of American Geographers* **70**, 199–206.

Hammond, K., Macinko, G. and Fairchild, W. (Eds) (1978). *Sourcebook on the Environment*. The University of Chicago Press, Chicago.

Higginson, J. (1979). Cancer and the environment: Higginson speaks out. *Science* **25**, 1363–1366.

Hunter, J. (1976). Aerosol and roadside lead as environmental hazard. *Economic Geography* **52**, 147–160.

Hunter, J. (1977). The summer disease: An integrative model of the seasonality aspects of childhood lead poisoning. *Social Science and Medicine* **11**, 691–703.

Hunter, J. (1978). The summer disease: Some field evidence on seasonality in childhood lead poisoning. *Social Science and Medicine* **12**, 85–94.

Interagency Task Force (1978). Environmental pollution and cancer and heart and lung disease. First Annual Report to Congress of Five-Agency Task Force, The Task Force, Washington, D.C.

Kagawa, Y. (1978). Impact of Westernization on the nutrition of Japanese: Changes in physique, cancer longevity and centenarians. *Preventive Medicine* **7**, 205–217.

Ling, G. (1981). Simple Markov Chain Model of smog probability in the South Coast Air Basin of California. *Professional Geographer* **33**, 228–236.

Mage, D. and Wallace, L. (1979). *Proceedings of the Symposium on the Development and Usage of Personal Monitors for Exposure and Health Effects Studies*. USEPA, Chapell Hill.

Manners, I. (1979). The persistent problem of the boll weevil: pest control in principle and practice. *Geographical Review* **25**–42.

Matanoski, G., Laundau, E., Tonascia, J., Lazar, C. and Elliot, E. (1980). Lung cancer mortality in proximity to a pesticide plant. National Technical Information Service, Springfield, Va.

Mrowka, J. (1978). Water and water quality. In *Sourcebook on the Environment* (Eds K. Hammond, G. Macinko and W. Fairchild), pp. 371–397. The University of Chicago Press, Chicago.

Muschett, F. (1981). Spatial distribution of urban atmospheric particulate concentrations. *Annals of the Association of American Geographers* **71**, 552–565.

National Cancer Institute and National Institute of Environmental Health Sciences (1978). Estimates of the Fraction of Cancer Incidence in the United States Attributable to Occupational Factors. Mimeo.

National Institute for Occupational Safety and Health (1977). The Development of an Engineering Control Research and Development Plan for Carcinogenic Materials. US Government Printing Office, Washington, D.C.

Office of Toxic Substances, USEPA (1975). Preliminary Assessment of Suspected Carcinogens in Drinking Water: Report to Congress. National Technical Information Service, Springfield, Va.

Olson, S. (1979). An ecology of workplace hazards. *Economic Geography* **55**, 287–308.

Page, G. (1981). A comparison of ground and surface waters for patterns and levels of contamination by toxic substances. *Environmental Science and Technology* **15**, 1475–1481.

Page, G. and Greenberg, M. (1983). A statistical approach to establishing maximum contaminant levels for toxic substances in water. *Environmetrics* (in press).

Pike, M., Gordon, R. Henderson, B. Merick, H. and Soo Hoo, J. (1975). Air pollution. In *Persons at High Risk of Cancer* (Ed. J. Fraumeni), pp. 225–239. Academic Press, New York and London.

Russell, C. (1978). *Safe Drinking Water: Current and Future Problems*. Resources for the Future.

Sawicki, E. and Westphal, D. (1961). *Symposium on the Analysis of Carcinogenic Air Pollutants*, 3 vols. National Technical Information Service, Springfield, Va.

Seskin, E. (1977). Air pollution and health in Washington, D.C. National Technical Information Service, Springfield, Va.

Sewell, W. (1980). Environmental decision-making: The unevenness of commitment. In *Environment and Health* (Ed. N. Trieff), pp. 605–624. Ann Arbor Science, Ann Arbor.

Shafer, S. (1979). An ecological history of coal refuse bank fires in Scranton, Pennsylvania. *Social Science and Medicine* **13D**, 327–341.

Smith, G. (1978). Solid waste and resource recovery. In *Sourcebook on the Environment* (Eds K. Hammond, G. Macinko and W. Fairchild), pp. 327–341. The University of Chicago Press, Chicago.

Smith, R. (1978). Dioxins have been present since the advent of fire, says Dow. *Science* 1166–1167.

Temple, T. (1979). Costle proposes new regulations. *EPA Journal* 5–6.

Tobacco Tax Council (1980). The Tax burden on tobacco. Vol. 15. The Council, Richmond, Va.

Tucker, W. (1978). Of mites and men. *Harper's*, 8 August.

US Environmental Protection Agency (1977). *Candidate List of Chemical Substances*, 3 vols. US Government Printing Office, Washington, D.C.

Whyte, A. and Burton, I. (Eds) (1980). *Environmental Risk Assessment*. John Wiley and Sons, New York.

Wilkins, J. and Comstock, G. (1981). Source of drinking water at home and site-specific cancer incidence in Washington County, Maryland. *American Journal of Epidemiology* **114**, 178–190.

Ziegler, D., Brunn, S. and Johnson, J. (1981). Evacuation from a Nuclear Technological Disaster. *Geographical Review* **71**, 1–16.

General references

Ann Arbor Science, Publishers, Ann Arbor, Michigan.
Environmental Science and Technology.

EPA Journal.
Journal of the Air Pollution Control Association.
Journal of the Water Pollution Control Federation.
National Academy of Sciences, Washington, D.C.
National Technical Information Service, Springfield, Virginia.
Science.
US Environmental Protection Agency, *Quarterly Abstracts.*
Wiley-Interscience, Publishers, New York.

Cardiovascular disease in Savannah, Georgia

Melinda S. Meade

Department of Geography, The University of North Carolina, Chapel Hill, North Carolina, USA

Causal factors

In the United States, most of the highest county death rates for cardiovascular disease (CVD) cluster on the south-eastern coastal plain in an area sometimes called the "stroke belt" or the "Enigma Area". Risk factors usually implicated, such as smoking, cholesterol, lack of exercise, "Type A" personality, blood sugar, explain less than half of the demographic incidence pattern and little of the spatial variation of incidence within the country. The known risk factors do not vary so sharply at the "Fall Line" between piedmont and coastal plain or cluster so differently in the aberrant counties. No explanation exists for the especially striking regionalization of strokes and hypertension. In the Enigma Area rates are elevated above national levels for blacks and whites, and for males and females.

Because of the strong coincidence with physical regions, geochemical factors have been suggested by many researchers. There is a large body of literature on the CVD associations with hard and soft water, and with nearly a score of trace elements implicated through the water as to either excesses or deficiencies. The constant interactions of trace elements, the changes brought about by water treatment plants, and the differing constituency of piping, are but a few of the complications that have arisen in studying "the water factor". Other researchers suggest soil and food chain involvement. The soils of the coastal plain are deficient in selenium, for example, as compared with the piedmont and mountain soils. Selenium not only appears to be an essential nutrient in blood enzymes, it also seems to block that activity of cadmium which can elevate blood pressure in animals. Some of the complexities of these associations and

GEOGRAPHICAL ASPECTS OF HEALTH
ISBN 0 12 483780 8

the difficulties of tracing any lines of causation are discussed elsewhere (Meade, 1980).

Whereas the most isolated counties in the south-east are integrated into the national marketing system, questions immediately arise concerning what form soil trace-element composition and human blood links could take. Even the most plausible links become stretched to breaking point when one considers that cities within the area also have high mortality rates. Furthermore, the physical regionalization of soil, climate and topography in the south-east is associated with very different agricultural systems, levels and types of industrialization, urbanization migration patterns and economic disparities. Any research examining the geochemical environment must control for these. Environmental conditions need to be ascertained, and then behavioural patterns of exposure need to be analysed before risks can be assessed.

Issues of scale

All approaches to analysis of the pattern and its physical or social associations have produced a literature replete with the complexities of scale. Early descriptions at state level were of higher mortality in the industrialized north-east and west coast. As data were developed and mapped at county level, the Enigma Area emerged (Sauer and Brand, 1971; Sauer and Parke, 1974). Maps showed that 84 of the 100 highest county rates occurred on the south-eastern coastal plain. The differences have been found to be real, and not due to variation in the judgements of physicians' classifications, or indices of medical care (Kuller et al., 1969). When mapped according to the regional mean, however, the pattern at county level is far less sharply demarcated (Meade, 1979). As new standardized procedures for measuring blood pressure have become available, interest has been renewed in the geographical variation within the country (Kotchen and Kotchen, 1978); blood pressure for whites and blacks, males and females, has been found to be significantly higher in the south (Department of Health, Education and Welfare, 1977). A study of three communities in high, medium, and low stroke mortality areas have found that the same trend does not hold for the risk factors of serum cholesterol, weight and height, or cigarette smoking (Stolley et al., 1977). Dietary factors have been associated with arteriosclerosis and hypertension on an international scale, but dietary data are not available at a county, or even state, scale within the US.

The association of soft water and high CVD, of one kind or another, has been found in 20 countries, but there is a wide range of scale of analysis, target elements, mortality data and findings. Sometimes water "hardness" is defined as carbonate in parts per million, but occasionally non-carbonate hardness is used. A few studies have also measured some of the 15–25 soluble substances derived from rock that vary in water: chrome, zinc and selenium are more variable than calcium or magnesium, and may be responsible for erratic findings where harness alone has been used. British studies may compare places with a carbonate hardness of 40 or 60 p.p.m., whereas in the United States a researcher may choose a local hardness level of over 200 p.p.m. Because it is not known if there is a dose effect, or if a threshold level has to be reached, such studies are hardly comparable.

There are various other coincidental factors associated with CVD and water patterns, factors which may turn out to be either spurious or more causal than anything in water. In Britain, the distribution of CVD varies not only with water hardness, but also with temperature, rainfall and elevation. In several multiple correlation studies, temperature has been more important than any water factor. Of course, settlement history, industry, density, blood type (from invasion and migration), and occupation also vary with precipitation, temperature, elevation and soil chemistry in Britain. Because CVD is high in the coastal south-east, US rates are also related to elevation, temperature and precipitation.

Various disease groupings, age classifications and mortality measurements and adjustments have been used. Despite such gross sources of error and confusion, epidemiologists such as Comstock assert that the general inverse association of water hardness and CVD mortality has been found with such frequency that it cannot be a merely spurious relationship, although it may be coincidental. As he notes when he affirms this, however, the more rigorous the analysis, the more local the scale, the weaker the pattern of associations (Comstock, 1979).

There is considerable evidence that "stress" increases the risk of CVD, and a massive literature concerned with psycho-social approaches to stress and human health has developed. One group of such studies is concerned with the stress induced by change itself, and the consequent need to adapt (Cassel and Tyroler, 1961). The remainder are largely concerned with the stress induced by low socio-economic status, discrimination, poor living conditions and visual blight or simply despair. Indicators such as crowding, housing quality, or simply poverty are used, and have been associated with infant mortality and alcoholism (Briggs and Leonard, 1977). Data are usually aggregated to city, or even state, level and analyses incur the risk of ecological fallacy. Associations of CVD with physical environmental variables has continually been made with no understanding or control of such socio-economic variations among places studied.

As a city within the Enigma Area, Savannah has a high death rate from stroke, has high blood pressure even among children and has a concerned community. The urban context makes the nature of any environmental hazards even more baffling. The city offers an unusual chance to study CVD at the intra-urban, interactive micro-scale. First, however, the spatial patterns of interactions between socio-economic factors and CVD needs to be illuminated. Study areas can then be matched for such effects, and any remaining variations due to physical factors can be studied. This study proceeds through three steps. First, it identifies the patterns and variations that exist within Savannah. Secondly, various statistical analyses are then used to explain the patterns through socio-economic and housing variation. Finally, tracts are matched according to explanation and risk parameters for further micro-scale study.

City-wide patterns

The Savannah metropolitan area comprises 54 census tracts that lie within Chatham County (Fig. 1). At its core lies an historic area of early eighteenth century planned "squares", waterfront wharves and merchants' shops of uncommon grace which are being preserved and renovated. The residential areas of the nineteenth century lie in a horseshoe around the historic district. Today they contain some of the most dilapidated housing, along with a few noteworthy mansions of the Victorian era. Many of the city's hospitals, golf clubs, larger parks and cemeteries also lie in this zone. In the twentieth century, the city proper expanded southward along a central boulevard, the line of fine residences now leading beyond the city limit to a major shopping mall, apartment complexes and professional offices. Hunter Airfield abuts the southwestern corner of the city proper, tied to a still very active army base. To the north-west, along the Savannah River, the wharves and warehouses were at first reinforced by railroad lines and later the municipal airfield. A container cargo dockyard, a large paper factory and various pipe, cement, quarrying, smelting, storing and shipping industries provide an economic base.

In the riverside industrial area, Garden City was developed as a partly planned settlement for workers, dating from the Second World War. Other, unplanned communities, docks and associated businesses, sprawl with generally poorer housing farther west along the river. At the eastern, Atlantic edge of the city lies Tybee Island, alias Savannah Beach.

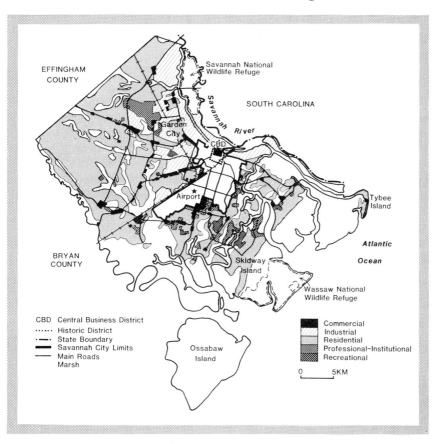

Figure 1. Greater Savannah in 1979.

The commercial area is a small town; along with the beach "cottages" of the rich from Savannah, it is highly seasonal. Based on restaurants, fishing and boating, the old river residential town of Thunderbolt on the tidal inlets is somewhat more permanent and substantial. The major change in recent times has been the development of the eastern and south-eastern tidal, inlet-infiltrated, marsh island areas for low-density residential areas. Once the site of rice plantations and once-malarious, the hinterland has been irrigated, drained and channelled, and offers today natural marinas and stately vegetation. The remainder of the county contains a few very small towns and old rural housing clusters where people still raise pigs and chickens. Most of southern Georgia is large covered by commercial pine, and so is the remainder of Chatham County. The county has a population of almost 200,000.

Savannah is not so clearly segregated spatially as most northern cities. Historically, segregation was a micro-scale phenomenon, often mixing races on the same block. Within the inner city, many of the fine old residences around the main parks and squares have remained prestigious and their tracts mixed in population. The city today has one of the most original programmes in the United States to prevent historic preservation and renovation from resulting in gentrification and the out-costing of the resident black population. Nevertheless, the older, inner city housing areas, especially those of the late nineteenth century, are predominantly black and the southward push and the recent movements to the islands have involved largely whites. Previously, the island areas had mainly a long-settled, rural fishing population of blacks. The unevenness of population distribution between the races makes data further broken down by age and sex difficult to analyse.

A few, predominantly black tracts in the inner city have almost ten per cent of their populations living at high room densities (>1·93 per room). So do Garden City and surrounding industrial tracts. The eastern and western suburbs have up to three per cent so living, and the remainder of the city less than one. As would be expected, the southern corridor of low room density and the eastern suburbs also have average family incomes (in 1970) of over $12,000, compared with an average in the inner city or industrial areas of less than $8,000. Residences within the city limits have municipal water and sewerage. Lead pipes have long since been replaced, but some lead-solder joints remain. As the city expanded southward in the 1960s, new areas were annexed to the municipal system. Garden City has a municipal water system in its planned areas, but some recent development there is not tied in. Lines are presently being expanded to the eastern and western suburbs, but some developments in these areas use their own deep wells. Although shallow wells remain widespread in Savannah, they are not supposed to be used for human consumption. In fact, they probably are rarely used except for lawns and livestock, as the demand of washing machines for fast flowing volumes of water was quite effective in converting domestic water sources to mains' supplies. The metropolitan area draws water for consumption from the Ocala aquifer which is broadly used across southern Georgia and northern Florida.

Stroke and blood pressure patterns are best described in Figs. 2–5. The Community Cardiovascular Council of Savannah has maintained a stroke register since 1973 (retrospective data to 1969) and a screening of the blood pressure of high school senior students since 1974. The reports

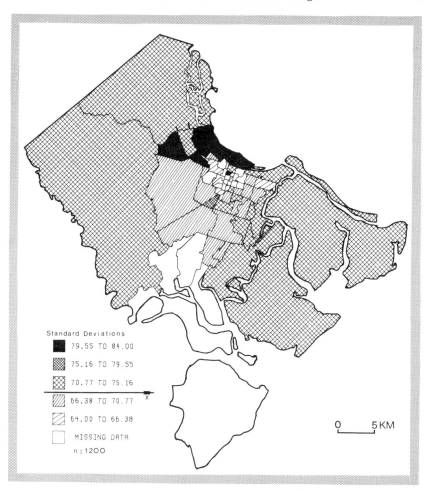

Figure 2. Locational quotients by census tract for strokes occurring to white males aged 45–64.

of high school seniors' blood pressure screening were sorted into census tracts using the US Census Bureau's computer program ADMATCH, and average values were mapped onto the Bureau's DIME geocoded base files using the computer mapping programs SYMAP and CALFORM. In the 1974–1979 period, a total of 9545 students (16–17 years old) were screened. Of these, 8·1 per cent had blood pressure elevated more than 140/90; 11·6 per cent of white males (Fig. 2) and 14·1 per cent of black males (Fig. 3). More than 2000 strokes were recorded in the stroke register from 1969 to

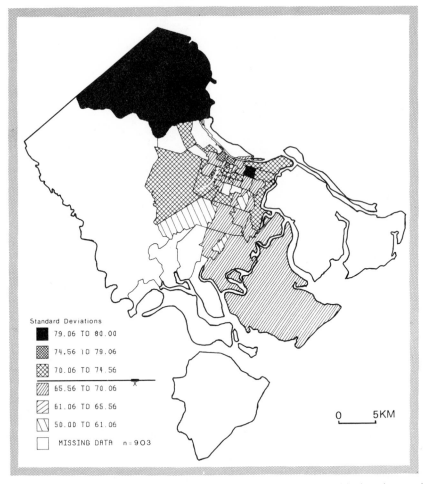

Figure 3. Locational quotients by census tract for strokes occurring to black males aged 45–64.

1978. Residence data for these were also sorted into census tracts. Because the 1970 census population data were too old to justify pretensions of great accuracy, locational quotients rather than mortality rates were calculated. The distribution of strokes relative to population for those aged 45–64 is presented in Figs 4 and 5.

Although the visual correlation of patterns of blood pressure, stroke and housing and socio-economic data is not complete, the major issue of concern is clear. There is enough micro-scale spatial variation within Savannah to encourage further analysis.

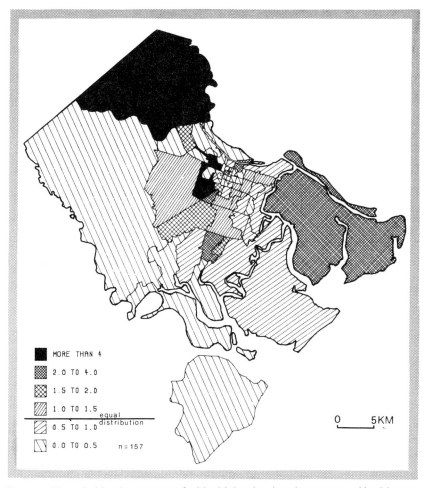

MORE THAN 4

2.0 TO 4.0

1.5 TO 2.0

1.0 TO 1.5

0.5 TO 1.0   equal distribution

0.0 TO 0.5   n = 157

0   5KM

Figure 4. Diastolic blood pressures of white high school seniors averaged by 54 census tracts of residence.

Associations and aberrancies

As data from the stroke register and the high school blood pressure surveys were mapped as well as such census (1970) variables as room density, average family income, families below the poverty line, rental units, plumbing, sewerage, water sources, educational levels, occupations, racial composition, etc., it became clear that whites and blacks had to be studied separately in all things. Males and females within each race are better correlated ($r^2 = 0.92$) and might be combined to increase the

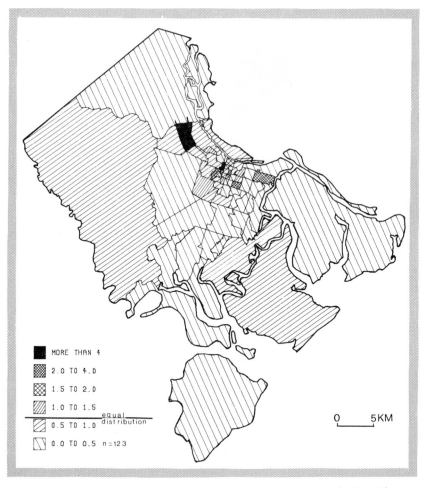

Figure 5. Diastolic blood pressures of black high school seniors averaged by 54 census tracts of residence.

numbers by tract if needed. After re-occurrences had been eliminated 1554 initial strokes and elevated blood pressures for over 2000 high school seniors were available. When these were broken down by 54 census tracts, race, sex and age, many cell values became very small, even zero. The uneven spatial distribution of each race exacerbates the problem, as does the chosen limitation to an age span of 45–64 for stroke analysis. For those aged older than 65, the diagnosis of stroke becomes more complicated and compromised as well as uncritically routine. For those aged less than 45, stroke even in Savannah is rare enough to add a large population not at risk to the denominator.

Originally, numerous multiple and stepwise correlations of regression analyses were carried out. Not worth including here, they indicated that municipal sewerage, plumbing and room density as well as average family income were significantly associated with stroke. To stratify the city into areas similarly associated with regard to socio-economic and housing conditions and cardiovascular conditions, canonical analyses were carried out for whites and blacks using the respective blood pressure and stroke data as the set of dependent variables and the census variables as the independent set. The redundancy (or explanation) of the morbidity variates (male and female strokes, systolic and diastolic blood pressure) was 37·1 per cent for whites in three variates, and 18·7 per cent for blacks in two. As the earlier correlation analyses indicated, the strongest loadings were for room density, plumbing conditions and municipal sewerage rather than income, education or occupation. Blacks shared more similar housing conditions, and for them white collar occupation and total number of black occupied units in each tract were more important.

These results in correlation and canonical analysis seemed plausible and were interesting, and the city was easily regionalized using canonical scores so that tracts which related similarly to the variates were grouped together. The analyses are not reproduced here because they are fallacious, as a closer look at the individual tract data shows.

Stroke and blood pressure data classified by tract, race and sex, fill 216 cells, and the stroke data is further broken down by age. The distributions and variance of these data are so different from that of the aggregate census data that the validity of a canonical analysis seems questionable. The nature of the data demands another approach, one suggested several times by McGlashan: mapping by deviation from a Poisson distribution (McGlashan and Chick, 1974).

Strokes by race for those aged 45–64 for the 54 census tracts were examined for their significant variation from what would be expected in a random distribution. The overall rate of strokes for the age category was multiplied by each tract population to produce an expected number of deaths. The difference between observed and expected was tested for its Poisson significance, the mean difference being lambda. The tracts for which strokes were significantly more or less than could occur by chance are shown in Figs 6–7. As can be seen, most of the variation in strokes could occur by chance.

To help classify tracts, another approach was tried. A factor analysis was carried out of the census socio-economic and housing variables for

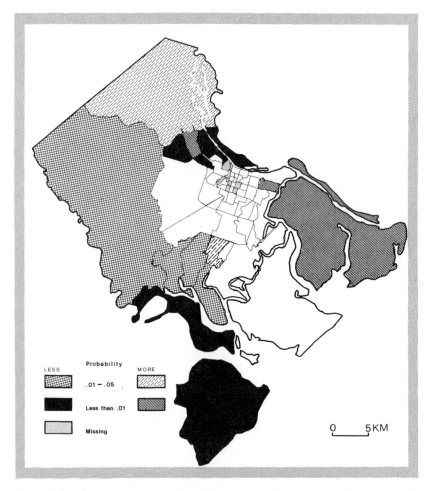

Figure 6. The probability of the number of strokes for white males aged 45–64 occurring more or less than could occur by chance in each of 54 census tracts. "Missing"/refers to local areas whose variation does not reach a significant level.

whites and blacks (Table 1). For whites, four factors had eigenvalues of over one, cumulatively accounting for 78·7 per cent of the variation. The strong first factor (45·3 per cent) was socio-economic, with strong loadings for average family income, both blue and white collar occupations, high school education and families below the poverty lines. Factor two was composed of public sewerage and public water; factor three of "all plumbing"; and factor four of high room densities. For blacks there was really only one unrotated factor, comprising socio-economic and housing

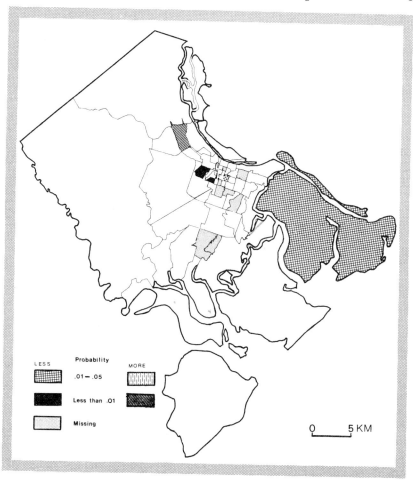

Figure 7. The probability of the number of strokes for black males aged 45–64 occurring more or less than could occur by chance in each of 54 census tracts. "Missing" refers to local areas whose variation does not reach a significant level.

variables. Equamax rotation removed blue and white collar variables from the housing on white factor one and combined it with high room density on factor three, and moved low room density and all plumbing to factor four. For blacks, rotation resulted in three substantial factors, two comprise income and education variables and poverty, factor three getting renters and high density as well as farmers, and factor one remaining a housing factor.

Stroke mortality for whites and blacks aged 45–64 and high school

Table 1. Principal axis factors

1970 Census variables[a]	White				Black		
	1	2	3	4	1	2	3
Average family income	0·915	-0·078	-0·288	-0·086	0·791	-0·506	0·241
% Blue collar	0·954	0·069	0·122	0·061	0·949	0·088	0·043
% Farmer	0·401	-0·056	0·504	0·337	0·326	0·195	0·611
% Families below poverty	0·649	-0·041	-0·227	-0·490	0·840	-0·265	-0·104
No. of occupied units	0·904	0·211	0·255	0·013	0·731	-0·578	0·244
% High school graduates	0·884	-0·070	-0·323	-0·120	0·953	0·210	-0·084
% Units <1·0 room density	-0·114	0·567	0·349	-0·448	0·926	0·126	-0·162
% Units >1·95 room density	0·509	-0·083	0·222	0·647	0·681	0·368	0·139
% Occupied with public sewage	-0·157	0·776	-0·371	0·302	0·819	0·183	-0·386
% Units with all plumbing	0·047	0·364	0·608	-0·349	0·869	0·190	-0·308
% Units with public water	-0·170	0·859	-0·283	0·157	0·935	0·127	-0·187
% Total population	0·983	0·068	0·031	-0·034	0·927	-0·244	0·172
% White collar	0·939	0·144	0·128	0·065	0·889	0·094	0·211
No. of renter occupied units	0·483	0·080	-0·438	-0·042	0·063	0·616	0·446
Eigenvalues	6·33	1·90	1·54	1·24	9·06	1·44	1·11
Portion	0·453	0·136	0·110	0·089	0·647	0·103	0·079
Cumulative portion	0·453	0·588	0·698	0·787	0·647	0·750	0·829
	Socio-economic	Water and sewerage	Plumbing	Density	Socio-economic Housing	Renter units	Farmers

[a]The variables listed were separate for whites and blacks, i.e. black average family income in one analysis and white average family income in the other; total black population in one, and total white population in the other.

seniors' blood pressure were converted into nominal data by classifying the lowest quartile as "low", the next 50 per cent as medium, and the highest quartile as "high". Discriminant analysis by race was carried out using the unrotated factor scores as the independent variables and the stroke rate as the dependent, thus relating socio-economic and housing variables to stroke by tract. The model developed for whites misclassified 29 per cent of tracts, only three of which were high or low quartiles classified as the opposite quartile; 69 per cent instead of 50 per cent were classified as being in the middle. For blacks, the model developed from black factor scores and strokes was less accurate, 43 per cent of tracts not being correctly classified. Mainly, high stroke tracts were misclassified as medium, but fully seven low tracts were classified as high, and two high ones as low. The tracts incorrectly classified by the discriminant model as high lay within the eastern and southern borders of the city limits, not in the suburbs.

These studies are not important for any level of explanation they achieved, but only as they elucidated patterns which could be used to frame a micro-level study within Chatham County.

Indicator tracts

Analysis of the pattern of land use, blood pressure, stroke and the ability of socio-economic and housing variables in a discriminant model to predict the level of strokes results in a micro-level understanding of the city's patterns and their anomalies. In particular, it allows a matched tract framework to be established for further analysis of geochemistry and behavioural exposure (Fig. 8). The characteristics of these indicator tracts are summarized in Table 2. For context, the reader is referred to the earlier description of city-wide patterns and Fig. 1.

Whites Tract—		Blacks —Tract
36·01	High stroke, well classified	18
39	Average stroke, well classified	33
108	Low stroke, well classified	111
42·02	High stroke, poorly classified	7
106·01	High stroke, poorly classified	106·01

The nature of stroke and blood pressure associations by tract can best be shown by a brief description of each of these indicator tracts.

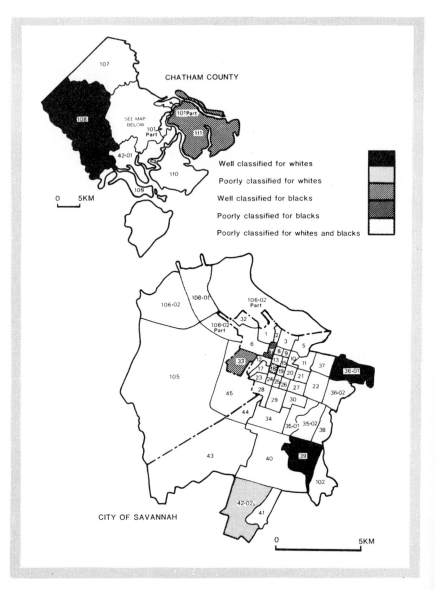

Figure 8. Census tracts designated to represent type areas of socio-economic and housing explanations for cardiovascular patterns.

Table 2. Characteristics of study tracts, 1970

	Tract 7	Tract 18	Tract 33	Tract 36-01	Tract 39	Tract 42-02	Tract 106-91	Tract 108	Tract 111
Population (45–64)									
White									
Male	—	—	0	342	3	337	465	482	213
Female	—	—	0	332	4	322	409	478	193
Black									
Male	1	172	418	35	0	—	33	50	145
Female	68	225	452	37	0	—	59	57	130
Strokes to Aged 45–64									
White									
Male	0	0	0	6	3	9	11	3	6
Female	0	0	0	9	4	5	9	1	6
Black									
Male	4	4	6	2	0	0	6	1	0
Female	4	10	4	2	0	0	5	0	0
Locational quotient									
Strokes all ages									
White									
Male	—	—	—	1·4	0·6	2·1	1·8	0·5	2·2
Black									
Male	10·6	1·0	0·6	2·4	—	—	7·7	0·9	—
Senior average									
Blood pressure (systolic/diastolic)									
White	—/—	—/—	—/—	115/65	118/73	116/69	115/73	119/73	121/71
Black	117/68	120/70	119/69	113/71	118/67	114/67	117/73	—/—	—/—
% Density >1·9	4·6	6·7	6·5	3·4	1·5	1·2	2·0	2·4	1·7
% Municipal sewerage	100·0	100·0	98·8	100·0	97·3	81·2	99·3	51·2	62·3
% Adult high school graduates	14·6	14·1	43·7	37·5	67·4	70·2	41·1	36·6	70·5
% Families below poverty	87·2	42·1	19·7	14·3	5·2	3·9	12·2	10·7	3·3
Average family income	2580	4601	7347	8524	12,441	11,168	9361	9210	12,990

36·01—This old urban tract, where all housing has municipal sewerage and water, is located at the north-eastern corner of the city, separated from the Savannah River by railroad sidings, warehouses and industrial land use. It is bounded on the northern, riverward side by a toll road.

There were a total of 40 strokes in the tract, 19 within the 45–64 study group: only three more than expected for blacks, but eight more ($p = 0.004$) than expected for whites. Blood pressure was a little lower than average for both groups. Yet the tract was moderately loaded on the white factors, being highest (0·6413) on the weak high density/occupation factor. On black factors, it loaded (0·6005) on housing. For whites it was correctly classified as being in the middle 50 per cent of the locational quotient for stroke range, whereas for blacks it was classified as being in the middle 50 per cent but in fact was in the highest quartile. It represents a high stroke for whites in the urban district with density, municipal plumbing, and housing associations that result in its being correctly classified in the discriminant model.

39—This tract lies in the south-eastern corner of the city. Traces of old rice fields may be seen just to the east. Half of the tract's area is a golf course, and it abuts on the south with a football stadium and large regional hospital. It has municipal sewerage and water, and relatively high income and educational levels.

There were a total of 18 strokes in the tract, seven to those aged 45–64; none, as expected, for blacks, and only one less than the number expected for whites ($p = 0.9$). Blood pressure was near average for both groups. The discriminant model correctly classified the tract both as being in the middle 50 per cent of the LQ range for whites and in the bottom quartile for blacks. For whites, its only important loading was on factor three, all plumbing (1·6302); for blacks, it loaded strongly on factor one, housing (−2·6495) and strongly on factor two, renting (0·6711). It represents the ordinary pattern of stroke in the city which is well predicted and classified by socio-economic and housing variables.

108—The tract is largely covered by pine woods and small, isolated residential clusters of old houses with one small town, although there are a few new residential subdivisions. There were 14 strokes, five within the age category: one less than could be expected for blacks, but six less than should have afflicted the white population. White blood pressure was higher than average, but none was taken for blacks. The discriminant model correctly classified the tract in the middle 50 per cent of the range for both whites and blacks. The socio-economic and housing variables were very important for this tract. For whites, loadings were very high (1·9100) on factor three, density, and high (−0·8200) on factor two, sewerage and water. For blacks, loadings were very high (−1·1852) on factor one, housing, and (1·7508) factor three, farmers. This tract was low for strokes, but well classified and explained by the socio-economic and housing variables. The strong weighting on lack of municipal sewerage and water is especially interesting with regard to the lower stroke incidence.

42·02—This tract is composed of suburban and office development to the immediate south of the city. The housing of this tract is characterized by the modern ranch-style of the 1960s and more recent, attractive apartment and condominium complexes.

There were 43 strokes in the tract, all happening to whites. This includes significantly ($p = 0·01$) more than the number expected to occur in the age group. Blood pressure was lower than average for whites and well below the mean for blacks. White strokes in the highest quartile of locational quotients and significantly so were not well predicted by the model. It was misclassified as being within the middle 50 per cent, and its only important loading was (1·2819) on plumbing. On the other hand, although there were no black strokes, the discriminant model classified the tract in the highest quartile. Loadings were very high (−3·1300) on black factor two, renter units, and high (0·9222) on the black housing factor. This tract represents a high stroke area for whites which is not well predicted by socio-economic and housing variables. This may be affected by the recency of its development and in-migration of population.

106·01—This tract had many more strokes than could be expected for both whites ($p = 0·0003$) and blacks ($p = 0·002$). There were a total of 65, the 31 among those aged 45–64 putting the tract within the highest quartile for both groups. Blood pressure was within one standard deviation of the mean for blacks and whites. The discriminant model for whites and blacks failed to classify the tract in the highest quartile, putting both into the middle 50 per cent. The only high factor loading for whites (1·2231) was on plumbing. None of the black factors had loadings over 0·6. This tract seems to be one of the most hazardous for everyone. It is a working class residential area surrounded on all sides by dock-yards, railyards, airports and the almost continual stench of the paper factory. It has municipal water. There is a mixture of house types, about half being of the asbestos-shingle, cottage style of the 1940s and 1950s and others older, with larger yards and gardens. It is largely a planned development, having its own schools and shopping, paved side roads and regular layout and upkeep, although substantial new fringe additions have occur-red. Its socio-economic and housing variables do not indicate its poor health conditions.

18—This predominantly black, inner-city tract has the typical land-scape of old, moderately maintained houses, but some are poorly maintained or even abandoned. Very little renovation is yet taking place.

In a total of 30 strokes, 14 were to blacks in the age category: more than could have occurred by chance ($p = 0.02$). There were no data on white blood pressure, but black high school seniors' blood pressure was average. The tract had a factor score of 0.8320 on black factor one, housing. It was correctly classified in discri-minant analysis as being in the middle 50 per cent range. The tract represents a high stroke environment strongly associated with old, unrenovated inner-city housing and plumbing, and high-density living that fits the model well.

33—This tract lies on the western edge of the city with industrial land to its immediate west. Among a total of 31 strokes, ten were within the age group 45–64, eight strokes less than expected ($p = 0.002$). Blood pressure was average for blacks and not taken for whites. It failed to load on the socio-economic factor for either blacks or whites, instead loading on the remaining weak factors. It had no locational quotient for white strokes, but was classified by discriminant analysis as belonging in the highest quartile. This tract is low average for blacks, and was correctly classified as being in the middle 50 per cent range.

111—This tract is a very distinctive one in the municipal area. Besides the expensive beach cottages and small resort town, there are over a dozen private residential developments. New settlement is low-density, often exclusive. Old settlement often houses many small-time fishermen and shrimp boat crews, as well as the people who service the resort trades. There were 38 strokes in the tract, 12 in the age category; more than could be expected for whites ($p = 0.004$) and less than expected for blacks ($p = 0.025$).

Blood pressure was high for whites and not taken for blacks. The tract was correctly classified for blacks as being in the lowest quartile, but for whites it was misclassified as being in the middle 50 per cent of the stroke range instead of the highest quartile. There was only one strong but surprising factor loading for whites (0·7654) on factor three, density. Loadings for blacks were very strongly negative (−2·2799) on factor one, housing. The striking inverse relation between stroke incidence for whites and blacks in this tract is not too surprising, given the contrast between types of home owning and employment here. The failure of the socio-economic and housing variables correctly to classify this high-stroke area for whites and their success in classifying it for blacks makes it interesting.

7—This tract is outside the renovation area, divided by freeways and urban construction projects, and is almost totally black. It had a total of 18 strokes, all to blacks, eight in the age category: six more than expected ($p = 0.025$). Blood pressure was average for blacks. The tract loaded (0·8039) on socio-economic/housing. On the basis of this, however, it was incorrectly classified by the discriminant model as being in the lowest quartile instead of the highest.

Basis for interpretation

One derives a sense out of all this that hypertension and blood pressure are associated at the micro-scale with the old, working city of Savannah. Old city housing, municipal water supply, high room density, wharves, warehouses and industrial surroundings repeatedly appear associated with high risk, and lower density, suburban, open areas with separate water seem associated with low risk. The areas that are unusually low for stroke and blood pressure are rapidly expanding into previously unurban environs; those that are unusually high have heavily industrial and business waterfront surroundings.

The first step toward analysing environmental risk has been taken by Tourtelot, a geologist with the US Geological Survey. On a fine sampling grid, he has taken soil samples and Spanish moss samples to monitor biologically-active elements of air-borne dust. Both materials are being analysed for a range of trace elements. Initial results, not yet complete for all elements, show a wide range of spatial concentrations of such elements as cadmium. The final results will be mapped and related to other distributions at census tract, and block, scale. (The Geological Survey has also borne most of the computer-time expenses for this study.)

The opportunity is ripe for a micro-scale integration of the varied associations found in diverse studies. Tap water constituency, blood pressure, blood chemistry, socio-economic condition, family and residential history, occupation, beverage consumption and home gardening and other behavioural aspects, can be derived from an interview survey within the indicator tracts. The trace element composition of air, water and soil can be related to these at a block-by-block level of analysis. City-wide patterns of death from hypertension and stroke can provide the backcloth for interpretation.

The use of patterns of covariation at different scales of analysis is a potent geographical tool. It has generally been assumed that a city with high rates of mortality lying within an area of high rates should be treated as a homogeneous, uniform entity. Intra-urban analysis of stroke in Savannah suggests that there in fact exists substantial variation. At such a scale, socio-economic factors can be controlled, environmental risks be determined, and behavioural exposure (micromobility, consumption) be ascertained for the first time. The integration of many factors such as is possible only at a micro-scale may suggest new, substantial research hypotheses for epidemiological and medical elaboration.

References

Briggs, R. and Leonard, IV, W. A. (1977). *Soc. Sci. Med.* **11**, 757–766.

Cassel, J. and Tyroler, H. A. (1961). *Arch. Env. Health* **3**, 25–38.

Comstock, G. W. (1979). In *Geochemistry of Water in Relation to Cardiovascular Disease*, pp. 46–68. National Academy of Sciences, Washington, D.C.

Department of Health, Education and Welfare (1977). *Vit. Health Stat*, Series 11, No. 203.

Kotchen, J. and Kotchen, T. A. (1978). *J. Chron. Dis.* **31**, 581–586.

Kuller, L. H. *et al.* (1969). *Am. J. Epid.* **90**, 537–578.

McGlashan, N. D. and Chick, N. K. (1974). *Aust. Geog. Stud.* **12**, 190–206.

Meade, M. S. (1979). *Soc. Sci. Med.* **13D**, 257–265.

Meade, M. S. (1980). In *Conceptual and Methodological Issues in Medical Geography* (Ed. M. S. Meade), pp. 194–221. Dept. of Geography, University of North Carolina Studies in Geography No. 15.

Robinson, V. B. (1978). *Soc. Sci. Med.* **12D**, 165–172.

Sauer, H. I. and Brand, F. R. (1971). *Geol. Soc. Amer. Mem.* **123**, 131–150.

Sauer, H. I. and Parke, D. W. (1974). *Amer. J. Epid.* **99**, 258–264.

Stolley, P. D., Kuller, L. H., Nefzger, M. D., Tonasica, S., Lilienfeld, A. M., Miller, G. D. and Diamond, E. L. (1977). *Stroke* **8**, 551–557.

Schizophrenia and ecological structure in Nottingham

John A. Giggs

Department of Geography, University of Nottingham, England

Elements in the ecological perspective

The identification of biological, social and environmental correlates of mental disorder constitutes a basic stage of aetiological research in psychiatry and related disciplines. Reviews of the extensive literature show that numerous enquiries have focused on the ecology of mental disorders, i.e. on their spatial patterning and areal correlates (Moos, 1976; Giggs, 1979, 1980; Smith, 1980). Most of the attention in ecological research has been given to analysing these phenomena at the intra-urban level.

The cumulative achievement represented by all this research is considerable. It is nevertheless also true that the potential inherent in the ecological method of analysing psychiatric disorders has not been fully realized. This situation has arisen because ecological psychiatry has not kept abreast of relevant conceptual and methodological developments in the social sciences. Furthermore, several social sciences have neglected this important area in human health studies. Geographers in particular have contributed only relatively recently and modestly to the subject. Nevertheless, they possess both the perspectives and the expertise to enhance considerably research in this field.

The present study examines recent developments in three important elements which are of central concern in the ecological perspective. The first concerns the problem of identifying accurately and comprehensively the social and physical environments of the city. The second involves determining and testing the significance of spatial variations in the incidence of schizophrenia within the present study area. The third

GEOGRAPHICAL ASPECTS OF HEALTH
ISBN 0 12 483780 8

element is the statistical testing of the relationships between the incidence of schizophrenia and the ecological structure of the study area.
Schizophrenia has been chosen for this particular enquiry because it is
significant in terms of its high incidence, chronicity and traditionally
central place in the literature of ecological psychiatry (Giggs, 1973a,
Moos, 1976).

Intra-urban ecological structure

Development of the subject

One of the first and most important technical stages in all psychiatric
ecological enquiries has been the selection of a set of spatial subdivisions
to form a framework for data analysis. Traditionally these units have
been quite large administratively defined entities, for which census data
are available. In the USA census tracts have customarily been employed
(e.g. Klee *et al.*, 1967; Lei *et al.*, 1974). In the UK electoral wards have been
most commonly used (e.g. Castle and Gittus, 1957; Hare, 1956a,b; Bagley,
et al., 1973; Dean and James, 1981). A few recent investigations have been
based on much smaller areal units, notably enumeration districts in
Britain (e.g. Giggs, 1973a; Taylor, 1974) and even street blocks in the USA
(e.g. Dear, 1977).

In the first major ecological study of mental disorder in an urban area,
Faris and Dunham (1939) analysed rates of mental illness for 120 "sub-
communities" in Chicago. These were contiguous groups of census tracts
possessing similar housing and demographic attributes. Seven variables
were used to identify these sub-communities and they were grouped
progressively to produce 11 areal types. These were termed "natural
areas" and were intended to characterize broadly the contrasting *milieux*
in which different forms and rates of mental disorders would be found.
This enquiry was clearly heavily influenced by the earlier "classical"
ecological research of the Chicago school (Park and Burgess, 1925).

Subsequent researchers in this field have endeavoured to improve the
theoretical and statistical bases of Faris and Dunham's pioneer investigation. In the USA the National Institute of Mental Health (NIMH) has been
particularly active. The "Social Area Analysis" technique devised by
Shevky and Bell (1955) has been used as the primary guideline by the
NIMH for the selection and analysis of census variables. The original
formulation has, however, been modified and elaborated to fit the
particular requirements of research in psychiatric epidemiology. The

NIMH has published several technical reports specifying the relevant census variables and techniques which are suitable for use in standardized analyses of residential sub-areas in American cities (e.g. Goldsmith *et al.*, 1968, 1975; Redick *et al.*, 1971; Goldsmith and Unger, 1972; Rosen *et al.*, 1975).

Theoretical and behavioural research in human geography has shown that the "family" of multivariate factor analytical methods provides results which are superior to those derived by Social Area Analysis *sensu stricto*. These methods have consequently been widely used in ecological and behavioural studies of cities since the early 1960s (Herbert and Johnston, 1976, 1980). Their application in specifically medical geographical contexts has, however, been surprisingly limited, as recent reviews of the literature have shown (e.g. Pyle, 1979; Phillips, 1981).

Factor analysis has been employed in very few ecological psychiatric enquiries (e.g. Giggs, 1973a; Taylor, 1974; Bagley and Jacobson, 1976; Bagley *et al*, 1976a,b; Dean and James, 1981). The present study therefore provides an opportunity to demonstrate the merits of the technique in the identification of the ecological areas in one large urban area. The study area is the region covered by the Nottingham Psychiatric Case Register. This is an administratively defined unit, consisting of the former Nottingham CB and the former Urban Districts of Hucknall, Arnold and Carlton (Fig. 1A). In 1971 the area had a total population of 405,661.

The ecological structure of the Nottingham Psychiatric Register Area

In the present study a total of 62 variables formed the data set (Table 1). These were derived from the 1971 census Small Area Statistics tables published by the Office of Population Censuses and Surveys (OPCS). These variables indexed all the major fields of social and environmental attributes which previous workers have shown to be relevant in the epidemiological study of mental illness and mental health care. The variables were calculated as rates or other appropriate measures for the 796 enumeration districts (EDs) located within the Nottingham PRA.

The first stage of the analysis consisted of a principal component analysis of the data set. This particular method was chosen for three reasons. First, it has been shown to produce results comparable to many other factoring procedures (Giggs and Mather, 1975; Davies, 1978). Secondly, no hypotheses need be made about the variables (Thurstone, 1947). Thirdly, the method does not necessitate making decisions about communalities (Giggs and Mather, 1975). Principal components analysis

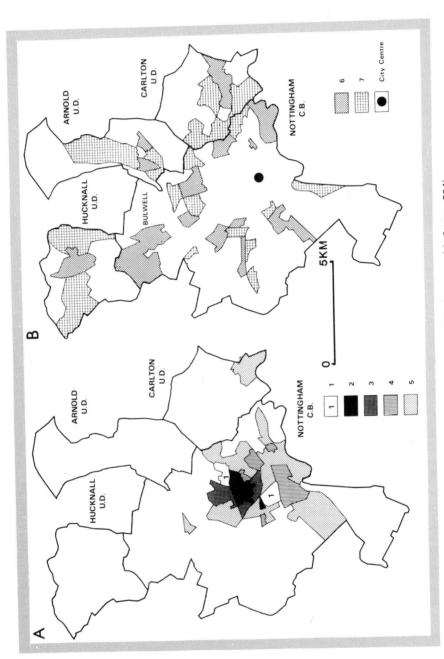

Figure 1. Inner city (A) and middle city (B) groups in Nottingham. (For key see table 2 on p. 204).

Table 1. Component loadings

Variables	Components				
	I	II	III	IV	V
Life-cycle					
1. Children		−0·476	−0·738	0·342	
2. Young adults			−0·541	−0·363	
3. Mature adults	−0·398		−0·649		
4. Middle aged			0·522		0·511
5. Elderly			0·922		
Family cycle					
6. Small adult	−0·563			−0·538	
7. Recently established			−0·546		−0·489
8. Longer established	−0·436	−0·516	−0·523		
9. Large adult households		−0·505	−0·494	0·476	
10. Older households			0·926		
Other household					
11. Single person	0·619	0·656			
12. Single pensioner	0·483		0·709		
13. Median size		−0·630	−0·624		
14. Large households		−0·687			
15. Lone parent households	0·588		−0·362		−0·355
16. Non-family		0·319			0·590
17. Unmarried adults	0·723	0·423			
18. Married females	−0·741				
19. Fertility ratio	0·484	−0·515		0·477	−0·315
20. Sex ratio (M/F)		−0·372	−0·486		
Labour force					
21. Economically active				−0·745	
22. Employed persons				−0·816	
23. Employed married females			−0·355	−0·580	0·373
24. Unemployed adults	0·880				
25. Sick workers	0·771				
26. Employed teenagers					0·592
Social status					
27. Professional/managers	−0·589	0·614			
28. Non-manual	−0·439	0·571			
29. Skilled		−0·690			
30. Semi-skilled	0·633	−0·392			
31. Unskilled	0·713				
Educational status					
32. Qualified		0·705	−0·304		0·393
33. Highly qualified	−0·400	0·744			
34. Students		0·724			
Car ownership					
35. One car	−0·897		−0·350		
36. Two car	−0·692	0·483			
Ethnic composition					
37. Irish	0·648	0·359			
38. Caribbean	0·598	0·363	−0·356		
39. South Asian	0·641	0·385	−0·303		
40. European		0·548			0·467

Table 1—*cont.*

Variables	I	II	III	IV	V
			Components		
41. Natives/New Commonwealth parents	0·762				
42. Natives/Other foreign			0·655		
Residential mobility					
43. Recent local movers	0·373			−0·454	−0·342
44. Recent new residents		0·586	−0·385		
45. Local movers	0·359			−0·435	−0·373
46. New residents		0·619	−0·447		−0·361
47. Unmarried movers	0·434	0·535		−0·406	
48. Married movers					−0·721
Household tenure					
49. Owner occupiers	−0·632	0·396		0·355	−0·321
50. Council tenants		−0·612		−0·528	
51. Rented unfurnished	0·541			0·446	
52. Rented furnished	0·520	0·654	−0·358		
Housing traits					
53. Dwelling size	−0·687			0·489	
54. Large dwellings		0·728			
55. Small dwellings	0·586	0·469	−0·313	−0·360	
56. Rooms/person	−0·338	0·599	0·659		
57. Serious crowding	0·778		−0·370		
58. Overcrowding	0·572	−0·545	−0·376		
59. Undercrowding		0·302	0·773	0·370	
60. Shared dwellings	0·540	0·518	−0·327		
61. Standard housing	−0·748			−0·425	
62. Substandard	0·617			0·502	
Per cent total variance	23·2	17·2	14·9	9·4	6·7

is thus the most appropriate factoring procedure in the present context, because all the information contained in the data matrix is employed and retained for the subsequent (i.e. classificatory) stage of the analysis.

Ten components emerged with eigenvalues exceeding unity. Collectively they accounted for 86·3 per cent of the total variance in the data matrix. Detailed interpretation of these results is unnecessary in the context of the present study and can be found elsewhere (Giggs and Mather, 1982). However, the loadings for the most important dimensions (i.e. Components I–V) are presented in Table 1. It is evident that these dimensions have important repercussions for mental health. Thus Component I is interpreted as being a *social and material resources* dimension. The variables with high positive loadings identify populations with limited social resources (i.e. atypical household/family types, low labour force participation, low social status and ethnic minorities). These vulnerable populations live in areas where limited material resources are most strongly concentrated (i.e. overcrowding and substandard, subdivided, privately rented dwellings). In contrast the variables with high negative loadings depict populations with good social and material resources.

Component II is also markedly bipolar and represents an intriguing blend of the *socio-economic status* and *urbanism/familism* dimensions found in many factorial ecologies (e.g. Herbert and Johnston, 1976). The variables with high positive loadings provide an unusual picture, for measures of high socio-economic status appear in association with many of the classic indicators of urbanism; low family status, high population mobility, ethnic minority status and "bedsit" accommodation. The variables with high negative loadings present a simpler picture. Here measures of low social status combine with variables depicting large and mature families. The public housing sector is also strongly represented. Component II is therefore interpreted as a *status-familism* dimension.

Component III is a *family/life-cycle* axis, differentiating areas with predominantly young and family-centred populations (negative loadings) from those with ageing populations and shrinking households (positive loadings). Component IV is labelled *economic participation*. It clearly represents an element of the family life cycle—the stages in which young, dependent, children are missing and where mothers have returned to work. Component V has been called *mobility status/life-cycle* because it picks out both high population turnover (negative loadings) and persons in the young–middle aged groups (positive loadings).

The results of the principal components analysis briefly presented here show that there are important sources of social and environmental differentiation within the study area. The spatial patterning of these attributes can be determined either singly, by mapping the scores for the individual components, or collectively, by synthesizing the results for all the dimensions. The latter course was adopted here, in order to produce an "optimum", multivariate, classification of the tracts within the study area. The weighted scores for the tracts on all 62 components were therefore grouped, using a non-hierarchical clustering technique (Mather, 1976). A detailed discussion of both the procedure and the results has been presented elsewhere (Giggs and Mather, 1982).

Table 2 shows that fifteen groups of tracts were derived from the cluster analysis. The average scores for these groups on Components I–V are presented so that their most important attributes can be determined. This can be done by comparing the sizes of the scores and the direction of their signs with the component loadings given in Table 1. The structure of the score profiles in Table 2 suggests that the 15 clusters form five distinct sets. Two of these sets are concentrated in central Nottingham (Fig. 1A). The first set has only one group and is labelled *inner city, high status-transient*. Its member tracts pick out Nottingham's two most

Table 2. Group means for component scores

Groups	Components				
	I	II	III	IV	V
Inner city, high status					
1. Transient	−0·68	35·61	−5·42	−10·41	0·72
Inner city, housing/social stress					
2. Immigrant/transient core	34·83	19·59	−17·51	−5·32	1·99
3. Immigrant/transient frame	19·72	11·44	−4·56	−0·93	0·98
4. Early family	23·51	−4·35	−4·06	8·67	−1·34
5. Ageing family	11.1	−0·22	5·82	1·87	1·28
Middle city, middle status					
6. Aged family/housing	−1·48	1·10	6·50	1·55	−0·92
7. Established/ageing family	−10·81	0·54	1·15	0·35	−0·43
Outer city, high status					
8. New/established family	−18·93	0·27	−12·95	2·69	−4·58
9. Ageing family	−17·78	11·87	1·99	4·07	0·35
10. Nottingham University	−8·55	31·44	−24·04	17·91	32·89
Outer city, council estates					
11. Low status/new family	9·77	−3·05	−8·20	−12·33	−9·40
12. Low status/mature family	5·88	−11·93	−1·32	−2·18	2·17
13. Low status/ageing family	1·17	−4·01	12·34	−3·37	1·74
14. Middle status/mature family	−2·45	−15·62	−11·52	−1·19	3·06
15. Middle status/mixed family	−7·89	−8·23	−2·34	−7·15	3·63

prestigious nineteenth century estates. The group is identified chiefly by a high positive score on Component II (i.e. *urbanism/high status*) and a high negative score on Component IV (i.e. *economic participation*).

The second set includes four groups which have high positive scores on Component I (Table 2) and are located almost entirely within 4 km of Nottingham's CBD (Fig. 1A). They are therefore collectively identified as an *inner city, housing/social stress* set. Variations in the sizes of the average scores on Component I and the other four dimensions reveal important secondary differences between the four groups. Thus groups 2 and 3, with high positive scores on Component II (urbanism) constitute the core and frame respectively of Nottingham's immigrant reception and transient ("bed-sitter") district. Figure 1A shows that all but one of the tracts in these groups are found in a single compact block on the northern fringes of the city centre. The tracts in group 4 (*early family*) contained most of Nottingham's oldest substandard small terrace housing. They are located mainly to the south and east of the city centre. The populations in these tracts are predominantly young and dependent families. The tracts in group 5 (*ageing family*) form an almost continuous ring around the city centre (Fig. 1A). Here the population and family cycle profiles are dominated by the elderly and older/single pensioner households.

Groups 6 and 7 form the third set. Table 2 and Fig. 1B reveal that these are *middle status* (Component I), *middle city* areas. The tracts which form group 6 (*aged family/housing*) are scattered in a discontinuous ring 3–4 km from Nottingham's city centre and in four clusters which represent the cores of Hucknall, Arnold and Carlton Urban Districts and of Bulwell village in north Nottingham. The distribution pattern for group 7 (*established/ageing families*) is similar to that for group 6 but is slightly more suburban in character. Table 2 shows that the populations in group 7 are slightly younger (Component III) and have superior social and material resources (Component I) to those living in group 6 areas.

The fourth set is composed of groups 8, 9 and 10, all possessing very favourable social and environmental attributes (Component I, Tables 1 and 2). They are located primarily in suburban areas (Fig. 2A) and are consequently labelled *outer city, high status*. The tracts in group 8 are almost all located on the northern and eastern fringes of the study area, in the zones where new private estate development has been greatest. The group has the best social and environmental attributes in the study area (Component I, Tables 1 and 2) and is called *new/established family* because of its high negative score on Component III. Group 9, in contrast, represents the rather older inter-war high status private suburbs. Most of the families here are found in the mature/declining stages of the life-cycle and the group is best described as *ageing family*. The single tract in group 10 has a very distinctive score profile because it contains the large campus of Nottingham University.

The fifth distinct set of clusters identifies the major suburban council estates in the study area (Fig. 2B) and is therefore labelled *outer city, council estates*. These housed a third of the total population in 1971 and consequently they have important differentiating attributes. These are mainly a function of variation in the timing of council estate building in different parts of the study area (Thomas, 1971). This fact helps to explain important variations between estates in terms of life-cycle, family cycle, economic status and other household characteristics. The five groups (11–15) in this set are therefore given titles which reflect the main variations in their social class and family life-cycle attributes (Table 2).

The results of the present analysis show that multivariate analytical methods (i.e. factor analysis and cluster analysis) produce comprehensive and objective characterizations of the system of "ecological" areas which existed in the study area in 1971. This system forms an objective framework for the analyses of variations in the incidence of schizophrenia and of its ecological correlates.

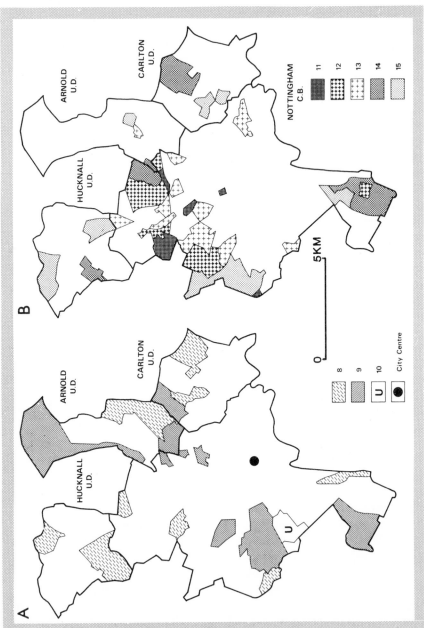

Figure 2. Outer city high status (A) and council estate (B) groups in Nottingham. (For key see Table 2 on p. 204).

Spatial variations in the incidence of schizophrenia

The data

A survey of the Nottingham Psychiatric Case Register revealed that 464 cases with a primary diagnosis of schizophrenia had been admitted to psychiatric units in the study area during the period 1969–1973. The diagnosis of "schizophrenia" here includes both schizophrenia *sensu stricto* (i.e. ICD 295) and paranoid states (i.e. ICD 297). Two groups of cases were then removed from the data set, namely persons aged 60 years and over and persons admitted from non-private addresses within the study area. The elderly cases (81 persons) have been excluded from this analysis because the schizophrenias of old age are frequently linked with other disorders associated with ageing (Mayer-Gross *et al.*, 1970). The 68 cases admitted from non-private addresses (i.e. from hostels and institutions, or having "no fixed abode" at the time of admission) have also been excluded because they are typically recent arrivals in the city and because most of the non-private accommodation is located in the central parts of the city (Hare, 1956b; Dean and James, 1981).

The case records of the 315 persons aged 15–59 admitted from private addresses were then consulted in order to determine their birthplace, marital status and family setting attributes at the time of first admission. Data on birthplace were included in the present investigation for two reasons. First, numerous studies in Britain, the USA and Australia have shown that foreign-born persons tend to have much higher rates of schizophrenia than native-born populations (CRE, 1976; Giggs, 1977, 1979). Secondly, foreign-born populations tend to be significantly over-represented in the central parts of large cities (Peach, 1975; Herbert and Johnston, 1976).

In both quantitative and spatial terms, therefore, ethnic minority groups are likely to exert important influences on the results of analyses of the social and spatial patterning of schizophrenia. This is certainly true of the present study area. In an earlier investigation of the incidence of schizophrenia in Nottingham CB during 1963–1969 it was shown that the average annual rates for new admissions among four immigrant groups were six to eight times higher than those for British-born persons (Giggs, 1973b). In the present study these "ethnic" groups have been aggregated into one set, using the best relevant 1971 census category, namely "residents (aged 15–59) with neither parent UK born". Table 3 shows that the spatial distribution of this relatively small population group was almost classically zonal in form, with the highest concentrations occurring in the central city and the lowest in the suburban tracts. Table 3 also

Table 3. Selected population data for the fifteen group solution

	Total population		Foreign parents	
	No.	%	Total population 1971 (%)	Total schizophrenics 1967–1973 (%)
Inner city, high status				
1. Transient	3,468	1·56	10·8	20·1
Inner city, housing/social stress				
2. Immigrant/transient core	4,725	2·12	36·8	47·6
3. Immigrant/transient frame	8,413	3·78	21·6	55·2
4. Early family	14,595	6·56	19·9	61·3
5. Ageing family	27,059	12·16	12·9	53·2
Middle city, middle status				
6. Aged family/housing	26,211	11·78	5·4	10·3
7. Established/ageing family	31,345	14·09	5·8	27·3
Outer city, high status				
8. New/established family	16,590	7·46	3·4	0
9. Ageing family	12,117	5·45	4·8	14·2
10. University	2,827	1·27	4·0	0
Outer city, council estates				
11. Low status, new family	5,562	2·50	8·7	0
12. Low status, mature family	12,772	5·72	3·0	13·3
13. Low status, ageing family	16,305	7·33	2·2	46·2
14. Middle status, mature family	23,443	10·54	3·0	9·1
15. Middle status, mixed family	17,031	7·66	2·2	5·6
Total	222,463	100·0	7·7	30·8

shows that, during 1969–1973, 30·8 per cent of all the first contact schizophrenics aged 15–59 were foreign-born. They were found in 12 of the 15 groups of census tracts identified earlier and in seven of these accounted for over 20 per cent of the total cases.

Data on marital status was included in the analysis because many studies have shown that the status of schizophrenic populations differs significantly from that of the "normal" (i.e. total) populations (e.g. Bastide, 1972). In the present investigation only two categories of marital status were employed, namely *married* and *unmarried* (i.e. SWD—single, widowed and divorced), because the small area tabulations of the 1971 census do not provide information for the three individual categories of non-married persons. The data for the schizophrenics revealed that married cases accounted for 33·3 per cent of all patients, 42·7 per cent of foreign-born cases and 29·4 per cent of "native-born" patients. In contrast, the 1971 census showed that married persons accounted for 69·9 per cent of all persons (i.e. aged 15–59 and living in private dwellings), 70·4 per cent of all foreign-born persons and 69·9 per cent of all native-born persons.

Data on the "family setting" of the schizophrenics at the time of admission were also collected, because previous workers have shown that this variable appears to have important repercussions *vis-à-vis* theories concerning both the onset and spatial patterning of the disorder (Gerard and Houston, 1953; Hare, 1956a,b). In the present investigation the classification of family setting adopted was (a) "in family setting": those living with parents, spouses, siblings, children or other persons; and (b) "out of family setting": i.e. those living alone. Analysis of the case notes showed that 37·8 per cent of the schizophrenics (i.e. 119 cases) were living out of a family setting at the time of first admission, compared with only 5·7 per cent of the total adult population in 1971. Unfortunately the cases could not be disaggregated into the native-born and foreign-born components because the 1971 census tabulations do not include the necessary population base statistics. This is regrettable, because the case note data for the schizophrenic population showed that there were substantial differences in family setting patterns between the two groups. Thus only 29·8 per cent of the native-born schizophrenics were living alone at the time of admission, compared with 55·7 per cent of the foreign-born cases.

The spatial variations

Nine illness variables (Table 4) were produced from the case notes. These differentiate the schizophrenic population in terms of birthplace, marital status and family setting attributes. These variables have been calculated as average annual admission rates per 1000 persons for the relevant "at risk" populations for the 15 ecological groups of EDs. The foreign-born population has not been subdivided into the two separate marital status categories because the numbers involved are too small to provide mean-ingful rates for statistical analysis over 15 areas. The consideration of sex differentials has also been omitted for the same reason.

The statistics presented in Table 4 show that there were marked spatial variations in the incidence of schizophrenia within the study area. The profile of admission rates for the total schizophrenic population (column 1) closely resembles the classic "gradient" pattern found in Chicago (Faris and Dunham, 1939). Figure 3A confirms this fact, for it shows that the rates fall sharply away from the city centre. However, the polynuclear character of the study area is reflected in the fact that small secondary peaks appear in four suburban locations. These are the cores of Hucknall,

Table 4. Average annual attack rates (per 1000 persons) and probability levels for schizophrenia

Groups	Total persons			Married		SWD[a]		Family setting	
	Total (1)	Foreign (2)	Native (3)	Total married (4)	Native married (5)	Total SWD (6)	Native SWD (7)	In family (8)	Alone (9)
Inner city									
1	0·288	0·536	0·259	0·114	0·000	0·468	0·512	0·071	1·247
2	0·889+++	1·149	0·737+++	0·247	0·000	1·567+++	1·347+++	0·362+	3·279++
3	0·689+++	1·760+	0·394++	0·277+	0·051	1·309+++	0·896++	0·355++	2·930+
4	0·425++	1·311	0·205	0·230+	0·079	0·797	0·442	0·249	2·951+
5	0·347+	1·434	0·187	0·227++	0·150+	0·606	0·263--	0·173	2·962++
Middle city									
6	0·298	0·565-	0·282+	0·182	0·170++	0·582	0·557	0·248	1·351
7	0·211	0·987	0·163	0·068--	0·027--	0·638	0·568	0·178	1·220
Outer city: high status									
8	0·181--	0·000--	0·187	0·114	0·118	0·540	0·555	0·171	0·826
9	0·231--	0·689	0·208	0·091	0·096	0·605	0·503	0·171	2·010
10	0·212	0·000	0·220	0·000	0·000	0·224--	0·231	0·000	0·222---
Outer city: council									
11	0·360	0·000-	0·386+	0·137	0·146	1·183+	1·318++	0·153	3·571+
12	0·235	1·061	0·210	0·094	0·049	0·518	0·529	0·172	2·266
13	0·160--	3·315++	0·088--	0·092	0·038	0·295--	0·187---	0·077---	2·198
14	0·188--	0·568	0·176	0·070-	0·060	0·513	0·493	0·165	1·676
15	0·211	0·535	0·204	0·116	0·102	0·445	0·453	0·168	2·485
Total	0·283	1·135	0·212	0·135	0·089	0·627	0·497	0·187	1·865

[a] SWD—single, widowed and divorced.

+++ Probability greater/less than 0·01; ++ probability greater/less than 0·05; + probability greater/less than 0·10.

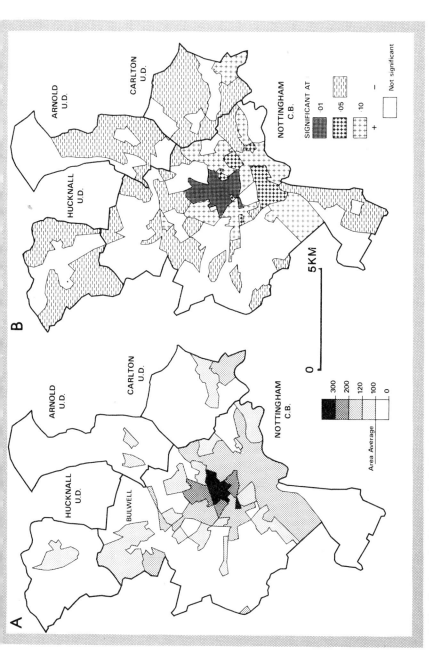

Figure 3. Distribution of schizophrenia in Nottingham. Standardized attack rates (A) where the area average is 0–283 cases per 1000 per annum (1969–1973). (B) Probabilities.

Arnold and Carlton UDs and the former village of Bulwell in north Nottingham (Figs 1B and 3A).

The distribution profiles of rates for the other eight variables (Table 4, columns 2–9) are quite variegated. This fact is confirmed by the correlation coefficients presented in Table 5. The profile for native-born married schizophrenics (column 5) is quite distinctive, because three of the five inner city groups have low rates. The profiles for five of the variables (columns 2, 3, 6, 7 and 9) also differ from that of the total schizophrenic population by virtue of the existence of high rates in some outer city locations. This feature is particularly marked in the case of schizophrenics living alone (column 9).

Testing the spatial variations

The data presented in Table 4 are important, because they confirm that the incidence of schizophrenia varied considerably within the study area. However, it may be the case that these variations could be statistically insignificant or could have arisen by chance. It is regrettable that very few of the studies of the spatial patterning of mental disorders which have been published to date have included statistical tests of the significance of the findings. In those investigations where tests *have* been employed the spatial units used have been crude and generally highly aggregated (e.g. Gerard and Houston, 1953; Jaco, 1954; Hare, 1956b).

The issue is an important one, because the testing of results is a key stage in epidemiological research. Thus Cooper (1973) has stated that: "The basic aims of epidemiology are to estimate rates of (disease) inception and prevalence in populations, *and to test for differences between the rates for defined subgroups*". In other (i.e. non-psychiatric) fields of human health research a few workers have attempted to explore the possibilities of this subject. Most have used the Poisson probability formula to map and test the variability of human morbidity and mortality for selected diseases at the intra-urban, regional and national scales (e.g. Patno, 1954; Choynowski, 1959; White, 1972; McGlashan, 1976; Ferguson, 1977; Pyle, 1979; Giggs *et al.*, 1980).

In the present study the Poisson probability test (Norcliffe, 1977) was applied to the raw data for each of the nine variables and the 15 area groups shown in Table 4. The test makes it possible to determine whether the incidence of schizophrenia in any of the 15 areas was significantly higher or lower than in the population of the study area as a whole. The key results of this analysis are also presented in Table 4. Although the 0·05

Table 5. Product-moment correlation matrix for the schizophrenia variables

	1	2	3	4	5	6	7	8	9
1. Total cases	1·000								
2. Foreign-born	0·169	1·000							
3. Native-born	0·898	−0·120	1·000						
4. Total married	0·793	0·310	0·556	1·000					
5. Native married	−0·201	−0·213	−0·185	0·264	1·000				
6. Total SWD	0·903	0·036	0·867	0·731	−0·001	1·000			
7. Native SWD	0·711	−0·227	0·857	0·449	0·017	0·902	1·000		
8. In family	0·792	0·166	0·646	0·831	0·157	0·813	0·606	1·000	
9. Alone	0·596	0·355	0·467	0·702	0·247	0·697	0·550	0·579	1·000

level of significance is conventionally adopted as the minimum acceptable for rigorous analysis, the present study also includes the 0·10 level for
both high and low significance, because this strategy results in better
knowledge of the spatial patterning of diseases (McGlashan, 1976; Pyle,
1979).

The most important finding produced by this analysis is the fact that,
for most of the areas, the incidence of schizophrenia did not differ
significantly from the frequency in the population as a whole. In some
localities, however, the incidence of schizophrenia *was* significantly
different. Figure 3B shows the resultant spatial pattern provided by
mapping the Poisson probabilities for all schizophrenics. Comparison
with the results of the analysis of the average annual attack rates (Table 4,
column 1 and Fig. 3A) is instructive. Figure 3B shows that three of the five
inner city areas (groups 2–4) had significantly more cases than expected.
These high rate areas are fringed by the discontinuous ring of tracts
comprising group 5. Here the probability level was +0·096. In contrast,
the incidence of schizophrenia in four of the eight outer city groups was
significantly lower than expected.

Given the comparative rarity of this particular form of mental disorder
and the substantial variations in the sizes of the populations at risk in the
15 sets of areas (Table 3), there is ample justification for suggesting that
the mapping of probabilities rather than absolute frequencies (or rates)
is the best strategy. Supportive evidence for this argument is provided in
Table 4 (columns 2–9) where the data for all schizophrenics are disaggregated into eight subsets. Thus among foreign-born schizophrenics (column 2) four of the five highest average annual attack rates were found in
the familiar inner city settings (groups 2–5). However, the results of the
Poisson probability test revealed that, for this important minority population, only one area had a significantly high incidence of schizophrenia
(i.e. exceeding the 0·05 level) and that was located in the outer city (group
13: council–low status/ageing family). Among native-born schizophrenics (column 3) only three of the 15 groups of areas had numbers
which were significantly higher or lower than in the native-born population as a whole. A weak gradient pattern is discernible, for the two areas
with significantly high incidence levels are located in the inner city
(groups 2 and 3) and the single set with a significantly low incidence level
is found in the outer city (group 13). However, two minor "high incidence" peaks also appear outside the inner city, for groups 6 and 11 had
probability values of +0·060 and +0·054 respectively.

The results of the tests for the marital status data (Table 4, columns 4–7)
are intriguing. For total married schizophrenics (column 4) the observed
numbers significantly exceed those expected on a random distribution

only in three of the 15 groups. These are all located in the inner city and the highest probability (+0·017) was recorded in the tracts of group 5. Figure 1A shows that this group constituted the *frame* of the inner city, rather than its "core". Among native-born married schizophrenics (column 5); only three area groups—5, 6, and 7—had significantly high or low numbers of cases. These were contiguous (see Figs 1A and 1B) and picked out the low–middle status middle city ring rather than the commonly expected core.

For schizophrenics who were not married (columns 6 and 7) there was a marked excess in two of the low status central city sets—groups 2 and 3. These constituted the core and frame respectively of the study area's immigrant reception and "bedsit" region (Fig. 1A). However, this would not appear to be the only "high risk" environment in Nottingham for unmarried schizophrenics. Thus the *low status, new family* milieux formed by the tracts which constitute group 11 also had a substantial excess of unmarried schizophrenics. Figure 2B shows that these apparently "high risk" new council flats estates are found chiefly in suburban locations.

The analyses of the schizophrenic populations by family setting produced results which appear to differ only in degree rather than kind from those for marital status. Among schizophrenics in family settings (Table 4, column 8) there was a significant excess of cases only in the small immigrant-reception and "bedsit" region (groups 2 and 3). The cases out of family setting, however, showed a marked excess in all four low status inner city areas and also in the new suburban council estates of group 11 (Table 4, column 9).

The results of the Poisson tests therefore show that the incidence of schizophrenia in some area groups is significantly different from that in the population of the study area as a whole. The overall incidence of schizophrenia (as measured by all cases—Table 4, column 1 and Fig. 3B) is high in the central area and diminishes progressively towards the suburbs. This pattern broadly resembles that found in other study areas (e.g. see Taylor, 1974; Moos, 1976).

The results of the tests for the eight subsets of the total schizophrenic population suggest that certain important social factors create this characteristic "gradient" pattern. The high incidence among foreign-born persons, unmarried persons and of cases living alone (Table 4, columns 2, 6 and 9) clearly contributes substantially to the non-random distribution of schizophrenia as a whole. The high incidence of schizophrenia among the large foreign-born population—which is concentrated chiefly in the inner city (Table 3)—obviously makes a particularly important contribution both to the overall pattern and to the results for the analyses of marital status and family setting (Table 4, columns 4, 6, 8 and 9). This evidence indicates that analyses of the social–ecological settings and correlates of schizophrenics should include separate studies of the foreign- and native-born cases if the roles of these factors are to be accurately determined.

Some of the tests produced results which have not been found in other studies. Thus the identification and analysis of the native-born married cases (column 5) revealed that it was the inner city–middle city *milieu*, rather than the central city proper, which apparently constituted the "breeding ground" for significantly large numbers of cases. Another important discovery was the fact that for five of the variables, significantly large numbers of cases were found in suburban locations. For foreign-born cases (column 2) the "high risk" *milieu* was formed by group 13 tracts (*council, low status-ageing family*). For native-born cases, unmarried cases and schizophrenics living alone (columns 3, 6, 7 and 9) and tracts identified belonging to group 11 (*council, low status-new family*).

Links between schizophrenia and urban ecological structure

Several authors have attempted to investigate the relationships between the incidence of schizophrenia and the contrasting ecological characteristics of areas found in urban settings (Giggs, 1973a; Dean and James, 1981). These studies form part of the wider tradition of what has been described as "associative analysis" in the particular context of medical geography (McGlashan, 1966, 1972; Pyle, 1976, 1977, 1979). In a recent detailed review of studies of neighbourhood effects on mental health, Smith (1980) has classified these particular investigations as *responsive* studies.

Reviews of the literature confirm that most of the work to date in this area has been conducted by non-geographers (Taylor, 1974; Giggs, 1979; Smith, 1980). In most of the early investigations authors explored the relationships between schizophrenia and only one or two explanatory variables. Thus, Hare (1956b) attempted to evaluate the role of family setting in Bristol by correlating the incidence of schizophrenia with the proportion of single person households, population density and the mean rateable value of private dwellings. More recent research in several disciplines, however, suggests that schizophrenia is the product of many interacting genetic, biological, social and environmental factors (Giggs, 1973a). In consequence, several geographers have attempted to explain the incidence of schizophrenia in terms of the contrasting multi-dimensional social and physical attributes of neighbourhoods found within large urban areas (Giggs, 1973a; Taylor, 1974; Dean and James, 1981). These newer approaches to understanding complex schizophrenia–environmental relationships necessarily involve the use of multivariate statistical methods. In an earlier study of the distribution of schizophrenia in Nottingham, Giggs (1973a) used an oblique factor analytical model to determine the relationship between the incidence of the disorder and a large array of social and environmental traits.

In the present investigation the "associative modelling process" (Pyle, 1979) is taken a stage further via a series of stepwise multiple regressions. The method is used here because it provides a means of exploring and measuring the relationships between each of the nine schizophrenia variables listed in Table 4 and complex sets of area traits. The independent social/environmental variables used here are the first five components identified earlier, in the ecological analysis of the study area. The group means for the 15 area types constitute the relevant data matrix (Table 2). These components form an ideal data base for regression analysis because they are independent, additive, readily interpretable, statistically derived summaries of the major sources of variation in a large matrix of relevant social and environmental variables.

Table 6 provides summary descriptions of the nine stepwise regression analyses performed on the variables listed in Tables 2 and 4. For the total schizophrenic population the amount of variation explained by the five components operating jointly was 83·2 per cent. Among the eight subsets of the schizophrenic population this proportion ranged between only 46·6 per cent (native-born married cases) and 80·9 per cent (total married cases). For schizophrenics living in family settings only four of the components entered into the equation. Component II—*status/familism*—was excluded by the default values used in the analysis ($F = 0·01$, $T = 0·001$).

An important feature of the results is the fact that the precise sequence in which the components entered the regression equation differed in every case for the nine dependent variables. The contributions to total explanation made by the components thus varied markedly between the schizophrenia groups. However, the analyses also show that Component I—*social and material resources*—was the single most important construct in the explanation of variations in the incidence of schizophrenia in the study area. In seven of the nine regression analyses Component I was the first independent variable to enter the equations. In an eighth (foreign-born cases) it was the second variable. The table also shows that the F for Component I was significant at 0·05 (or better) in seven of the regression equations.

Table 6. Stepwise multiple regression results

Variable	Components	R^2
Total cases	I Social—material resources	0.710^a
	II Status—familism	0.785
	V Mobility status—life-cycle	0.804
	III Family—life-cycle	0.829
	IV Economic participation	0.832
Foreign-born	III Family—life-cycle	0.371^a
	I Social—material resources	0.559^b
	V Mobility status—life-cycle	0.649
	II Status—familism	0.650
	IV Economic participation	0.651
Native-born	I Social—material resources	0.457^b
	III Family—life-cycle	0.606
	IV Economic participation	0.684
	II Status—familism	0.733
	V Mobility status—life-cycle	0.751
Total married	I Social—material resources	0.599^b
	V Mobility status—life-cycle	0.719^b
	IV Economic participation	0.770
	II Status—familism	0.801
	III Family—life-cycle	0.809
Native married	V Mobility status—life-cycle	0.263
	IV Economic participation	0.373
	II Status—familism	0.429
	I Social—material resources	0.464
	III Family—life-cycle	0.466
Total SWD	I Social—material resources	0.542^a
	V Mobility status—life-cycle	0.619^b
	III Family—life-cycle	0.750
	II Status—familism	0.773
	IV Economic participation	0.773
Native SWD	I Social—material resources	0.274
	IV Economic participation	0.453
	III Family—life-cycle	0.642^b
	V Mobility status—life-cycle	0.727
	II Status—familism	0.738
In family	I Social—material resources	0.395^b
	V Mobility status—life-cycle	0.520
	IV Economic participation	0.574
	III Family—life-cycle	0.591
Alone	I Social—material resources	0.550^a
	V Mobility status—life-cycle	0.723
	II Status—familism	0.752
	IV Economic participation	0.769
	III Family—life-cycle	0.774

[a] Significant at the 0·01 level ⎫ determined by F values.
[b] Significant at the 0·05 level ⎭
[c] SWD = single, widowed or divorced.

Component V—*mobility status/life-cycle*—was the second most important construct in the explanation of variation in schizophrenia. In the regression equation for native-born married cases it emerged as the first explanatory variable and in four other equations it appeared second. However, in only two equations (for total married cases and total SWD cases) was the F for Component V significant at the 0·05 level.

In the equation for foreign-born cases Component III—*family/life-cycle*—emerged as the first and most significant explanatory variable (F significant at 0·01). Thus the highest rates of schizophrenia for foreign-born cases were found in areas with ageing populations and declining households (Table 1). Component IV also emerged quite early in the analyses of the data for native-born cases and both the SWD variables. For native-born unmarried cases, however, the dimension was the only one significant at the 0·05 level.

Two of the components made only modest contributions to the explanation of the variation in schizophrenia. Component II—*status/familism*—entered the equation for total cases in second place and the equations for native-born married cases and cases living alone in third place. Component IV—*economic participation*—entered two equations in second place (for native-born married and SWD cases) and three equations in third place (native born-cases, married cases and cases living in family settings). In none of the nine equations did these two components have F values significant at the 0·05 level.

Conclusions

The findings of the present study confirm that geographers can make novel and useful contributions to ecological psychiatry. Conceptual and methodological developments in urban social geography over the past two decades can be profitably adapted to suit the particular requirements of that field. It has been shown that factor analysis and cluster analysis can be used to identify and characterize accurately and objectively the contrasting social and environmental *milieux* found within large urban areas. This system of residential sub-areas can then be profitably used in a wide range of psychiatric investigations. Examples of the more important kinds of applications would include: the identification of areas with different potentials for both mental health and ill health (e.g. Redick *et al.*, 1971); the analysis of the distribution patterns of specific psychiatric disorders; the identification of "disease–environmental" relationships at both the ecological and behavioural levels; and the analysis and evaluation of both existing and proposed mental health service systems and their utilization patterns (Dear, 1977; Giggs, 1979; Smith, 1980; Dean and James, 1981).

In the present study it has been shown that the ecological "system" of Nottingham forms a useful spatial framework within which both the distribution and socio-environmental correlates of schizophrenia can be analysed. This enquiry has confirmed that there are statistically significant variations in the incidence of schizophrenia (measured by nine variables) among 15 different kinds of socio-environmental areas. Multiple regression analysis subsequently revealed that there were strong, but varied, links between the incidence of the nine schizophrenia variables and the five leading components identified in the ecological analysis of the study area. The character and significance of these results is now being investigated via detailed study of the case notes of the individual patients. Similar work in other urban areas is now clearly required in order to determine the generality (or uniqueness) of the results for Nottingham.

Acknowledgement

The author gratefully acknowledges that this research was funded by a grant from the Social Science Research Council.

References

Bagley, S. and Jacobson, S. (1976). *Psychol. Medicine* 6, 423–427.
Bagley, S., Jacobson, S. and Palmer, O. (1973). *Psychol. Medicine* 3, 177–187.
Bagley, S., Jacobson, S. and Rehin, A. (1976a). *Psychol. Medicine* 6, 417–421.
Bagley, S., Jacobson, S. and Rehin, A. (1976b). *Psychol. Medicine* 6, 429–438.
Bastide, R. (1972). *The Sociology of Mental Disorder*. Routledge and Kegan Paul, London.
Castle, I. M. and Gittus, E. (1957). *Sociol. Rev.* 5, 43–64.
Commission for Racial Equality (1976). *Mental Health among Minority Ethnic Groups: Research Summaries and Bibliography*. CRE, London.
Cooper, B. (1973). *Psychol. Medicine* 3, 401–404.
Choynowski, M. (1959). *J. Amer. Stat. Ass.* 54, 385–388.
Davies, W. K. D. (1978). *Canadian Geogr.* XXII, 273–297.
Dear, M. (1977). *Annals.Ass. Amer. Geogr.* 67, 588-594.
Dean, K. G. and James, H. D. (1981). *Trans., Inst. Brit. Geogr.* 6(1), 39–52.
Faris, R. E. and Dunham, H. W. (1939). *Mental Disorders in Urban Areas*. University of Chicago Press, Chicago.
Ferguson, A. G. (1977). *J. Trop. Geogr.* 44, 23–32.
Gerard, D. L. and Houston, L. G. (1953). *Psychiat. Quart.* 27, 19–37.
Giggs, J. A. (1973a). *Trans., Inst. Brit. Geogr.* 59, 55–76.

Giggs, J. A. (1973b). *Nursing Times* 1210–1212.

Giggs, J. A. (1977). In *Australia 2000: The Ethnic Impact* (Ed. M. Bowen), pp. 256–266. University of New England, Armidale.

Giggs, J. A. (1979). In *Social Problems and the City: Geographical Perspectives* (Eds D. T. Herbert and D. M. Smith), pp. 84–116. Oxford University Press, Oxford.

Giggs, J. A. (1980). In *Environmental Medicine* (Eds G. M. Howe and J. A. Loraine), pp. 281–305. William Heinemann Medical Books Ltd., London.

Giggs, J. A. and Mather, P. M. (1975). *Econ. Geogr.* **51**, 366–382.

Giggs, J. A. and Mather, P. M. (1982). Report Series on Applied Geography, No. 2. Department of Geography, University of Nottingham.

Giggs, J. A., Ebdon, D. S. and Bourke, J. B. (1980). *Trans., Inst. Brit. Geogr.* **5**, 229–242.

Goldsmith, H. F. and Unger, E. L. (1972). Laboratory Paper No. 37. Mental Health Study Center, National Institute of Mental Health, Adelphi, Maryland.

Goldsmith, H. F., Stockwell, E. G., Munsterman, J. T., Lee, S. Y. and Unger, E. L. (1968). Laboratory Paper No. 22. Mental Health Study Center, National Institute of Mental Health, Adelphi, Maryland.

Goldsmith, H. F., Unger, E. L., Rosen, B. M., Shambaugh, J. P. and Windle, C. D. (1975). DHEW Publication No. (ADM) 76–262. National Institute of Mental Health, US Government Printing Office, Washington, D.C.

Hare, E. H. (1956a). *Brit. J. Prev. Soc. Med.* **9**, 191–195.

Hare, E. H. (1956b). *J. Ment. Sci.* **102**, 753–760.

Herbert, D. T. and Johnston, R. J. (Eds) (1976). *Social Areas in Cities*, Vols I and II. John Wiley and Sons, London and New York.

Herbert, D. T. and Johnston, R. J. (Eds) (1980). *Geography and the Urban Environment: Progress and Applications*, Vol. III. John Wiley and Sons, London and New York.

Jaco, E. G. (1954). *Amer. Sociol. Rev.* **19**, 567–577.

Klee, G. D., Spiro, E., Bahn, A. K. and Gorwitz, K. (1967). In *Psychiatric Epidemiology and Mental Health Planning* (Eds. R. R. Monroe, G. D. Klee and E. B. Brody), pp. 107–148. Psychiatric Research Report No. 22. The American Psychiatric Association, Washington, D.C.

Lei, Tzuen-Jen, Rowitz, L., Mcallister, R. J. and Butler, E. W. (1974). *Amer. J. Ment. Defic.* **79**, 22–31.

Mather, P. M. (1976). *Computational Methods of Multivariate Analysis in Physical Geography.* John Wiley and Sons, London and New York.

Mayer-Gross, W., Slater, E. and Roth, M. (1970). *Clinical Psychiatry.* Bailliere, Tindall and Cassell, London.

McGlashan, N. D. (1966). *Int. Pathol.* **7**, 81–83.

McGlashan, N. D. (Ed.) (1972). *Medical Geography: Techniques and Field Studies.* Methuen and Co. Ltd., London.

McGlashan, N. D. and Harington, J. S. (1976). *The South African Geogr. Journ.* **58**, 18–24.

Moos, R. R. (1976). *The Human Context: Environmental Determinants of Behavior.* John Wiley and Sons, New York.

Norcliffe, G. B. (1977). *Inferential Statistics for Geographers.* Hutchinson and Co. Ltd., London.

Park, R. E. and Burgess, E. W. (1925). *The City.* University of Chicago Press, Chicago.

Patno, M. E. (1954). *Publ. Hlth Rep.* **69**, 705–715.

Peach, C. (Ed.) (1975). *Urban Social Segregation.* Longman, London and New York.

Phillips, D. R. (1981). *Contemporary Issues in the Geography of Health Care.* Geo. Books, Norwich.

Pyle, G. F. (1976). *Econ. Geogr.* **52**, 95–102.

Pyle, G. F. (1977). *Soc. Sci. and Med.* **11**, 679–682.

Pyle, G. F. (1979). *Applied Medical Geography.* W. H. Winston and Sons, Washington, D.C.

Redick, R. W., Goldsmith, H. F. and Unger, E. L. (1971). Mental Health Statistics Methodology Report No. 3, Series C. National Institute of Mental Health, Chevy Chase, Maryland.

Rosen, B. M., Lawrence, L., Goldsmith, H. F., Windle, C. D. and Shambaugh, J. P. (1975). Mental Health Statistics Methodology Report No. 11, Series C. National Institute of Mental Health, Washington, D.C.

Shevky, E. and Bell, W. (1955). *Social Area Analysis.* Stanford University Press, Stanford.

Smith, C. J. (1980). In *Geography and the Urban Environment: Progress in Research and Applications* (Eds D. T. Herbert and R. J. Johnson), pp. 363–416. John Wiley and Sons, London and New York.

Taylor, S. D. (1974). The Geography and Epidemiology of Psychiatric Disorders in Southampton. Unpublished Ph.D. thesis, University of Southampton.

Thomas, C. J. (1971). *East Midl. Geogr.* **5**, 119–132.

Thurstone, L. L. (1947). *Multiple Factor Analysis.* University of Chicago Press, Chicago.

White, R. R. (1972). In *Medical Geography: Techniques and Field Studies* (Ed. N. D. McGlashan), pp. 173–186. Methuen and Co. Ltd., London.

Health-care problems in north-west Sutherland: a peripheral region of Scotland

Sheila Bain

Department of Geography, University of Aberdeen, Scotland

Introduction

North-west Sutherland is one of the most isolated regions of the British mainland. Cape Wrath which forms the north-western tip of the region is 130 miles north of Inverness and nearly 300 miles north of Edinburgh. An investigation into the health-care problems of the area was undertaken as part of a much larger study into public transport (Farrington *et al.*, 1981).

Physical environment

The major portion of the area is upland, covered in peat, thin soils, screes and rocks, and it experiences a high degree of exposure to severe climatic conditions especially in winter. The lowlands with better soils and a less harsh climate are confined to the coastal belt and the straths (broad mountain valleys) which penetrate the area north-west and west of Lairg, and south from the north coast. The coastline is highly indented by sea lochs, and these present considerable difficulties for surface communications between the coastal lowlands round the periphery of the area. Large sections of the area are occupied by mountain masses with rugged terrain, and the road network reflects these physical limitations as well as the distribution of settlement, itself largely a product of the environmental limitations of much of the area. Land use on these upland areas is restricted to extensive activities such as peat cutting, forestry, grouse moor, deer forest and seasonal rough grazing. More intensive agriculture

GEOGRAPHICAL ASPECTS OF HEALTH
ISBN 0 12 483780 8

is restricted to lowland strips around the coasts, and to the larger straths. Thus, the agriculture of the area is characterized by crofts (smallholdings), small farms and large sporting estates. The wild beauty and relative emptiness of the area attracts tourists and sportsmen on a national and international scale.

Communications

Roads

Three main routeways give external access to and from the area; eastwards along the north coast towards Thurso and Wick, south-eastwards from Lairg towards Bonar Bridge, Dingwall and Inverness, and southwestwards to Ullapool, Dingwall and Inverness (Fig. 1). It is relevant to note that of the total route mileage of 334, only 57 miles are of twin track road, the remainder being single track with passing places. In the words of the Highland Regional Council's Department of Roads and Transport:

Single track roads are the bane of the whole system, since it is a characteristic of such roads that the level of service (speed, comfort and general ease of travel afforded) falls way abruptly as soon as traffic flows rise above more than a very low level. . . . In addition, it has been established that the new larger commercial vehicles to be permitted under E.E.C. Regulations will be unable to reach many parts in the north and west of the Region (Highland Regional Council, 1980).

Although much work has been done to improve the area's road network, most of it has been carried out on the western stretches of the coastal route. Along the north and west coasts many settlements (often crofting townships) are located on favourable lowlands near the shore or in the straths, and these are connected to the main road network by miles of single track roads with variable surface qualities. Such routes with low levels of population, and the physical limitations of the roads themselves are only feasible for post-bus operations (combining the distribution of mail and the carriage of passengers), rather than conventional bus transport.

Ferries

The only ferry of significance in the context of large-scale public use and access is that operated by the Highland Regional Council between

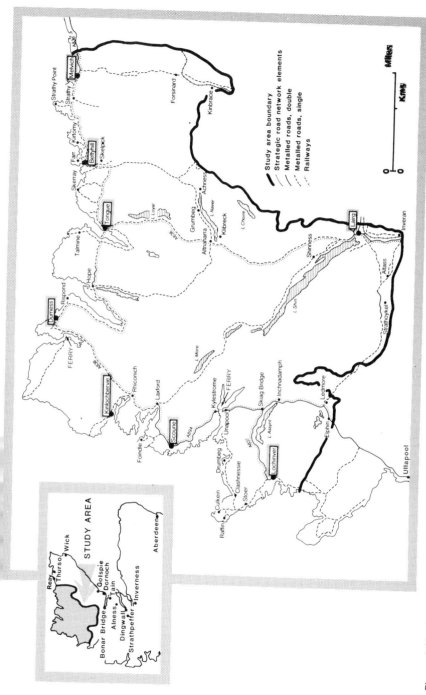

Figure 1. North-west Sutherland: roads, railways and settlements in the study area.

Unapool and Kylestrome. As well as fulfilling an important local function, it also provides a vital link in the coastal route between the Kinlochbervie area and Inverness, via Ullapool. It is planned to replace the ferry by a bridge in the next few years.

The other ferry operating in the study area is the privately owned Kyle of Durness ferry, giving access from Keoldale (near Durness) to Cape Wrath, with its important lighthouse.

Railways

The former Highland Railway's line from Inverness to Wick and Thurso impinges on the area in two lengths, providing three stations with passenger facilities; Lairg, Forsinard and Kinbrace. The route is quite heavily graded and sinuous, but has advantages in winter when weather conditions adversely affect movement by road; occasionally even rail movements are brought to a halt by drifting snow.

Airports

There are no airfield facilities in the area suitable for fixed-wing aircraft operating public services.

Socio-economic characteristics

The socio-economic characteristics of a population play a large part in affecting the level of accessibility experienced by the people. In particular, factors such as car ownership rates, household structures, employment and proportions of groups such as the elderly act as constraints with a direct bearing on accessibility needs and levels (Hillman *et al.*, 1973; Moseley *et al.*, 1977). The last Census of Population from which data is readily available is that conducted in 1971 and the information is too dated to be used as a basis for analysis. However, a useful source of recent information is the Community Survey Reports produced by the Highland Regional Council's Department of Planning in April, 1980. Further information on a wide range of demographic, social and economic data was obtained by a questionnaire survey of approximately 10 per cent of the population which was undertaken in connection with an investigation into public transport in north-west Sutherland (Farrington *et al.*, 1981).

Population

The pattern of settlements (Fig. 1) shows a clear peripherality with the main concentrations being in the south-east, including Lairg, and along parts of the north and west coasts, particularly Lochinver, Scourie, Kinlochbervie, Durness, Tongue, Bettyhill and Melvich. Large tracts in the central part of the area have a sparse population and a consequent lack of transport facilities. The total population resident in north-west Sutherland in 1971 was 4569, and the average population density was approximately 5·2 persons per square mile. This low density in itself highlights some of the difficulties in providing a socio-economic infrastructure.

The distribution of the young and elderly members in the population are indicated in Fig. 2. Concentrations of high proportions of those over retirement age (men 65 and over; women 60 and over) are to be found in some coastal areas, including Drumbeg and Culkein (north of Lochinver), Sheigra and Oldshoremore (north-west of Kinlochbervie), and in Talmine and Skerray on the north coast. The other area with over 30 per cent of the population in this age group was Strathnaver (south of Bettyhill). Over most of the area, less than 20 per cent of the population is below the age of 15.

In recent years the number of elderly persons in the area has increased due to the purchase of "second homes". Many visitors and tourists are so attracted by the wild scenery of the area, the slower pace of life, the friendliness of the indigenous population, that they return to live permanently in the area upon retirement. Added to this group of elderly incomers, must also be the group of persons who were born in the region, but for reasons of employment, marriage, etc., moved south in their young and middle years, but upon retirement return to their birthplace.

Car ownership

Car ownership is naturally a vital factor in influencing levels of mobility and accessibility. The basic measure of this factor, the ratio of cars to households, is shown for each enumeration district (Fig. 3). Concentrations of lower car ownership are to be noted in the areas near Kylestrome, north of Kinlochbervie, Talmine, Skerray, Strathy Point and Melvich—all coastal areas with average car ownership rate of 0·69 cars per household or less. To emphasize the variability of car ownership within the area, districts with the largest number of cars per household are shown south of Drumbeg, north of Kinlochbervie, south of Talmine and south of Strathy Point.

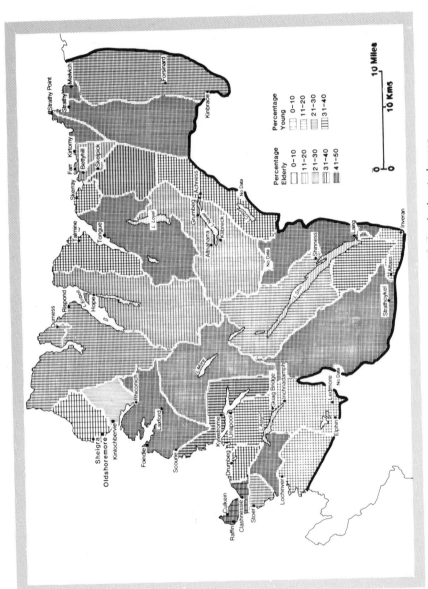

Figure 2. Distribution of the young and elderly members of the population in the study area.

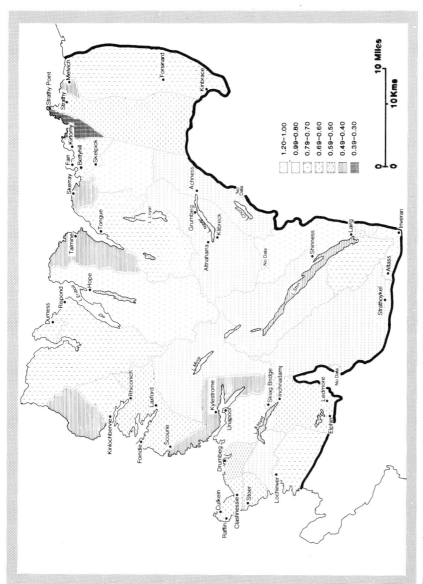

Figure 3. Average numbers of cars per household in the study area.

The level of total dependence was highly variable through the area, though in the five enumeration districts in the north and west coastal areas of the lowest ratio of cars to households, more than 41 per cent of the population was totally dependent on public transport. Over the area as a whole, the investigation indicated that 29 per cent of households were totally dependent, 45 per cent of households were partially dependent, and only 26 per cent of households were independent of public transport. Or, to express it differently, nearly 1000 out of 4569 persons in this area are found to be dependent upon public transport.

Health services

Background

The 1909 Royal Commission on the Poor Law found evidence of "a large amount of suffering in the remote Highlands unrelieved by medical or nursing attendance". The Highlands and Islands Medical Services Committee (Dewar Committee) set up in 1912 resulted in the establishment of the Highlands and Islands Medical Service Fund. This provided grants for doctors, nursing services, hospital and ambulance, telegraph and telephone services. The National Health Service Act of 1948 and the subsequent reorganization in 1974 have only marginally altered the form and location of primary medical and nursing services in the Highlands. In 1967, an enquiry into the current provision of general medical services in the Highlands, suggested that transport and communications, integration of services, conditions of service and remuneration were some of the major problems. The investigation noted that:

> the chief threat to the efficiency of the medical services . . . is the professional isolation of the doctor. The doctor who is cut off by distance from his colleagues in general practice and in hospital, by the same token carries an inescapably greater degree of personal responsibility; yet in the smallest and most remote practices this is associated with a very light volume of routine medical duties. This provides an extraordinarily difficult basis for the continuing provision of satisfactory medical care. It may also make personal relationships difficult: neither the patient nor the doctor has in practice the free choice that is so carefully provided for in the regulations relating to the NHS (Birsay Report, 1967).

Provision and distribution of services

The main health facilities in the area are provided by the six resident General Practitioners with surgeries and branch surgeries as follows:

Lairg
Lochinver (regular visits to Stoer and Inchnadamph)
Scourie (branch surgery at Kinlochbervie)
Durness
Tongue
Armadale (branch surgeries at Melvich and Bettyhill)

All the GPs except the Lairg doctor dispense drugs for their own patients (Fig. 4).

The average list size for single-handed practices in the Highland Region is 1445 persons as compared with an average list size for the whole of Scotland of 1856 persons. However, small lists in the Highlands do not necessarily mean a leisurely way of life for the doctor. First, there is the summer tourist trade, and in the autumn, the influx of sportsmen and both these groups will add to the demand on the time of the local GPs. Secondly, the Scottish Medical Practices Committee have operated a rule-of-thumb formula such that in the 1960s, £100 of mileage payment was considered roughly equivalent to 60 extra patients. A small patient list scattered over a wide area can thus mean a work load not greatly below the city average.

The geographical distribution of practices has changed hardly at all since the inception of the NHS and the present locations seem to reflect fairly accurately the distribution of the population and lay-out of the road system. One major problem exists, however, for both patients and doctors in the Highland Region, and that is the lack of any real choice. Doctors in solo practice, especially, where they are a long way from other practices—a common situation in this area—also have to treat friends, neighbours and their own families. Doctors themselves who may become ill, will also face the considerable problem of "calling in" their nearest colleague, who may be located at least 20 miles distant.

In the day-to-day running of the practices, problems do arise, when the doctor may be called to an emergency case at some distance from his main surgery, and then a second emergency occurs. A considerable amount of decision-making often has to rest with the doctor's receptionist, but through close involvement with their community, both doctors and receptionists come to have an insight into the lives, habits and personal idiosyncracies of their patients.

Maternity care is also a major problem for the doctors in the Highland Region. With the trend towards 100 per cent hospitalization, general practitioners have largely lost the obstetrical skills they once had. Thus the doctor has to weigh the risk of sending the patient to hospital too late against the cost to the woman and her family of a two-weeks' "unproductive" wait at a distant hospital. A further development consequent upon

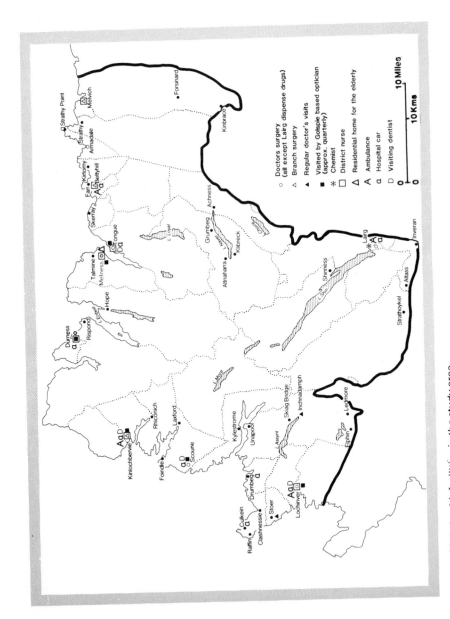

Figure 4. Main health facilities in the study area.

the closing of so many "cottage" hospitals, has been the increasing number of deliveries made in ambulances en route to the main hospitals.

Doctors in the area also have to commit themselves to difficult decisions regarding terminal cases. Often they are faced with the alternative of sending an elderly person to the main hospital in Inverness where up-to-date care and medical treatment can be provided, but this has to be considered in relation to the problem that members of the family will experience in visiting the patient. Elderly persons in some parts of the Highlands may never have left their immediate environment or neighbourhood during their lifetime, and to remove them to a large hospital at a great distance from their families and friends may not be the most humane decision. Thus in some cases, general practitioners need to consider carefully that, in the patient's interest, it may be better to leave them at home and to attempt to relieve pain and suffering by medical means.

Certain problems do exist with regard to the recruitment of doctors to the area. First, general practitioners can find it difficult to obtain the services of a locum if, for personal reasons, they must absent themselves from the area. Secondly, if they are family men with children, there are no secondary school facilities in the area, and this can be an important consideration for the doctors and their families (as it is for everyone else in the area).

District nurses play a crucial role in the area, and complement the general practitioners in several important ways. They have an extensive knowledge of the members of the local community, and in many cases have lived there for a long period. They often carry out preliminary diagnosis in so far as they are asked by patients, whether what they have "is worth troubling the doctor with". Occasionally, when the general practitioner is unavailable, they may treat emergency cases. District nurses are based at Melness, Tongue, Bettyhill, Melvich, Durness, Kinlochbervie and Lochinver.

There are no hospitals in the area. There are general hospitals at Golspie (23 beds, resident consultant surgeon, emergency maternity service, out-patient department) and Dingwall (40 beds, resident medical officer, out-patient department, maternity service), with out-patient clinics in all specialities, but many patients from north-west Sutherland requiring in-patient treatment must be admitted to the general and mental hospitals in Inverness. Specialist maternity units are located at Thurso, Inverness and Dingwall. Thurso also provides general and specialist facilities for the north-eastern part of the area. The Nicolson MacKenzie Hospital, just west of Dingwall, at Strathpeffer (15 beds) treats rheumatology patients from all parts of the Highlands.

Geriatric hospitals are at Wick, Bonar Bridge (about five miles south-east of Inveran) and The Mound, and residential homes for the elderly are located at Melness, Golspie, Thurso and Wick, and the Church of Scotland maintains homes at Reay and Dornoch. A new local authority home is to be built in Ullapool. At present, the only sheltered housing scheme in the area is that at Melness with four units plus "temporary care" accommodation for four more persons. Similar projects are being considered for other parts of the area. Seven units are due to be completed in Lochinver in 1982, and a Regional Council Day Care Centre in the same place is due for completion in 1984. This will cater for the elderly and others needing locally-based short-term care.

The area is served by ambulances based at Lochinver, Lairg, Bettyhill and Kinlochbervie. These ambulances are operated on a contract basis, whereby the contractor provides 24-hour cover and staff with a basic knowledge of first-aid. The service is supported by a large number of hospital service cars which are controlled, co-ordinated and financed by the Ambulance Service. Hospital cars are used where a patient, on medical grounds, cannot travel by public transport but does not require an ambulance. This allows ambulances to be used for accident and emergency patients. Hospital cars are located at Lochinver, Culkein, Bettyhill, Drumbeg, Lairg, Tongue, Durness, Scourie and Kinlochbervie. If necessary, ambulances or hospital car assistance can be provided from the contract centre at Ullapool and the full-time service stations at Golspie, Wick and Thurso. Backloading of ambulances and hospital cars returning from hospitals to the area forms a large part of the ambulance service commitment. Hospital authorities notify Ambulance Control 48 hours in advance of patients being discharged to the more remote parts of the area, and this enables control to co-ordinate home journeys and eliminate unnecessary mileage.

The resources of the ambulance service in north-west Sutherland are frequently stretched, mainly due to the long distances involved to the main hospitals at Thurso, Wick, Golspie and Inverness, and to the lack of public transport which, even when available, patients are reluctant to use because of the unsuitability for hospital appointment times.

The only chemist in the area is located at Lairg. However, the fact that the general practitioners dispense medicines does, of course, mean that patients in these remote areas have relatively easy access to medicines. Nevertheless the range of medicines available is somewhat restricted and where a GP does not have a required drug in stock, a prescription must be sent or taken to Lairg and this adds considerably to the cost. The local stores only carry a very limited range of proprietary preparations.

The work of the primary care teams is complemented by the special skills of dentists and opticians. These professions have a contractual relationship with the NHS which provides them with a nationally determined fee for each item of service but which does not, as in the case of the GPs and nurses, guarantee a minimum living income. As a result, members of these professions are more likely to practise in densely rather than sparsely populated areas so that professional overheads can be spread over a larger number of patients. Areas of low population density like this area therefore, have always had difficulty in attracting and retaining these professionals.

While many people in the area are relatively close to their GP, this does not hold for their proximity to opticians and dentists. For those living in the area, requiring these services usually means a period of waiting until one of the visiting practitioners has a session in the locality. Alternatively, whilst on holiday outside the area, they will arrange to visit some of these services.

The optician who serves the area is based at Golspie on the east coast of Sutherland (Fig. 1). Visits by the optician at three to six month intervals are made to the following settlements: Tongue, Melness, Durness, Scourie, Kinlochbervie and Lochinver. There are also opticians at Dingwall, Alness and Tain just outside the area.

Before 1974 the responsibility for providing dental care in the Highlands was, as elsewhere, divided. Local authorities provided preventive and curative care for school children and also gave dental care to expectant and nursing mothers, and young children. For other patients the dentist obtained payments from the NHS at a nationally determined fee for each item of service. Thus, as with opticians and pharmacists, this did not help to attract dentists to settlements as scattered as those in this area, because a large and easily accessible population was necessary to generate sufficient income. Dentists tended to settle in the towns on the east coasts of Sutherland and Caithness, and those who moved on were often hard to replace. There is the other problem connected with dentists who do not stay long in a practice, and that is the difficulty the local people have in building up a regular relationship with the dentist, when they are on the variable fringe of distant practices and when posts remain unfilled for periods of time.

The pattern of dental services is in a state of flux in 1982. Until 1979 the area was served by a two-man practice based in Dornoch on the east coast of Sutherland. One or other of the dentists visited one day each month in Melness, Tongue, Durness, Scourie, Kinlochbervie and Lochinver. One of the dentists retired and the remaining one could not maintain the schedule, and also plans to retire. The successor has decided to visit only Tongue, Scourie, Kinlochbervie and Lochinver and for smaller periods of time. Thus as has happened with optical problems, the population of the area use the far-flung network of emigrated relatives to arrange dental treatments for them in settlements outside the area, and these visits are often arranged during a holiday period. One outcome of this difficulty of obtaining dental care, is that the total tooth loss rate is much higher in this area than in other parts of Scotland (Adult Dental Health Survey, 1974). Complete clearances of teeth of also high in this area, but this is due in part to the difficulties of repeat visits to the dentist and to the fact that the preservation of natural teeth is not rated very highly by many people in the area. Problems also arise with the replacement of dentures. The tolerance of defects in false teeth, like the tendency to opt for extraction rather than filling, is a sign of the difficulties in making repeat visits to the dentist.

Conclusion

In the last two decades, centralization of health facilities has been pursued in many rural areas in Britain with the aims of providing more specialist facilities, and saving on resources (including staff), to the detriment of the accessibility of these services enjoyed by rural communities. As far as this particularly remote area is concerned, there has not been large-scale reduction, partly of course, because facilities were always sparse within the area. Of the hospitals serving the area, only the 14-bed General Pope Hospital in Helmsdale has been closed recently (1977) while general medical practices, though always reviewed on becoming vacant, have been maintained, and facilities for elderly people within the area are actually being increased.

There are nevertheless three types of problems which may be noted in connection with access to health facilities in north-west Sutherland. First, with regard to dental care, there is the physical difficulty experienced by the dentist in Dornoch in covering the area and the fact that many persons in the area are dependent on visiting dentists as far south as Edinburgh or Glasgow. Secondly, with optical services, again the problem is one of physical coverage by one practice of this vast area, and the fact that there is no grant scheme for patients visiting the optician.

One solution to both these problems would of course be to establish an optician and a dentist within the area, at Lochinver or Kinlochbervie, with heavy subsidies to meet the shortfall in income due to the small numbers involved. Naturally this could be expensive and the present economic climate is not conducive to such a step. Another approach would be to subsidize at a greater rate the visits of these practitioners to the area. This method of subsidizing facilities to come to the people rather than obliging people to travel is a direct alternative to the need for public transport felt by people without access to cars. A problem arising is that by taking more services into the area, fewer people are likely to travel by public transport (itself already subsidized) to places outside the area for the facilities they require. It should be noted that the Highland Health Board already effectively subsidized dental and optical services in their area to a total of £10,700 per year.

The third type of problem related to access to health facilities concerns both the patients themselves and also their visitors during hospital stays. The ambulance service is intended to be provided only on a medical certificate for those who are not fit to travel to a hospital by any other means. The expense which can fall on patients in the Highlands using public and private transport to travel between home and hospital is acknowledged in the Scottish Home and Health Department's Highlands and Islands Travelling Expenses Scheme for Hospital Patients. Patients who have to travel more than 30 miles to a hospital, and their escorts where required, are entitled to reclaim all but the first £1 of their travelling expenses. Unavoidable overnight expenses can also be reclaimed. In addition to this scheme, any person whose attendance at hospital involves financial difficulty can approach the Department of Health and Social Security for assistance.

Thus there is a "safety-net" which should ensure that no-one suffers financially through hospital attendance as a patient or escort. Difficulties arise, however, from the size of the study area and the pattern and timing of public transport. It has already been explained that many patients from the area have to go to Inverness. In 1978, approximately 20 per cent of in-patients from the area were in Inverness hospitals. A return journey between the study area and Inverness is only possible by rail, but bus services connecting with the trains do not allow onward same-day return trips. Only those patients or hospital visitors within reach of Lairg, Kinbrace or Forsinard stations by some means other than public transport can catch an early enough train to make the return journey possible. For most of the study area, an overnight stay is inevitable if public transport is used to make a trip to hospital as patient or as visitor, and the latter of course, cannot reclaim reimbursement of expenses or time lost.

Hospital visitors using public transport to and from Inverness therefore incur hardship in respect of time and money spent in travelling and overnight stays, and patients incur time losses in the same way (unless transported by ambulance or hospital car) though being reimbursed for travelling expenses (Figs 5 and 6). Added to all these problems are the adverse weather conditions in the winter and early spring, and the crowded roads in the tourist season. It might be argued that these are inevitable aspects of life in the Highlands, and that people adapt to this

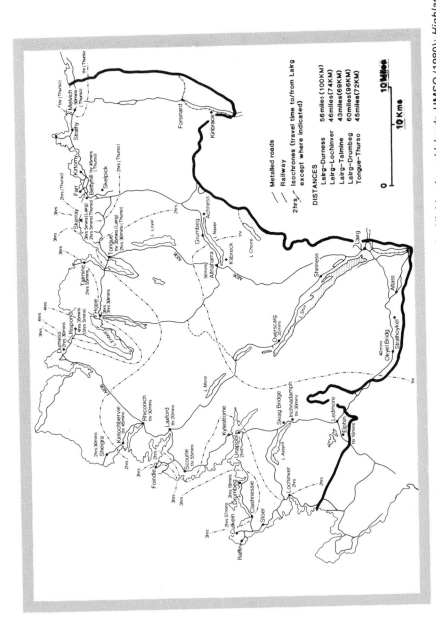

Figure 5. Distance/time relationships in the study area. Sources: *Getting Around the Highlands and Islands*, HMSO (1980); *Highlands Omnibus Timetable* (1980); *Post Office Postbus Timetable* (1980) AA Handbook (1979); O.S.½ʳ Map Sheet 3.

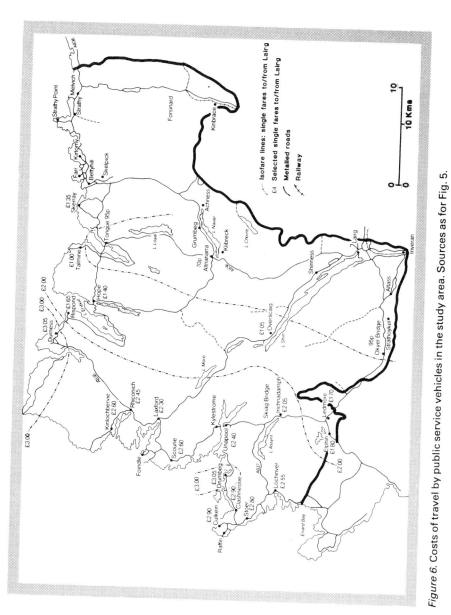

Figure 6. Costs of travel by public service vehicles in the study area. Sources as for Fig. 5.

inevitability, either by bowing to it and accepting the penalties of time and cost involved, or by arranging private transport through friends and relatives. The very scale of the study area, and the distances involved in reaching facilities which are well outside the area, would seem to indicate that any improvement in the future would be difficult to achieve.

References

Birsay Report (1967). *General Medical Services in the Highlands and Islands*. HMSO, Edinburgh.

Farrington, J. H., Stanley, P. A. and Bain, S. M. (1981). *Public Transport in North West Sutherland*. Department of Geography, University of Aberdeen.

Highland Regional Council (1980). *Transport Policies and Programmes, 1980–85.* Highland Regional Council, Inverness.

Hillman, M., Henderson, I., and Whalley, A. (1973). Personal Mobility and Transport Policy. PEP Broadsheet No. 567.

Moseley, M., Harman, R. G., Coles, O. B. and Spencer, M. B. (1977). *Rural Transport and Accessibility*, 2 vols. Geo Books.

Office of Population (1974). *Adult Dental Health in Scotland*. Censuses and Surveys. HMSO, Edinburgh.

Cigarette Smoking among New Zealanders: evidence from the 1976 census

L. D. Brian Heenan

Department of Geography, University of Otago, Dunedin, New Zealand

Smoking as a health hazard

There is a consensus in the medical literature that the habit of smoking, especially cigarettes, presents or is suspected of presenting a significant risk factor for a spectrum of diseases. Current evidence points to higher rates of general mortality among smokers compared with non-smokers, and in particular to their greater susceptibility to chronic respiratory symptoms, emphysema and lung cancer. Smokers too are more likely than non-smokers to suffer from myocardial infarction, coronary heart disease and sudden death, and in addition pregnant women who smoke cigarettes tend to produce large proportions of babies affected by lower foetal birth weight and reduced foetal breathing movement (O'Donnell, 1978).

In effect, while the hazards to human health associated with smoking are understood with some certainty, much less is known about the characteristics of those who smoke, where they live, why they do so, and effective means of preventing the habit. In the search for answers to these questions, medical geographers appear to have made little contribution so far. Yet clearly the geographer has a role to play, if one accepts the proposition that medical geography is or can be the spatial analysis of problems related to most aspects of human health (Pyle, 1979), and, more specifically, that a primary concern of the medical geographer is to elucidate where diseases and their known and suspected causative agents are occurring (McGlashan, 1967).

GEOGRAPHICAL ASPECTS OF HEALTH
ISBN 0 12 483780 8

Thus the present essay was inspired by the contention that New Zealanders who smoke cigarettes are differentially distributed through the population in terms of both where they live and their socio-demographic characteristics. The contention is evaluated through an examination of the 1976 census data on the broad regional distribution and national (i.e. total population) age–sex, ethnic and occupational affiliations of respondents classified as current cigarette smokers.

Health-related questions in the New Zealand census

With a small number of notable exceptions (e.g. Borman, 1980), the modern population census has not developed as a particularly rich source of data for research in medical geography. The census itself is not widely, regularly or intensively used to collect health-related information. One reason for this is that competing claims for information on other topics makes it difficult to justify more than one or perhaps two, if any, such questions in the census questionnaire. More importantly perhaps are doubts about the quality and usefulness of self-reported health-related data obtained from the census. For instance, some eligible respondents might not answer the relevant question(s) at all, while others may do so, but in a way which does not fit specifications which guide data processing.

An added problem is that of misreporting. Although comparable data are not yet available for New Zealand, there are indications that census under-reporting of smoking habits can be substantial, perhaps as high as 30 per cent in many countries (Cherry and Forbes, 1979). They argue that under-reporting is likely to be particularly marked among 15–19 year-olds (as much as 70 per cent in Canada), because their smoking habits are often reported on the census form by the head of household acting in a proxy role.

Health-related questions have been included in the personal schedule used in each of the last three New Zealand censuses. The earliest, in 1971, sought information on methods of treatment from respondents "under care for diabetes". This question was replaced in 1976 by one on current cigarette smoking, including the number smoked "yesterday", that is the day before the census. A similar question was again included in the 1981 census.

Respondents to the question in 1976, and aged 15 years or older, were distributed among four major categories. The first included those who had never smoked cigarettes regularly or at all; the second, persons who "do not smoke now, but used to smoke regularly (one or more cigarettes per day)"; the third, respondents who "now smoke regularly (one or more cigarettes per day)"; and, finally, those who did not supply sufficient information to qualify for inclusion in one or other of the above three smoking practice categories.

Although "not specified" cases represented only 3·2 per cent of the total population, there was considerable variation between sub-groups. For example, by ethnic status (as defined in Table 1, footnotes d–f), the lowest proportion was for the European group (3 per cent), followed by the Maori (5·3 per cent), then the Pacific Island Polynesian (6·7 per cent). Proportions for each sex were similar. By age, "not specified" was most frequent among those in their late teens (15–19 years), but again with a marked discrepancy between the European (3·5 per cent) and each of the principal Polynesian groups (Maori, 8·6 per cent; Pacific Island Polynesian, 9·0 per cent). Unless otherwise stated, the analysis presented below is confined to specified cases of cigarette smoking as recorded on the 1976 census personal questionnaire.

General incidence of cigarette smoking

A total of 758,550 persons, that is 35·6 per cent of the total (specified) population, declared themselves to be regular cigarette smokers at the 1976 census. A further 353,627 (16·6 per cent) indicated that they had smoked regularly in the past but no longer did so, while the remainder (1,017,942, or 47·8 per cent) maintained that they had never smoked regularly or at all. In other words, given the known health risks associated with the smoking habit, over half of the specified total population were currently directly exposed or had been in the past.

Marked differences exist in smoking practice between the sexes however. Fully two-fifths (39·6 per cent) of the men were current smokers in 1976, whereas among women the figure was less than a third (31·7 per cent). Nevertheless, proportionately more males (21·7 per cent) than females (11·6 per cent) had once smoked regularly but were not current smokers at the 1976 census. These figures suggest that males are much more likely than females to break the habit, an interpretation supported by more or less comparable sample statistics from the 1981 census. Between 1976 and 1981 the proportion of males who had once smoked regularly, but who had recanted before the 1981 census, rose from 21·7 to 23·8 per cent, while over the same period the number of current regular smokers declined from 39·6 to 34·6 per cent. Comparable figures for women were 56·4 and 56·7 per cent, and 31·7 and 29·4 per cent respectively.

Table 1. Total (crude) and age–sex adjusted current smoking rates, by ethnic group and sex, census 1976

Ethnic group	Male				Female			
	TSR^a	ASR^b	% Dev.^{c}	χ^2	TSR^a	ASR^b	% Dev.^{c}	χ^2
European^d	383	—	—		299	—	—	
New Zealand Maori^e	561	829	+116·5	**	594	1096	+267·1	**
Cook Island Maori^f	455	547	+40·1	**	314	464	+55·5	**
Samoan^f	447	537	+27·1	**	177	93	−220·2	**
Niuean^f	465	487	+47·3	**	287	259	−13·4	*
Tokelauan^f	506	565	+91·1	**	299	278	−6·8	
Tongan^f	554	732	+102·3	**	226	153	−48·7	**
Pacific Island Polynesian^{f,g}	462	775	+42·8	**	243	177	−40·8	**

^{a} Total smoking rate: number of current cigarette smokers per 1000 total population (specified only).
^{b} Age-adjusted smoking rate (with European age-specific smoking rates as the standard).
^{c} Per cent deviation above (+) or below (−) the European average.
^{d} Comprises persons not included as either New Zealand Maori or Pacific Island Polynesian.
^{e} Includes persons who specified themselves as half or more New Zealand Maori, plus those who indicated that they were persons of the Maori race of New Zealand but did not specify the degree of Maori origin.
^{f} Persons of half or more descent except for half Pacific Island–half New Zealand Maori persons who have been included in the New Zealand Maori grouping.
^{g} Also includes small numbers of persons of Polynesian ethnic groups additional to those listed.
Note: χ^2 (1 df.) significant at 95 (*) or 99 (**) per cent.

Cigarette smoking among ethnic groups

Statistics on smoking practice from the 1976 census were made available for two major ethnic fractions of the population, namely, New Zealand Maori and Pacific Island Polynesian. The latter comprised five sub-groups more or less defined by island(s) of origin, those being Cook Island Maori, Samoan, Niuean, Tokelauan and Tongan. However, by subtracting figures for the New Zealand Maori and Pacific Island Polynesian groups from those for the New Zealand total population it is possible to obtain data for a third major ethnic category, the so-called European component described in Table 1. The vast majority in this group are of European stock, together with small numbers of Chinese, Indians, and so on.

Total (crude) and age–sex adjusted (using the European rates as the standard) rates for the several ethnic groups are presented in Table 1. Concerning males, the principal point to be made is that both total (TSR) and age-adjusted (ASR) smoking rates for each polynesian fraction are much higher than the standard (European) rate. Moreover the ASR is invariably statistically significant ($p < 0.01$). For two groups, the Maori and Tongan, the incidence of regular cigarette smoking is more than twice the occurrence among Europeans, and not much less than twice in a third, namely the Tokelauan.

The pattern of relationships among women is more complicated but several remarkable points emerge from Table 1. One is the sharp contrast drawn between the exceptionally high TSR and ASR for Maori women, and the below average (i.e. the European standard = 298·6) rates recorded for females in each of the Polynesian groups apart from the Cook Island Maori. Indeed the crude (TSR) and standardized smoking rates for Maori women are in fact higher than comparable rates for males in every ethnic group listed in Table 1. Furthermore, Samoan women are evidently much less addicted to cigarette smoking than are other Polynesian females, a finding also consistent with the comparatively low incidence among Samoan men in New Zealand (Table 1).

Age–sex distribution of current smokers

The smoking habit is found among European and Polynesian New Zealanders in all age–sex categories, but to varying degrees within and between the three major ethnic groups (Fig. 1, Table 2). Several noteworthy features emerge from Fig. 1. First, at every age, rates for Pacific Island Polynesian males, together with both Maori men *and* Maori women,

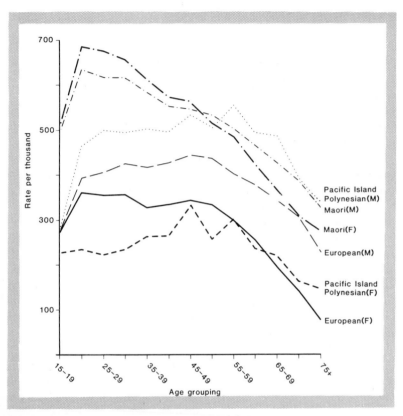

Figure 1. Age–sex specific rates of current regular smoking for major ethnic groupings, 1976 census.

exceed the comparable rate for European men (and for that matter European women as well).

A second point is the unusually heavy frequency of cigarette smoking among young adult Maori men and women, such that peak rates are much higher and reached earlier than in almost every other ethnic grouping. Indeed, as indicated by a percentage conversion of the rates in Table 2, over half (two-thirds among women in their twenties) of Maori males and females in each age grouping from 20–24 to 55–59 and 15–19 to 50–54 years, respectively, were smoking cigarettes regularly at the 1976 census. In contrast, age-specific rates for European and, especially, younger Pacific Island Polynesian women, appear abnormally low.

Thirdly, the unusual pattern of cigarette smoking among Maoris is reinforced by the peculiar relationships between rates of smoking for younger male and female adults. Unlike any other ethnic group, the

Table 2. Age and sex specific current smoking rates by ethnic group, census 1976

Ethnic group	Age-specific rates per 1000 (rounded)													
	15–19	20–24	25–29	30–34	35–39	40–44	45–49	50–54	55–59	60–64	65–69	70–74	75+	Total
	Former smokers													
European male[a]	53	105	151	184	208	240	275	324	353	367	403	423	425	225
European female[a]	65	114	137	140	130	131	135	143	151	152	150	127	92	125
Maori male[b]	74	103	133	143	152	158	171	179	195	211	211	261	247	133
Maori female[b]	83	106	144	111	111	128	121	121	126	145	148	153	150	110
Pacific Is. Polynesian male[c]	59	92	88	90	115	120	129	151	109	121	142	254	196	97
Pacific Is. Polynesian female[c]	55	77	60	55	56	69	61	82	119	98	80	129	149	66
	Current smokers													
European male[a]	275	394	407	425	418	428	443	435	401	380	345	305	239	383
European female[a]	275	362	356	358	329	337	346	334	299	255	198	142	78	299
Maori male[b]	496	637	619	619	584	552	546	534	502	467	428	389	329	561
Maori female[b]	512	685	678	659	611	573	562	514	487	423	368	308	276	594
Pacific Is. Polynesian male[c]	285	465	500	494	503	498	534	507	555	497	489	394	333	462
Pacific Is. Polynesian female[c]	228	236	222	235	263	266	333	256	301	238	221	164	149	243

[a] Comprises persons not included as either New Zealand Maori or Pacific Island Polynesian.

[b] Includes persons who specified themselves as half or more New Zealand Maori, plus those who indicated that they were persons of the Maori race of New Zealand but did not specify the degree of Maori origin.

[c] Persons of half or more descent except for half Pacific Island–half New Zealand Maori persons who have been included in the New Zealand Maori grouping.

frequency of cigarette smoking among women is the greater of the two at every age from 15–19 to 45–49 years (Fig. 1).

The age–sex specific curves of current smoking depicted in Fig. 1 for Pacific Island Polynesians are closely followed, broadly speaking, by those for each of the component ethnic sub-groupings. However, as one might anticipate given their above-standard (European) ASR, the rates for Cook Island Maori women are generally higher, and in addition, the occurrence of regular cigarette smoking among Tokelauan men aged 45–49 to 55–59 years is of exceptional frequency (45–49, 655 per 1000 specified cases; 50–54, 762; 55–59, 846), but the samples involved are small ones.

One further point well captured in Table 2 is the apparently greater reluctance of Maoris and Pacific Island Polynesians to forsake the smoking habit compared with Europeans. This is certainly so overall as well as in most age–sex groupings. The contrast presumably reflects interactions between a number of influences, among them the recency of the cigarette smoking habit among Pacific Island Polynesians, perhaps as a concomitant of immigration and consequent urbanization; the very low incidence of the custom among Pacific Island Polynesian women; and, among Maoris, the probability that the health risks associated with heavy cigarette smoking take their toll in mortality before the habit is broken.

Cigarette smoking among male occupations

Information on cigarette smoking practice gathered at the 1976 census was made available for a range of qualitative attributes linked to the total national population only, rather than cross-tabulated with the different systematic (e.g. ethnic groupings) and spatial (e.g. statistical and urban areas) sub-categories of the population defined by the census. Qualitative attributes covered included head of household and type of dwelling, fertility (number of children born to ever-married females aged 16 years and over), religious profession, income, hours worked, occupation and geographical location. Limited space precludes consideration of all of these aspects, and for this reason the discussion is confined to two only, namely, current regular smoking among males aged 15 years and older by occupational grouping, and place of residence represented by the 13 statistical areas into which the country is divided for census purposes.

Total (TSR) and age-adjusted (ASR) rates of current regular smoking for each major occupation grouping are presented in Table 3. These suggest that, generally speaking, cigarette smoking is much less popular in three (Table 3: 0/1, 2, 3) of the four so-called white collar groupings than one

Table 3. Total (crude) and age adjusted current smoking rates for major occupation groups, males only, census 1976

Major group code	Occupation group	TSR[a]	ASR[b]	% Dev.[c]	χ^2
0/1	Professional, technical and related	270	179	−53·2	**
2	Administrative and managerial	270	240	−37·4	**
3	Clerical	380	363	−5·2	**
4	Sales	416	420	+9·8	*
5	Service	477	584	+52·5	**
6	Agricultural, etc., workers	371	346	−9·6	**
7/8/9	Production, etc., workers	486	592	+54·6	**

[a] Total smoking rate: number of current cigarette smokers per 1000 total population (specified only).
[b] Age-adjusted smoking rate (with European age-specific smoking rates as the standard).
[c] Per cent deviation above (+) or below (−) the European average.
Note: χ^2 (1 df.) significant at 95 (*) or 99 (**) per cent.

finds in blue collar jobs. This is especially so of those in Service or classified as Production, etc., workers (major groupings 5 and 7/8/9), contrasted with the much lower rates recorded for men employed in Agriculture (major grouping 6).

Although direct evidence from the census is lacking, the occupationally-related cigarette smoking rates for males are undoubtedly weighted to some extent by a Maori/Pacific Island Polynesian ethnic factor. In so far as both ethnic groupings were in 1976 largely urbanized, they are under-represented in the low-rate white collar occupation groupings (0/1, 2, and 3 (as well as 4)), and over-represented in unskilled or semi-skilled manual positions with work descriptions which place them in the high-rate occupation groupings, Service (5) and Production, etc., (7/8/9).

Moreover it should be recognized that considerable differences in rates of current regular cigarette smoking among males may and clearly do occur within the major occupation groupings listed in Table 3. The point is very well documented by rates for minor occupation groupings comprising one low-rate major grouping, 0/1: Professional, technical and related workers (Table 4), and one high-rate major grouping, 5: Service workers (Table 5). Of particular note in the low-rate case are the abnormally high, statistically significant ($p < 0.01$) rates for Composers and Performing Artists (minor grouping 1711–1799) and Athletes and Sportsmen (minor grouping 1801–1809). This last finding begins to raise serious questions about the impact on the frequency of cigarette smoking among sportsmen in this country, of now commonplace sponsorship

Table 4. Total (crude) and age adjusted current smoking rates for occupation minor groups comprising occupation major group 0/1 (professional, technical and related workers), males only, census 1976

Minor group code	Occupation group	n	TSR[a]	ASR[b]	% Dev.[c]	χ^2
0110–0149	Physical scientists	835	248	148	−61·4	**
0211–0390	Architects, engineers	7973	268	177	−53·7	**
0411–0430	Aircraft and Ship's Officers	1034	476	370	−3·3	**
0511–0549	Life scientists	922	246	148	−61·4	**
0611–0799	Medical, dental, veterinary	3404	291	207	−46·0	**
0810–0849	Statisticians, mathematicians, etc.	482	272	180	−52·9	**
0901–0909	Economists	164	258	159	−58·6	**
1101–1109	Accountants	2454	249	152	−60·4	**
1211–1290	Jurists	898	259	166	−56·7	**
1311–1399	Teachers	5376	234	134	−65·1	**
1411–1490	Workers in religion	340	122	36	−90·5	**
1510–1599	Authors, journalists	816	382	365	−4·6	
1610–1639	Sculptors, painters, etc.	1034	344	290	−24·2	**
1711–1799	Composers and performing artists	814	453	539	+40·8	**
1801–1809	Athletes, sportsmen	401	473	618	+61·3	**
1911–1990	Other	1364	328	262	−31·5	**
Major group 0/1		28,311	270	179	−53·2	**

[a] Total smoking rate: number of current cigarette smokers per 1000 total population (specified only).
[b] Age-adjusted smoking rate (with European age-specific smoking rates as the standard).
[c] Per cent deviation above (+) or below (−) the European average.
Note: χ^2 (1 df.) significant at 95 (*) or 99 (**) per cent.

of sporting events by New Zealand tobacco producing and marketing firms.

Useful information from the census on cigarette smoking practice by occupation does not end there however; it also provides evidence of the existence of major differentiation between related workers in the same minor groupings of occupation. For example, also using 1976 census data, Hay (1980a,b) found sharply contrasted proportions of current regular cigarette smokers among doctors and nurses (occupation minor grouping 0611–0799). Nurses in general, men and women together, exhibited very high proportions of smokers, the habit being most prevalent among those in community and psychiatric work (Hay, 1980b). Among doctors on the other hand a much smaller percentage declared themselves to be regular smokers (Hay, 1980a). This outcome is not unexpected, given an earlier decline in cigarette smoking among New Zealand doctors documented by independent survey data (Christmas and Hay, 1976), which in turn is consistent with recent British experience (Doll and Peto, 1976).

Table 5. Total (crude) and age-adjusted current smoking rates for minor occupation groups comprising major group 5 (Service workers), males only, census 1976

Minor group code	Occupation group	n	TSR[a]	ASR[b]	% Dev.[c]	χ^2
5001–5009	Managers (catering, lodging services)	1114	512	625	+63·1	**
5101–5109	Working proprietors	1702	465	508	+32·7	**
5201–5209	Housekeeping, etc., supervisors	132	478	534	+39·5	
5311–5329	Cooks, waiters, bartenders	3887	587	898	+134·3	**
5401–5409	Maids and related	400	550	746	+94·8	**
5510–5529	Building caretakers, etc.	2921	418	529	−38·2	**
5601–5609	Launderers, etc.	545	531	701	+83·1	**
5701–5709	Hairdressers, etc.	492	467	542	+41·4	**
5811–5899	Protective service workers	9595	457	525	+37·0	**
5911–5999	Other	1899	472	562	+46·7	**
Major group 5		22,687	477	584	+52·5	**

[a] Total smoking rate: number of current cigarette smokers per 1000 total population (specified only).
[b] Age-related smoking rate (with European age-specific smoking rates as the standard).
[c] Per cent deviation above (+) or below (−) the European average.
Note: χ^2 (1 df.) significant at 95 (*) or 99 (**) per cent.

Cigarette smoking by region of residence

Data on cigarette smoking practice from the 1976 census of New Zealand was made available for two kinds of area unit, these being the 13 major regions represented by statistical areas (SA), as mapped in Fig. 2, and the 24 urban areas. It is differences in current regular smoking rates among males and females (both total population and Maori) in SA which are of concern here.

The differences in cigarette smoking practice between males and females which emerged in the earlier discussion are sufficiently large to justify the separate treatment of the sexes in considering the regional incidence of the habit as documented in Table 6. Clearly, while the two distributions are broadly similar, important differences occur in detail. Whether one takes the TSR or ASR set, the male rate is invariably higher than the female, but the extent to which regional ASR alone vary above or below the appropriate standard rate (European male 383 per 1000 specified cases; European female 298·6) is much greater among females than it is among males.

Nevertheless the location of high (above standard) and low (below standard) incidence regions is similar among males and females. Thus rates are lowest in the centrally situated more or less contiguous regions

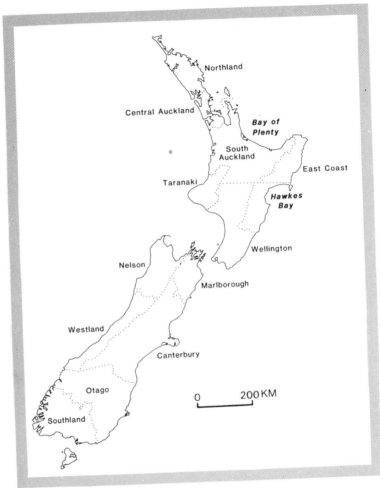

Figure 2. Statistical areas (SA) used for the New Zealand population census, 1976.

of Wellington (males only), Marlborough, Nelson and Canterbury, and they tend to increase to both the north and south of these SA. For both sexes, regular cigarette smoking is most frequently practised in the East Coast SA, but female rates in particular remain very high over most of the North Island. This in turn enables one to draw a general distinction between that island and the South Island where noticeably lower above- or below-average female ASR prevail. A similar pattern is apparent among males, except that the incidence among Southland men is second only to the male rate for the East Coast.

Table 6. Total (crude) and age–sex adjusted current smoking rates for statistical areas (SA), census 1976 total population

Statistical area	TSR[a]	ASR[b]	% Dev.[c]	χ^2	TSR[a]	ASR[b]	% Dev.[c]	χ^2
	Male				Female			
Northland	395	397	+3·6		323	345	+15·6	**
Central Auckland	395	394	+2·8		322	372	+24·7	**
South Auckland	405	427	+11·5	**	337	372	+24·5	**
East Coast	426	473	+23·6	**	361	434	+45·2	**
Hawkes Bay	416	451	+17·8	**	331	367	+10·6	**
Taranaki	400	417	+8·9	**	308	317	+6·2	*
Wellington	398	367	−4·1	**	328	357	+19·3	**
Marlborough	368	356	−7·1	*	282	268	−10·2	*
Nelson	376	370	−3·4		280	264	−11·7	**
Westland	393	411	+7·2	*	314	330	+10·4	*
Canterbury	373	364	−5·0	**	281	267	−10·7	**
Otago	398	418	+9·0	**	303	312	+4·4	**
Southland	423	465	+21·4	**	312	323	+8·3	**

[a] Total smoking rate: number of current cigarette smokers per 1000 total population (specified only).
[b] Age-adjusted smoking rate (with European age-specific smoking rates as the standard).
[c] Per cent deviation above (+) or below (−) the European average.
Note: χ^2 (1 df.) significant at 95 (*) or 99 (**) per cent.

In effect, the general geographical pattern among both males and females tends to be bi-modal, with incidence peaks lying toward the south of the South Island and in the east and north of the North Island. An obvious question raised by the spatial arrangement of frequency rates for the total population is the extent to which the level of those rates is influenced by cigarette smoking among Maoris. In as much that the age–sex adjusted (ASR) rates for SA are almost invariably twice as high as the equivalent standard population rate (Table 7), then it may be said that the Maori factor tends to raise the total rate, though this influence will vary according to the relative importance in each SA of Maori compared with non-Maori (European) current regular smokers.

Thus the impact of the Maori factor is greatest in the four North Island SA (Northland, Central Auckland, South Auckland and the East Coast) in which most Maoris live. For instance, when Maoris are excluded from the calculations, ASR for men and women (female figures in brackets) change as follows: Northland: total, 396·8 (345·3), non-Maori, 354·3 (266·8); Central Auckland: total, 393·8 (372·2), non-Maori, 370·8 (332·1); South Auckland, total, 427·0 (371·6), non-Maori, 384·6 (290·9); East Coast, 473·5 (433·6), non-Maori, 295·3 (308·5). In other words, in the East Coast case in particular, the sex-specific ASR are elevated well above the standard rate as a consequence of cigarette smoking practice among Maoris. On the other hand total ASR for males and females living in other SA, especially

Table 7. Total (crude) and age–sex adjusted current smoking rates for Maori population in each statistical area (SA), census 1976

Statistical area	TSR[a]	ASR[b]	% Dev.[c]	χ^2	TSR[a]	ASR[b]	% Dev.[c]	χ^2
		Male				Female		
Northland	526	668	+74·4	**	541	892	+198·8	**
Central Auckland	578	834	+117·8	**	618	1124	+276·5	**
South Auckland	555	808	+111·1	**	590	1216	+307·1	**
East Coast	515	696	+81·6	**	532	920	+208·3	**
Hawkes Bay	561	828	+116·2	**	567	998	+234·3	**
Taranaki	557	816	+112·9	**	580	1062	+255·8	**
Wellington	568	859	+124·2		619	1179	+294·8	**
Marlborough	505	668	+74·5	**	564	998	+234·2	**
Nelson	572	850	+121·9	**	626	1226	+310·6	**
Westland	578	868	+126·7	**	621	1197	+300·7	**
Canterbury	569	861	+124·8	**	605	1132	+279·2	**
Otago	591	909	+137·2	**	601	1126	+276·9	**
Southland	627	1004	+164·4	**	618	1182	+295·7	**

[a] Total smoking rate: number of current cigarette smokers per 1000 total population (specified only).
[b] Age-adjusted smoking rate (with European age-specific smoking rates as the standard).
[c] Per cent deviation above (+) or below (−) the European average.
Note: χ^2 (1 df.) significant at 95 (*) or 99 (**) per cent.

those in the South Island, are to a greater extent determined by cigarette consumption among non-Maoris. This is so in Southland, where the non-Maori male ASR (447·8) is just 3·7 per cent less than the figure of 465·0 for the male total population. Hence the explanation of cigarette smoking practice among Southland men must be sought in parameters other than those of an ethnic (i.e. Maori/Polynesian) character.

Conclusion

Data drawn from the New Zealand census of 1976 confirm the existence of substantial differentiation in current cigarette smoking practice among New Zealanders. The selection of topics examined in this essay reveals intriguing and often large disparities between male and female, by age and ethnic identity, among the various male occupation groupings, and from one region to another. Perhaps one of the most essential and unhealthy facts documented is the high frequency of cigarette smoking among Maori females and Maori and Pacific Island Polynesian males generally, and in particular among younger Maoris of both sexes. Clearly, the implied health risks are potentially very serious, and for Maoris at least there is strong circumstantial evidence to the effect that the hazards are being realized. That they, compared with non-Maoris, are to varying degrees more frequently afflicted with virtually all of the health risks identified in the first paragraph of this essay, is well documented in a succession of studies over the last two decades (se, for example, Rose, 1960; Borrie *et al.*, 1973; Heenan, 1976; Pomare, 1980).

Precise knowledge on the nature of variation in cigarette smoking habits between different segments of the population is of course a critical requirement if effective preventive intervention programmes are to be developed. In pursuit of such knowledge the information provided by the census has considerable actual or potential utility as a starting point in the search to identify those groups most at risk, and those which should become the target of health education and related intervention strategies. In this regard, as the present essay demonstrates, the medical geographer has a worthwhile contribution to make. Because of the particular analytical tools at his disposal, and the peculiar nature of his disciplinary perspective he is well placed to work with health and related personnel in seeking to identify those who smoke cigarettes, why they do so, and where they live.

References

Borman, B. (1980). Diabetes mellitus morbidity in New Zealand: a geographic perspective. *Soc. Sci. Med.* **14D**, 185–189.

Borrie,J., Rose, R. J., Spears, G. F. S. and Holmes, G. A. (1973). *Cancer of the Lung in New Zealand*. New Zealand Dept. of Health, Special Report No. 42, Wellington.

Cherry, W. H. and Forbes, W. F. (1979). Cigarette smoking in New Zealand. *N.Z. Med. Jl.* **89**, 448.

Christmas, B. W. and Hay, D. R. (1976). The smoking habits of New Zealand doctors: a review after 10 years. *N.Z. Med. Jl.* **83**, 391–394.

Doll, R. and Peto, R. (1976). Mortality in relation to smoking: 20 years observation on male British doctors. *Br. Med. Jl.* **2**, 1525–1536.

Hay, D. R. (1980a). Cigarette smoking by New Zealand doctors: results from the 1976 population census. *N.Z. Med. Jl.* **91**, 285–288.

Hay, D. R. (1980b). The smoking habits of nurses in New Zealand: results from the 1976 New Zealand census. *N.Z. Med. Jl.* **92**, 391–393.

Heenan, L. D. B. (1976). Differential general and respiratory disease mortality among birthplace groupings in New Zealand. *Jl. Chron. Dis.* **29**, 759–771.

McGlashan, N. D. (1967). Geographical evidence on medical hypotheses. *Trop. & Geogr. Med.* **19**, 333–343.

O'Donnell, T. V. (1978). Smoking and New Zealand health. *N.Z. Med. Jl.* **88**, 62–65.

Pomare, E. W. (1980). *Maori Standards of Health: A Study of the Period 1955–1975*. Medical Research Council of New Zealand, Special Report Series, No. 7, Auckland.

Pyle, G. F. (1979). *Applied Medical Geography*. John Wiley and Sons, London.

Rose, R. J. (1960). *Maori–European Standards of Health*. New Zealand Dept. of Health, Special Report No. 1, Wellington.

Scale in the relationship between behaviour and disease

Robert W. Roundy
Department of Human Ecology,
Rutgers University, New Brunswick, New Jersey, USA

Lynn M. Roundy
John F. Kennedy Medical Center, Edison,
New Jersey, USA

and

Ted Nawalinski
Smith Kline Animal Products, West Chester,
Pennsylvania, USA

Introduction

Medical geographers and other social scientists are in the habit of assuming that normative (i.e. typical or average) community behaviour plays a major role in the transmission and prevalence of a disease. We assume that higher prevalence rates result from theoretically conducive behaviour; i.e. that those who do the most to protect themselves from disease will achieve the greatest protection while those who place themselves most at risk will suffer the most.

Behaviour and disease in medical geography

This essential assumption is inherent, at various scales of inquiry, in the classic studies of human behaviour–disease ecology interaction published in medical geography since the Second World War (May, 1950, 1958, 1961; Audy, 1965, 1972; Learmonth, 1965) and continues to be made

GEOGRAPHICAL ASPECTS OF HEALTH
ISBN 0 12 483780 8

in the more recent medical geographical studies of communicable diseases, for example Roundy (1976, 1978, 1979, 1980). Valued accounts of specific disease problems either have been generated by this assumption or have drawn this conclusion.

There are retrospective geographical studies of epidemics that diffused through susceptible populations that both hypothesized and legitimately concluded that human behavioural patterns influenced the speed and direction of the epidemic spread. Hunter and Young (1971) showed the significance of community factors (e.g. social and economic interaction) and household factors (e.g. room density and economic well-being) to the success and spatial patterns of an influenza epidemic transmitted from person to person. Pyle (1969) and Stock (1976) independently modelled the diffusion pattern of cholera epidemics, Pyle showing the importance of community behaviour, especially the development and use of communication and transport systems in nineteenth century cholera epidemics in the United States, and Stock showing the relevance of behaviours at the community, family and individual level to cholera in West Africa in more recent years.

Infectious hazards also possess a human behaviour component to their success. Examples of such endemic-like hazards include a number of disease agents that obligatorily alternate between human and non-human hosts through their life-cycle. Most of the examples in Hughes and Hunter's (1970) classic review of economic development activities in Africa and resultant increased disease hazards are of diseases possessing obligatory non-human hosts. Field or review studies also exist specifically for schistosomiasis (Dalton, 1976; Dalton and Pole, 1978; Kloos *et al.*, 1980–1981), malaria (Prothero, 1965; Fonaroff, 1968; Learmonth, 1957), onchocerciasis (river blindness) (Hunter, 1966, 1980; Bradley, 1976), the trypanosomiases (Knight, 1971; Prothero, 1963; Matzke, 1979; Van Wettere-Verhasselt, 1969–1970; Haddock, 1979) and various mosquito-borne filariae (Dunn, 1976).

There are also endemic environmental infectious hazards without obligatory non-human hosts associated at some scale with human behaviour. Behaviour such as defaecation habits, personal hygiene, and food preparation and handling can be relevant to the transmission of the geohelminths, intestinal parasites such as hookworm, *Ascaris lumbricoides*, and *Trichuris trichiura* that spend a part of their life-cycle as eggs and larvae in the soil. Although not well studied in the geographical literature (however, see Gaál and Márton, 1980; Takemoto *et al.*, 1981), researchers in cognate fields have shown reasonably reliable associations between infection and behaviour in selected environments (Dunn, 1972; Kochar *et al.*, 1976).

Besides infectious diseases, the occurrence of diseases of other aetiologies such as nutritional deficiencies (Wilson, 1979; Newman, 1980) and toxic disorders (Hunter, 1976, 1978) are also assumed to be associated with human behaviour. Diseases of unknown aetiologies, such as some cancers, have been investigated with varying success by geographers with the underlying assumption that certain behaviours in specific environments are highly influential in determining the distribution of the cancer and who, either as individuals or as groups within given communities, are most likely eventually to show evidence of the cancer (Armstrong, 1976; Armstrong *et al.*, 1978; McGlashan, 1972, 1977).

All of these studies succeeded to some degree in showing the significance of the interaction between human behaviour, local environments, and causative agents, parasitological or otherwise, in generating spatial, temporal and social disease patterns. But it is not clear that human behaviour always dominantly explains disease occurrence. Furthermore, in a reiteration of the notion of the ecological fallacy, it is possible in some circumstances that it is not normative behaviour that is responsible for disease patterns, but rather individual, discrete events and activities of a fortuitous nature that lead to infections. While large-scale and retrospective studies may explain how infected people came to be at risk, small-scale and concurrent studies may not be able to explain which individual is now, or will be, at risk.

The significance of normative behaviour

We can illustrate the question of the significance of normative behaviour with the results of a study in peninsular Malaysia which is unique in several ways: (a) the pathogenic intestinal protozoa studied are not commonly considered in the geographical literature; (b) these species do not disrupt, and were not reported by, the human population, indicating either low levels of virulence and pathology or an acceptance of any discomfort; and (c) recent social, economic, cultural and technological changes in the study communities tend to jeopardize the success of the disease system.

The study project

The project lasted from December, 1976 until late 1978. It represents the collaborative efforts of a geographer, parasitologist, medical technologist and field and laboratory assistants.

Two pairs of Malay villages were studied. One pair, Kampong Lubok Kelubi and Kampong Masjid, are located about 40 km by good road south from Kuala Lumpur in Ulu Langat Subdistrict of Selangor State.

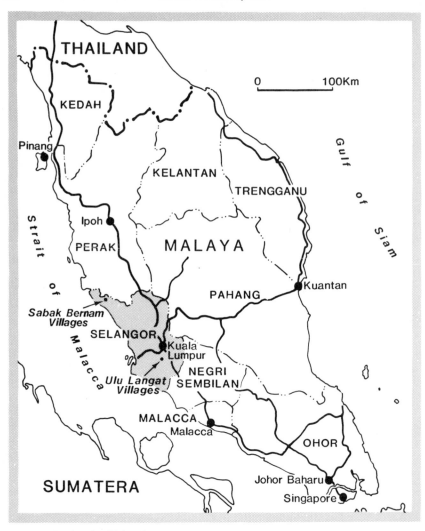

Figure 1. Peninsular Malaysia.

The second pair, Kampong Tok Khalifah and Kampong Parit 9, are about 128 km by good road north-west of Kuala Lumpur in Sabak Bernam District of Selangor State (Fig. 1).

The inhabitants of the two Ulu Langat villages are predominantly Malays of Sumatran descent, one village being predominantly Minangkabau, the other Kerenchi. Both villages have similar mixed economies with individuals and families engaged in farming and gardening, smallholder rubber production, and salaried positions in manufacturing, offices and services. All ages and both sexes are highly mobile, moving commonly throughout their local sub-district and further for markets, jobs, education, entertainment and social visits. A high proportion of households are served with or have access to electricity and piped water. Both villages have good access to schools and government health clinics.

The inhabitants of the contrasted Sabak Bernam villages are Malays of predominantly Javanese descent. Both villages are smallholder agricultural communities, Kg. Tok Khalifah depending primarily on coconut groves and Kg. Parit 9 on irrigated *padi*. Neither population is very mobile beyond its village's production area, although school children commonly and adults occasionally go to nearby villages or the local town of Sungai Besar. Minimal services exist in these two villages. Few houses have electricity though some use lorry batteries to run televisions for a few hours each night. During the study some households received a piped water supply. Schools and health centres are available and used, but they are less accessible than in most other parts of Selangor State.

The four settlements were censused with the aid of updated Malaria Eradication Programme maps. One-third to half the households were randomly selected to form the sample for intensive study. All selected households were asked to cooperate with our study with those refusing to cooperate being replaced with randomly selected alternatives. Each sample household was to contribute to the three basic parts of the study.

(1) Each household member was to provide a faecal sample each month for about a year which would be analysed for helminthic and protozoal infection.
(2) About midway through the year one member of each household would answer a questionnaire on household and individual health, hygiene, water use, food use, occupations and other activities.
(3) Each household would be subject to periodic visits and observations by the geographer and field assistants.

Satisfactory standards of information were collected from 300 people from 72 households in the four study villages. This sample is small relative to the analyses attempted and findings reported should be read as suggestive rather than definitive. Eight species of protozoa were identified in the study population, including *Entamoeba histolytica*, *Giardia lamblia*, *Dientamoeba fragilis*, *Entamoeba hartmanni*, *Entamoeba coli*, *Endolimax nana*, *Iodamoeba butschlii* and *Chilomastix mesnili*. All of these protozoa are transmitted orally and may serve as indicators of faecal contamination of water, food, utensils, clothing, bodies and/or personal surroundings.

Table 1. Protozoa prevalence for the four study settlements

Source			Kg. Masjid	Kg. Lubok Kelubi	Kg. Parit 9	Kg. Tok Khalifah	Totals
Households surveyed			24	20	14	14	72
Population surveyed			94	79	63	64	300
Population with at		#	61	45	13	18	137
least one protozoa		(%)	64·9	57	20·6	28·1	45·7
	G.l.	#	24	13	1	1	39
Population		(%)	25·5	16·5	1·6	1·6	13
with	D.f.	#	3	1	4	6	14
pathogenic		(%)	3·2	1·3	6·3	9·4	4·7
protozoa	E.h.	#	7	5	2	0	14
		(%)	7·4	6·3	3·2	0	4·7

Key: Pathogenic Protozoa: G.l., *Giardia lamblia*; D.f., *Dientamoeba fragilis*; E.h., *Entamoeba histolytica*.
Source: Field collection of stools and questionnaire data.

Only the first three, *E. histolytica, G. lamblia* and *D. fragilis*, are potentially pathogenic and therefore of direct public health importance. *G.
lamblia* is transmitted primarily in contaminated water; all others except
for *D. fragilis*, are usually food-borne, although they may also be present
in contaminated water. The precise transmission medium for *D. fragilis*
is unknown. All three pathogenic species may be classified as both
water-borne and water-washed organisms (White *et al.*, 1972), implying
the value of both pure water for consumption and copious quantities of
water for hygiene to their prevention. Results for each settlement are
given in Table 1.

The assessment

Using these data, we shall now assess if behaviours presumed to
associate positively or negatively with intestinal protozoa infections,
especially those of pathogenic protozoa, really do so associate. These
presumed associations will be sought primarily at the scale of the
household and the village. Occasionally, villages too will be compared to
one another. These are the scales most commonly sought in geographical
and similar social science disease-oriented research. From the standpoint
of medical geography we are testing the assumption that hazardous acts
yield dangerous results for parasites that are endemic, non-catastrophic
in most cases, and presumably associated with simple, everyday
behaviours that everyone must engage in. Specifically, behaviours
associated with water supply, household member interaction, hygienic
behaviour, toilet facility use and food and beverage consumption in the
four study villages are to be tested.

Water source and infection

One assumption concerning intestinal protozoa is that people with access to pure water will exhibit lower prevalences of infection; that water piped directly to the house should be safest, followed by water from standpipes, with "open" water from streams, ponds and wells the most hazardous. The safety of water collected from metal roofs is unclear, although given the year-round rainfall and its consequent cleansing of roofs, such water is probably safe. Their lower prevalences (Table 1) imply that Kg. Parit 9 and Kg. Tok Khalifah have the safest water supply, which is not supported by the data (Table 2). Thus one set of assumptions concerning normative behaviour and its influence upon disease appears unfounded.

It could be, however, that infection is influenced by norms acting within a household rather than at the village level. In Kg. Masjid, 15 of 24 households had high protozoa prevalences (50 per cent or more of members infected) including five of the seven (71·4 per cent) households with piped water and ten of the 17 (58·8 per cent) using standpipes. Three of five households with a high prevalence of pathogenic species have piped water, two use standpipes; 34 cases of infection with the pathogens *E. histolytica, G. lamblia* and *D. fragilis* occurred in 16 of the 24 households. *G. lamblia* was found in at least one household member in two of the seven households (28·6 per cent) with piped water and 12 of the 17 households (70·6 per cent) with standpipe sources. *E. histolytica* was found in four of the seven piped water households (57·1 per cent) and two of 17 standpipe households (11·8 per cent). *D. fragilis* infection was rare, occurring in one of seven piped households (14·3 per cent) and two of 17 standpipe households (11·8 per cent).

Conclusions at this household scale are, therefore, somewhat mixed. *G. lamblia* was more common in households getting water from standpipes,

Table 2. Domestic water sources for the four study settlements by household

Source	Number of Households			
	Kg. Masjid	Kg. Lubok Kelubi	Kg. Parit 9	Kg. Tok Khalifah
Piped to house	7	3	—	—
Standpipe	17	12	$1\frac{1}{2}$	3/2
Stream	—	5	—	—
Well or pond	—	—	2 + 2/2	8 + 4/2
Roof	—	—	8 + 3/2	1 + 3/2
Totals	24	20	14	14

Note: Households with two separate sources of water are tallied as $\frac{1}{2}$ for each source.
Source: Questionnaire data.

but more households with piped water showed high protozoa prevalence, high pathogenic protozoa prevalence, and *E. histolytica* infection in at least one member.

In Kg. Lubok Kelubi, 12 of the 20 surveyed households including two of three households with piped water supply (66·7 per cent), seven of 12 using standpipes (58·3 per cent), and three of five drawing water from streams (60 per cent) had a high protozoa prevalence. Only two of the 20 households, one with piped water, the other with a stream source, showed high pathogenic protozoa prevalence. We identified 19 infections with pathogenic species in ten households. *G. lamblia* was found in two of three piped water (66·7 per cent), six of 12 standpipe (50 per cent), and two of five stream households (40 per cent). *E. histolytica* was found in two piped water (66·7 per cent), two standpipe (16·7 per cent), and one stream household (20 per cent). *D. fragilis* was found in only one household supplied by a standpipe.

In Kg. Lubok Kelubi, the prevalence of infection was so low that it could not be correlated to water supply. In general, however, households with piped water had the highest prevalence. A few households should be investigated further for individual and group behaviours.

In Kg. Parit 9 only two of 14 households had a high prevalence of all protozoa species and one had a high prevalence of pathogenic species, with four of its eight members positive. In Kg. Tok Khalifah, five of 14 households (35·7 per cent) had a high prevalence of all protozoa but only one, with a pond as its water source, was classified as having a high prevalence of pathogenic species.

These data on water source and protozoa prevalence lead to the conclusion that the evidence when assessed either at the village level or for households within a settlement yields no major trends. If normative behaviour resulted in infection, we should find specific settlement and household patterns. Instead, such correlations as do exist most frequently go against expectations. Rather than verifying the assumed importance of normative trends, the value of this phase of the study seems to be in identifying discrete households that should be investigated further at a more intensive scale.

Household multiple infections

Intestinal protozoa are transmitted person to person. Is there, therefore, any evidence from household scale data that infections are likely to be transmitted within the family? For this inquiry the data are of limited utility. Households vary in size (in this study from one to ten members) and not all members of households provided stool samples. Thirty-five of the 72 households had at least one member infected with a pathogenic protozoa species; 15 of these had more than one member infected, six households with two, six with three, two with four, and one with five infected members.

Most multiple infections for a specific pathogen were for giardiasis, with eight households in Kg. Masjid or Kg. Lubok Kelubi showing such multiple infections. *Dientamoeba* and amoebiasis appeared as multiple infections in no more than one household each per settlement.

No trend appears at the household scale to indicate pathogenic protozoa are habitually transmitted from one household member to another. There are some households that stand out with group data, such as households in Kg. Masjid with five and three members respectively with giardiasis, but no normative evidence explains why these households and others with two members with the same infection should exist. Most households with two or more members with infections of giardiasis reported piped or standpipe water as their domestic water source and all of these households are on water distribution systems with households reporting single or no cases.

Hygienic behaviour

As water source tells us little about likely infection, is it possible normative water use traits will explain infection patterns? What is done with water to make it safe to use? How is water used to improve local hygiene?

Virtually all study households reported boiling water before drinking it. This was observed to be likely in the home as most directly consumed water was drunk in a hot beverage, most especially tea. If done properly, boiling should kill any protozoal cysts in the water.

People in all four study communities showed a high level of personal hygiene. Every household had a bathing site, ranging from a special bath house to some nearby body of water. No type of bathing site could be associated with the presence or absence of pathogenic infections. All respondents reported bathing two or more times per day except for one household in Kg. Parit 9 whose members reported bathing once per day. Hands were washed three or more times per day in all households. With high levels of personal hygiene so common, no pattern of exposure leading to infection can be shown. Indeed, neither of two people in the one household reporting only one bath per day had any pathogenic protozoa infection.

Faeces disposal

A common assumption is that villages and households with the best faecal waste disposal will have the lowest rates of infection with intestinal

Table 3. Household toilet in the four study settlements

Type of Toilet	Number of Households			
	Kg. Masjid	Kg. Lubok Kelubi	Kg. Parit 9	Kg. Tok Khalifah
Pour flush	$1 + \frac{1}{2} \male$	5	2	5
Pit latrine	—	—	10	9
Platform over water	—	1	2	—
None-into water	$22 + \frac{1}{2} \female$	13	—	—
None-onto ground	—	1	—	—
Totals	24	20	14	14

Note: In one household in Kg. Masjid the type of toilet used is divided by sex.
Source: Questionnaire data.

protozoa. The type of facility used as a toilet by members of households in our study area is given in Table 3. Using pour-flush toilets and pit latrines which carry faeces away into a deep pit where organic hazards can be broken down before groundwater systems bring the material back for possible human contact should be protective. On the other hand, defaecating on the ground or from platforms into surface waters should yield high levels of water-borne infection. These assumptions seem to be supported by the data. In the two villages of Sabak Bernam with low infection rates, 86–100 per cent of the study households had sanitary toilets, but only 6–25 per cent of the households of the two Ulu Langat settlements with a high prevalence had sanitary toilets.

However, these data have to be assessed and the apparent normative connection between behaviour and hazard then becomes less clear. In the case of Kg. Tok Khalifah, where all households had pour-flush toilets or pit latrines, nearly all such facilities had been constructed in the year or so prior to the stool examination. The low protozoa prevalences might historically and inexplicably have been associated with inadequate toilets and the ground and running water disposal system used prior to toilet construction.

For Kg. Parit 9, ten of the households reported using pit latrines in answer to the questionnaire. We later found most reports were misidentifications. Structures resembling outhouse privies constructed on low pillars with the faeces deposited onto the surface of the ground rather than into pits were used. A supposed sanitary system was really not all that protective, yet it was used by households with low levels of infection.

In the two Ulu Langat villages, both with high levels of infection, 94 per cent of the households in Kg. Masjid and 70 per cent in Kg. Lubok Kelubi used nearby streams or ditches as toilets. This implies a hazard to those using these streams for domestic water, as do five study households in Kg. Lubok Kelubi. However, only one of these gathered its water near a known defaecation site; all others gathered their water upstream from any defaecation site or from a stream so large and so far downstream from other uses as to be protected by dilution and aeration. The one household that gathered water near a defaecation site had a high prevalence of infection (four people with two cases of *G. lamblia*, one of *E. histolytica*, and three other identified, non-pathogenic species).

Food and beverage sources

For all four settlements, most food and beverages are prepared and consumed at home. In some cases, home-prepared food is consumed at a worksite or at school.

In Kg. Masjid and Kg. Lubok Kelubi, salaried workers (mostly males) will sometimes take meals at small restaurants or workplace canteens. Adult males also tend to consume beverages at coffee shops, adult females at neighbours' homes. School-age children get occasional snacks and beverages from the carts of itinerant peddlers. In Kg. Parit 9 and Kg. Tok Khalifah, food or beverages are rarely consumed away from the home except for a few adult males or school-age children who may visit a coffee shop, a school canteen or an itinerant peddler.

Because food supplies, in most cases, come from the home, members of a family are exposed primarily to one common potential source of infection. Households with some members eating or drinking away from home showed prevalence rates similar to those with less mobile members, yielding no specific grouped evidence that wider ranging food and beverage sources are consistently associated with different infective patterns.

Conclusions

As stated at the outset, medical geographers tend to assess health hazards and their likely patterns in a community through aggregates of data. We assume that there are some general trends of behaviour, especially trends in exposure to hazard, that yield reliable patterns of infection. Aggregates of behaviour do explain patterns of vector-borne diseases, some non-vectored diseases, such as schistosomiasis, and diseases transmitted in epidemics, whether from person to person or *via* some biological intermediary. But for some diseases, it is not so easy to show a direct relationship between exposure and disease burden. Our evidence indicates a need for assessing disease hazard at various scales depending on the specific problem under examination.

In this particular study we are dealing with a problem of varying prevalence and presumptively low incidence. From the stool data for protozoa we find a hazard exists, but at a low prevalence for pathogenic species. When we add the evidence from the discovery of non-pathogenic protozoa in the stools we find that faecal contamination in these communities is fairly common, evidenced by the appearance of protozoa in one-half to nearly all of the households in each community and in 15–60 per cent of the individuals in each area. Regardless of the possibility for faecal contamination, there seems to be little hazard of direct transmission among members of a household as witnessed by the uncommonness of household multiple infections.

Transmission of faecal-borne protozoa occurs seemingly infrequently, but how infrequently is as yet unclear. Individual protozoal loads in a person cannot be quantified. One, two or many infections with a given protozoa yield the same evidence of infection. For geohelminths, however, average parasite loads can be quantified. The proportion of people showing worm eggs in their stools indicates the population exposed to parasite ingestion. As excreted worm eggs are produced by specific adult worms, the density of eggs in the stool may be used to indicate the number of worms in the intestinal tract, which in turn may roughly suggest the frequency of exposure to geohelminth infection for the individual. For the four study villages, the prevalence of geohelminths *Trichuris trichiura* and *Ascaris lumbricoides* from the same stools from which the protozoa data are derived is given in Table 4. These results, especially for *T. trichiura*, indicate high prevalences of faecal-borne agent transmission in all four villages. Based upon egg counts in the stools, the worm burden in almost every infection was light, indicating that almost all infected persons carried very few worms in their intestinal tract. As these two intestinal helminths may both survive and produce eggs in periods measured in months to years, this implies the reasonably uncommon ingestion of infective agents, yielding a state of moderate to high prevalence concurrent with very low incidence, an implication which may also hold for protozoa.

One must conclude that normative behaviour data may not necessarily correlate well with disease occurrence. Traditional survey techniques may not identify sub-populations at risk because the infections identified here are most likely to be the result of discrete events that may or may not be normative. Protozoal, or even helminthic, agents are rarely present in food or in water or on unclean bodies or clothing, even though faecal contamination of these items may be nearly universal.

Table 4. Geohelminth prevalence in the four study settlements

Source		Kg. Masjid	Kg. Lubok Kelubi	Kg. Parit 9	Kg. Tok Khalifah	Totals
Population		95	86	64	63	308
Positive for *Trichuris trichiura*	#	77	50	61	55	243
	(%)	88·1	58·1	95·3	87·3	78·9
Positive for *Ascaris lumbricoides*	#	16	10	46	43	115
	(%)	16·8	11·6	71·9	68·3	37·3

Note: "Population surveyed" results vary from those in Table 1 because some stools were analysed only for protozoa or for helminths because of the size or condition.
Source: Field and laboratory data.

Low incidence of transmission may be of recent occurrence to these populations. Post-independence improvements in preventive and curative health care plus improved understanding and implementation of environmental hygiene may have decreased the potential for transmission. Whatever the cause, low prevalence has made normative behaviour irrelevant as a device to explain transmission of faecal-borne protozoal infections. What appears to be happening is that environment, not human behaviour, is exercising the major influence on parasite prevalence. Indeed, the relevance of human behaviour to the success of the parasite may vary with the role of the local environment.

We should thus recognize the possible futility of attempting to improve health situations by encouraging seemingly safe normative behaviour. We may be making a valueless investment or actually decreasing the prevalence of good health. Kg. Parit 9, where most of the households used to obtain their domestic water supplies from rain water running off metal roofs, showed very low rates of pathogenic protozoa infection. Apparently, transmission then was a rarity in this village. By the time the questionnaire was given to the community most households were receiving piped domestic water supplies from private water taps in their compounds. If that system were to become contaminated through pollution of the source or mechanical breakdown, it could expose a previously safe population to a concentrated hazard of infection.

What all this leads to is the recognition in medical geography that scales of analysis should vary in association with the problem at hand. As geographers look at diseases with low incidence (i.e. low rate of new cases over time), which might include some infectious diseases, some toxicological hazards, and some diseases of as yet unknown aetiology, they need to identify more precisely the precise moment and situation of transmission. Aggregate data may not be adequate to indicate what the precise moment might be. Intensive behavioural investigations of a few individuals at risk might be necessary to identify the significant behaviours and habitats that together produce a pathogenic response in some community members.

Acknowledgements

The fieldwork reported here was supported by the University of California International Center for Medical Research (UC-ICMR) through research grant AI 10051 to the Department of International Health, School of Medicine, University of California, San Francisco, from the National Institute of Allergy and Infectious Diseases, National Institutes of Health, US Public Health Service. It has also been approved by the University of California Committee on Human Research, Protocol No. 17081-01. Research was undertaken in affiliation with the Malaysian Institute for Medical Research, Kuala Lumpur. Support for the production of the current report came from a Rutgers University Research Council grant for the study of rural change and health.

Appreciative thanks are given to villagers from the four kampongs who agreed to take part in this study, including their village leaders and local health and government personnel. Our assistants, Modh. Shahir bin Lajis, S. Thavaranchitham, and C. K. Chandrasekaran, also made this study possible. Special thanks go to Dr George F. de Witt, Director of the Malaysian Institute for Medical Research, for his personal and professional support and for permission to publish this study.

References

Armstrong, R. W. (1976). The geography of specific environments of patients and non-patients in cancer studies, with a Malaysian example. *Economic Geography* **52**, 161–170.

Armstrong, R. W., Kannan Kutty, M. and Armstrong, M. J. (1978). Self-specific environments associated with nasopharyngeal cancer in Selangor, Malaysia. *Social Science and Medicine* **12D**, 149–156.

Audy, J. R. (1965). Types of human influence on natural foci of disease. In *Theoretical Questions on Natural Foci of Disease* (Eds B. Rosicky and K. Heyberger), pp. 245–253. Publishing House of the Czechoslovak Academy of Science, Prague.

Audy, J. R (1972). Aspects of human behavior interfering with vector control. In *Vector Control and the Recrudescence of Vector-Borne Diseases*, pp. 67–82. Pan American Health Organization Scientific Publication No. 238, Washington, D.C.

Bradley, A. K. (1976). Effects of onchocerciasis on settlement in the Middle Hawal Valley, Nigeria. *Transactions of the Royal Society of Tropical Medicine and Hygiene* **70**, 225–229.

Dalton, P. R. (1976). A sociological approach to the control of *Schistosoma mansoni* in St. Lucia. *Bulletin of the World Health Organization* **54**, 587–595.

Dalton, P. R. and Pole, D. (1978). Water-contact patterns in relation to *Schistosomiasis haematobium* infection. *Bulletin of the World Health Organization* **56**, 417–426.

Dunn, F. L. (1972). Intestinal parasitism in Malayan aborigines (Orang Asli). *Bulletin of the World Health Organization* **46**, 99–113.

Dunn, F. L. (1976). Human behavioural factors in the epidemiology and control of *Wuchereria* and *Brugia* infections. *Bulletin of the Public Health Society (Malaysia)* **10**, 34–44.

Fonaroff, L. S. (1968). Man and malaria in Trinidad: ecological perspectives of a changing health hazard. *Annals of the Association of American Geographers* **58**, 526–556.

Gaál, L. and Márton, M. (1980). Human geohelminthiases and the epidemiological situation of the direct spreading of enteral parasitoses in Szabolcs-Szatmár County—In the view of socio-economic changes. *Geographia Medica* **10**, 97–106.

Haddock, K. C. (1979). Disease and development in the tropics: A review of Chagas' disease. *Social Science and Medicine* **13D**, 53–60.

Hughes, C. C. and Hunter, J. M. (1970). Disease and "development" in Africa. *Social Science and Medicine* **3**, 443–493.

Hunter, J. M. (1966). River blindness in Nangodi, Northern Ghana: a hypothesis of cyclical advance and retreat. *Geographical Review* **56**, 398–416.

Hunter, J. M. (1976). Aerosol and roadside lead as environmental hazard. *Economic Geography* **52**, 147–160.

Hunter, J. M. (1978). The summer disease: some field evidence on seasonality in childhood lead poisoning. *Social Science and Medicine* **12D**, 85–94.

Hunter, J. M. (1980). Strategies for the control of river blindness. In *Conceptual and Methodological Issues in Medical Geography* (Ed. M. S. Meade), pp. 38–76. Studies in Geography No. 15, Department of Geography, University of North Carolina at Chapel Hill.

Hunter, J. M. and Young, J. C. (1971). Diffusion of influenza in England and Wales. *Annals of the Association of American Geographers* **61**, 647–653.

Kloos, H., Higashi, G. I., Schinski, V. D., Mansour, N. S., Polderman, A. M., Aklilu Lemma and Murrell, K. D. (1980–1981). Human behaviour and schistosomiasis in an Ethiopian town and an Egyptian village: Tensae Berhan and El Ayaisha. *Rural Africana* **8–9**, 35–65.

Knight, C. G. (1971). The ecology of African sleeping sickness. *Annals of the Association of American Geographers* **61**, 23–44.

Kochar, V., Schad, G. A., Chowdhury, A. B., Dean, C. G. and Nawalinski, T. (1976). Human factors in the regulation of parasitic infections: cultural ecology of hookworm populations in rural West Bengal. In *Medical Anthropology* (Eds F. X. Grollig and H. B. Haley), pp. 287–312. Mouton Publishers, The Hague.

Learmonth, A. T. A. (1957). Some contrasts in the regional geography of malaria in India and Pakistan. *Transactions and Papers, Institute of British Geographers* **23**, 37–59.

Learmonth, A. T. A. (1965). *Health in the Indian Sub-Continent 1955–64: A Geographer's Review of Some Medical Literature.* Occasional Paper 2, Department of Geography, Australian National University, Canberra.

Matzke, G. (1979). Settlement and sleeping sickness control—A dual threshold model of colonial and traditional methods in East Africa. *Social Science and Medicine* **13D**, 209–214.

May, J. M. (1950). Medical geography: its methods and objectives. *Geographical Review* **40**, 9–41.

May, J. M. (Ed.) (1958). *The Ecology of Human Disease.* MD Publications, New York.

May, J. M. (Ed.) (1961). *Studies in Disease Ecology.* Hafner Publishing Company, Inc., New York.

McGlashan, N. D. (1972). Food contaminants and oesophageal cancer. In *Medical Geography: Techniques and Field Studies* (Ed. N. D. McGlashan), pp. 247–257. Methuen and Co., London.

McGlashan, N. D. (1977). The oesophageal carcinoma problem in Transkei. *South African Journal of Science* **73**, 294–299.

Newman, J. L. (1980). Dietary behavior and protein–energy–malnutrition in Africa South of the Sahara: some themes for medical geography. In *Conceptual and Methodical Issues in Medical Geography* (Ed. M. S. Meade), pp. 77–92. Studies in Geography No. 15, Department of Geography, University of North Carolina at Chapel Hill.

Prothero, R. M. (1963). Population mobility and trypanosomiasis in Africa. *Bulletin of the World Health Organization* **28**, 615–626.

Prothero, R. M. (1965). *Migrants and Malaria in Africa.* University of Pittsburgh Press, Pittsburgh.

Pyle, G. F. (1969). The diffusion of cholera in the United States in the nineteenth century. *Geographical Analysis* **1**, 59–75.

Roundy, R. W. (1976). *Hazards of Communicable Disease Transmission Resulting from Cultural Behavior in Ethiopian Rural Highland-Dwelling Populations: A Cultural-Medical Geographic Study.* Ph.D. dissertation in Geography, University of California at Los Angeles.

Roundy, R. W. (1978). A model for combining human behavior and disease ecology to assess disease hazard in a community: rural Ethiopia as a model. *Social Science and Medicine* **12D**, 121–130.

Roundy, R. W. (1979). Human behavior and disease hazards: spatial perspectives on rural health. *GeoJournal* **3**, 579–586.

Roundy, R. W. (1980). The influence of vegetational changes on disease patterns. In *Conceptual and Methodological Issues in Medical Geography* (Ed. M. S. Meade), pp. 16–37. Studies in Geography No. 15, Department of Geography, University of North Carolina at Chapel Hill.

Stock, R. F. (1976). *Cholera in Africa.* International African Institute, London.

Takemoto, T., Suzuki, T., Kashiwazaki, H., Mori, S., Hirata, F., Taja, O. and Vexina, E. (1981). The human impact of colonization and parasite infestation in subtropical lowlands of Bolivia. *Social Science and Medicine* **15D**, 133–139.

Van Wettere-Verhasselt, Y. (1969–70). The geographical environment and ecology of the tsetse-fly (*Glossina palpalis*) in Bas-Congo. *Geographia Medica* **1**, 7–19.

White, G. F., Bradley, D. J. and White, A. U. (1972). *Drawers of Water: Domestic Water Use in East Africa.* University of Chicago Press, Chicago.

Wilson, C. S. (1979). Food-custom and nurture. *Journal of Nutrition Education* **11** (Suppl. 1), 212–264.

Some reflections on the ecology of dengue haemorrhagic fever in Thailand

Hella Wellmer

Heidelberger Akademie der Wissenschaften,
Geomedizinische Forschungsstelle,
Heidelberg, West Germany

Introduction

Dengue is an old and widespread tropical disease. Besides high fever, the patients complain of aching and severe pain in muscles and joints.

This chapter deals with a disease which is clinically totally different from classical dengue. It had come as rather a surprise when, in 1960, Hammon identified dengue fever in the Philippines. The new disease was given the name Dengue Haemorrhagic Fever (DHF). Similar epidemics occurred and the virus was isolated during the following years in Bangkok (1958), Singapore (1960), South-Vietnam (1961), Malaysia (1962), Calcutta (1963/64), and Indonesia (1968/69). All these early epidemic outbreaks were first concentrated in harbour cities, and only later spread to inland areas. In Thailand DHF became the infectious disease with the highest number of deaths per year.

The disease and its epidemiology

The following theory about the evolution of the disease is accepted by most authors today. When a person first comes into contact with dengue virus, the result will either be a classical dengue of varying severity, or the infection will not even be recognized at all. When, after a certain interval of time, a second infection with another dengue virus subtype occurs the

GEOGRAPHICAL ASPECTS OF HEALTH
ISBN 0 12 483780 8

result will be DHF. The special immunological status of childhood may play a role in the pathogenesis. As most people in south-east Asia come in contact with dengue virus during their lives, young infants will have dengue antibodies from their mothers for a certain period after birth. This may explain its relatively low incidence in infants. DHF is a disease of children and only rarely affects persons over the age of 14, the dominant age group being 4–9 years old. Whilst there is no obvious connection to nutritional status or race, it is very unlikely that a foreign child will be infected twice unless it is born in an Asian country or lives there for a very long time.

The disease begins with uncharacteristic fever and abdominal symptoms. In severe cases the disease shows toxic features abruptly on the second or third day, which is when hospital admission usually occurs. Vomiting and haemorrhages occur including bleeding in the skin and mucous membranes or with blood appearing in the stools. This stage may develop into a shock syndrome and was responsible for the fatal outcome of 10 per cent of the cases during the early epidemics, when treatment was not as developed as it is today. If this crisis is overcome the patient will recover completely in as short a period as two days.

The virus

The virus of dengue is an arbo-virus (arthropod-borne virus) borne by mosquitos. So far four subtypes are known. The virus multiplies in the vector without damaging it. When a mosquito bites, virus is transmitted to a vertebrate host. In classifying arbo-viruses dengue virus is grouped with the viruses of yellow fever and central European encephalitis in the largest group, group B. With few exceptions, arbo-virus diseases depend for diffusion totally on their vectors, as transmission from man to man impossible. Thus the distribution of arbovirosis always closely parallel the distribution of its vector.

The vector

Even during the early epidemics the spatial connection of DHF and the mosquito, *Aedes aegypti*, was obvious, although dengue virus is borne by other mosquitos as well. Entomologists agree that *Aedes aegypti* was introduced into Asian countries only at the end of the last century. When its distribution pattern was investigated in the early years of this century in spite of careful search further inland, it was only found at the sites coastal harbours. It was found inland for the first time in 1914, in Kuala Lumpur, 27 miles from the coast. The most common dengue vector in south-east Asia then was *Aedes albopictus*, a mosquito species with quite different living conditions and habitat requirements.

The following history of the invasion of Asia by *Aedes aegypti* is likely (Smith, 1956). In early days, dengue was a zoonosis of monkeys, borne by jungle living mosquitoes. Where man and his mosquito, *A. albopictus*, came in close contact with the jungle ecosystem, *A. albopictus* became the link between the jungle disease and man, biting both monkeys and men. In the course of time, dengue became a common disease but with a high rate of immune persons in the population. It thus became a children's disease. With the development of large cities, mainly along the coast, *A. albopictus*, which prefers natural waterbodies and bites only out of doors, lost its breeding places in these surroundings. The result was a low immunity in the city populations when, at the end of the last century, *A. aegypti* arrived by ship from Africa. As this species actually prefers the artificial surroundings provided by man and is an excellent dengue vector as well, severe epidemics at once occurred in the ports of Asia. Yet later, however, the city population regained immunity and no further epidemics were reported after 1930. Dengue became a children's disease again with *A. aegypti* established as its vector in the urban habitat.

In the 1950s a new disease, haemorrhagic fever, began to spread in epidemics throughout south-east Asia. Two main theories have been put forward: possibly the virus itself mutated in the new vector to a more virulent subtype, or possibly haemorrhagic fever is the result in the immune system to a second infection with another subtype during childhood. So far international scientists are still in disagreement upon these points.

The ecology of DHF in Thailand

In Thailand, a system of regular DHF reports for all 72 provinces was established in 1962. Before that date, DHF cases, though common, were only recorded in Bangkok from 1958 and adjacent provinces from 1960. It can easily be shown that the first provinces reporting any considerable incidence before 1970, were those situated along the main railway lines (Fig. 1). That matches McDonald's observation in Malaysia, where *A. aegypti* was spread by people using trains. Indeed all three vector stages can be spread by this mechanical means: eggs, larvae and adults. This mode of mechanical spread seems to have been the main one, as within very short distances the same author observed villages infested with *A.*

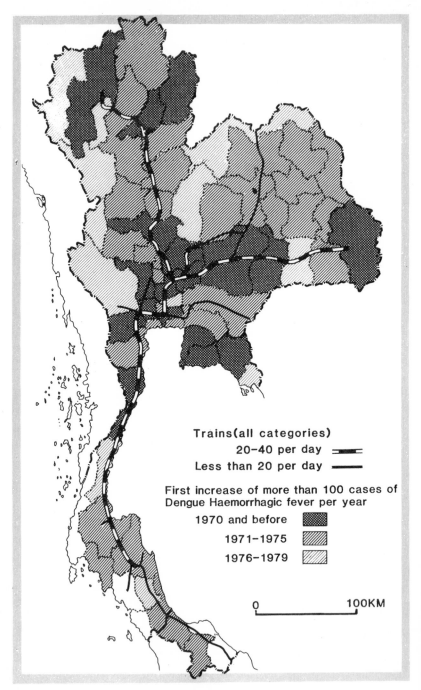

Figure 1. Railways and the onset of epidemic spread of dengue haemorrhagic fever in Thailand (by provinces). Sources: Freitag (1977) and Wellmer (in press).

aegypti and only two miles away villages completely free of this mosquito. That means that the flight of the mosquito itself does not play a significant role. Also, McDonald's (1956) experiments proved that it is very difficult to establish *A. aegypti* in a village where the population density is low and the breeding places inadequate.

Methods and findings

The Ministry of Health, Bangkok, provided weekly records of reported DHF cases for all 72 provinces for the ten-year period from 1970 to 1979 (see Table 1). Population numbers were based on the 1971 census. By computer mapping it was possible to follow the main centres of high incidence of DHF during this decade and areas with constantly low incidence could also be shown. As a first step the monthly and annual data were mapped by provinces on a frequency distribution, and obvious break points were used to allocate areas to incidence classes. This resulted in six categories of incidence rates of DHF per 10,000 population. As a second step the maps were transformed to isolines. Maps of population density, density of doctors and incidence of DHF per doctor

Table 1. Total DHF numbers for Thailand 1958–1979

Year	Bangkok + Thonburi (after Avril)	Thailand (after Avril)	Thailand (Min. of Health)
1958	2418		
1959	127		
1960	1742		
1961	418		
1962	4187	6078	
1963	1644	3070	
1964	5358	9020	
1965	1253	3466	
1966	1986	5845	
1967	358	2060	
1968	779	6032	
1969	1385	8613	
1970	574	2840	2,743
1971			11,296
1972			23,560
1973			8,283
1974			8,112
1975			17,440
1976			9,445
1977			38,664
1978			12,042
1979			11,412
1980			>48,000

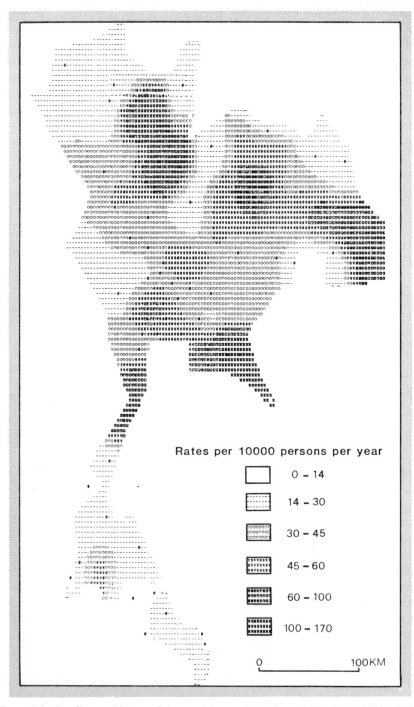

Figure 2. Isoline (isomorb) map of dengue haemorrhagic fever in Thailand, 1970–1979.
Source: GEOMAP Version 5c, University of Waterloo, Ontario, Canada.

were mapped as well. Figure 2 provides an example of the computer mapped distribution of DHF incidence in Thailand for the decade 1970–1979. In years with a high number of reported cases, the most infected areas were the northern and southern central plain, the Khorat plateau and the south-east. Less infected generally were the northern and western mountains, the hills surrounding the Khorat plateau and the south. In years of low incidence the disease distribution was more or less even over the whole country.

The question arose whether in Thailand the highest incidence occurred predominantly in urban areas. As the data were based on provinces, problems of scale arose when only urban centres were considered, because every province has its urban area. A possible solution was provided by the consideration that the growth rate of a city influences the quality of vector breeding places.

A. aegypti, in contrast to the indigenous vector, *A. albopictus*, prefers artificial containers for breeding, where the eggs can be deposited on the side of the container about the water surface. The eggs hatch immediately after the next rain, when water fills the container. In Bangkok, *A. albopictus* almost completely disappeared because of the dearth of natural waterbodies with dense vegetational surroundings.

With the rapid growth of cities in Asia water supply and waste disposal were unable to keep pace. Besides clearing the vegetation, the result has been an increase of all sorts of water containers for drinking and household use, and a wide range of tins, shells and plastic containers around the huts and houses. Thus *A. aegypti* is not only provided with its favourite breeding places but also with the proximity of its favourite vertebrate host to feed on, man.

In Thailand, the provinces with most rapid growth of urban population during the years 1960 to 1972—when DHF spread to all provinces—were shown to be those which reported DHF above the national average (calculated as rates). Out of nine urban centres with growth of more than 30,000 inhabitants each between 1960 and 1972, seven are situated in provinces where the DHF incidence is above the national average. The two remaining cities are both situated in the south of the country and these can be explained on climatic grounds (Fig. 3).

The climate, of course, is a very important factor in DHF transmission as it is in arthropod-borne diseases. When temperatures fall below 18°C, *A. aegypti* stops biting. Additionally larvae need temperatures above 15–20°C for their development; therefore, the 20°C isotherm forms the limit for *A. aegypti*. One example of the importance of this is that in the mountains of northern Thailand, mean monthly temperatures fall below 22°C regularly for one to two winter months each year. That means that temperatures at night will certainly fall below the 18°C limit mentioned.

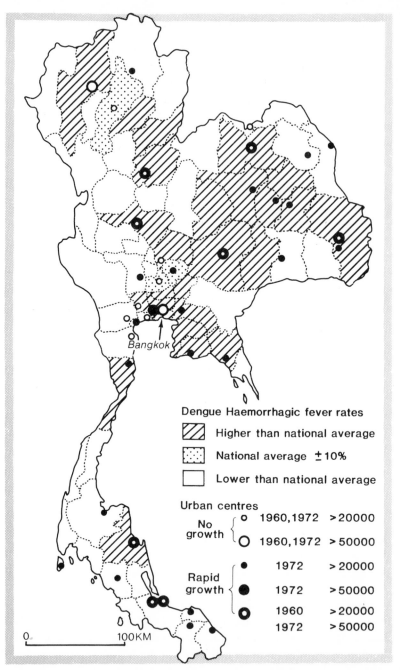

Figure 3. Dengue haemorrhagic fever and urbanization (urban centres with rapid growth between 1960 and 1972 and dengue haemorrhagic fever cases by Provinces compared to the national average, 1970–1979). Source: *Thailand, The Environment of Modernization* (1976). McGraw, Sydney.

This fact is reflected in the seasonality of DHF in the northern provinces, where the peak in July is never very high, and where almost no cases are reported in winter (Fig. 4).

The situation in the central provinces and on the Khorat plateau is quite different. Temperatures are fairly constant throughout the year and there is a marked dry season. Although a steep increase of DHF cases follows the onset of the SW-monsoon in May or June (see Fig. 4 for the Central Plain area and Bangkok), the fact of there being a dry season may add to the high endemicity in these provinces. Here people use water containers to gather every drop of rain during the dry season. Water butts with a capacity of up to 200 litres are situated next to the houses collecting water from the roofs and so provide breeding places throughout the year. The butts are rarely completely empty. These are the very provinces which report DHF all the year round, though with a sharp increase in May–June and a high plateau from July to October.

The south of Thailand is formed by the northern part of the Malaysian peninsula with 12 humid months a year. A central hill range, running from north to south provides the eastern coast with heavy rains during the NE-monsoon period and the western part with rains in the SW-monsoon. Despite these differences in the seasonality of rainfall the seasonality of DHF on both sides of the hill range is the same. This effect is still quite unexplained but it might relate to an inborne cycle of activity of *A. aegypti* which is modified by rainfall.

The seasonal DHF curve in the southern provinces is similar to the north, with a slight peak in July and almost no cases in the NE-monsoon period.

Prospects

As the climate of the Malaysian peninsula has no time of the year at which the life support conditions of *A. aegypti* are not fulfilled, and as these remote provinces were reached late by the disease, it is probable that a marked increase will occur in these southern areas in the future. The more so as the province of Trat is a very interesting exception to the general pattern. This province in the far south-east of Thailand on the eastern side of the gulf has the same climatic conditions as the main Malaysian peninsula but is much closer to the densely populated areas round Bangkok and had reported considerable numbers of cases even before 1970. In Trat province the disease is reported throughout the year, without the raised incidence during the SW-monsoon, but with a sharp peak in July. Compared to the relatively small number of 94,119 inhabitants of this province (Census 1970) the peak in July is the highest for the

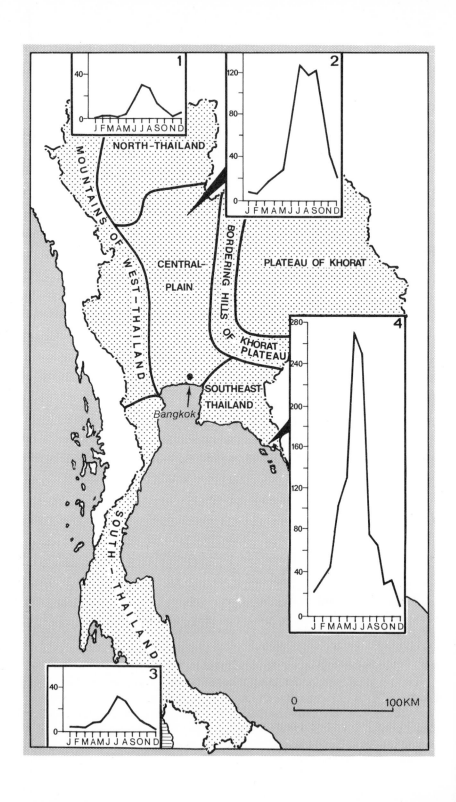

whole country with a monthly mean of 27 cases per thousand inhabitants for July (during 1970–1979) every year.

As a result of these observations an endemic area of DHF in the Central Plain and Khorat Plateau can be assumed. For reasons of climate the situation in the north is not likely to change much, whereas, for the south, any prediction at all would be very insecure.

For the country as a whole, reported DHF cases had a biennial rhythm in the first decade (1958–1968), but since then no pattern can be detected beyond a general increase of case numbers (see Table 1). These increasing numbers are difficult to assess because a high number of unreported cases might even exceed those reported. Although many cases may not be serious and are treated as unreported out-patients or without seeing a doctor or a health worker at all, the number of hospitalized patients has certainly been reported more conscientiously during the time since the reporting system started. Furthermore, those patients who are not hospitalized are also more fully reported because blood tests became more common and health workers became more aware of the necessity of reports. In spite of these difficulties, the spatial dynamics of DHF in Thailand and its clear and differing patterns of seasonality can now be reliably defined from the case reports. It is also clear on the ecological evidence that an increase of DHF can be confidently expected in every growing urban area and, perhaps, even more seriously, throughout the whole of the south of the country.

Acknowledgements

First I express my gratitude to Professor H. J. Jusatz, Director of the Geomedical Research Centre in Heidelberg, who initiated this study. The collaboration of the Ministry of Health, Bangkok, which provided the regular weekly DHF reports and the Department of Meteorology, which provided the recent climatological data is greatly appreciated.

I thank Professor M. Domrös, Mainz, for most of the climatological data and Professor U. Freitag, Berlin, for the gift of some maps from his Atlas of Thailand. Professor W. Fricke, Director of the Department of Geography, Heidelberg, generously permitted the use of the Geomap Computer Program.

Last but not least, the valued help of Professor Ouay Ketusinh of Bangkok during my stay in Thailand is deeply appreciated.

Figure 4. The average monthly incidence of dengue haemorrhagic fever per 1000 inhabitants, 1970–1979, for four natural regions of Thailand. Source: Natural regions according to W. Maas. Hinterindien (1963). 1. Northern Provinces; 2. Central Plain and Khorat Plateau; 3. South Thailand; 4. Trat Province.

284   Hella Wellmer

References

Aiken, S. and Leigh, C. H. (1978). Dengue haemorrhagic fever in south-east Asia. *Trans Inst. Brit. Geogr.* **3**, 4, 476–497.
Avril, W. (1972). Dengue Hämorrhagisches Fieber in Südasien. *Diss. reihe des Sudasien-Instituts der Univ. Heidelberg*, Bd. 14.
Cheong, W. H. (1967). Preferred *Aedes aegypti* habitats in urban areas. *Bull. WHO* **36**, 586–589.
Freitag, U. (1977). *Atlas of Thailand.* Thai Survey Department, Bangkok.
Halstead, S. B. (1966). Epidemiological studies of Thai haemorrhagic fever 1962–1964. *Bull. WHO* **35**, 80–81.
Halstead, S. B. (1980). Dengue haemorrhagic fever—a public health problem and a field of research. *Bull. WHO* **58**, 1, 1–21.
Halstead, S. B. and Yamarat, C. (1965). Recent epidemics of haemorrhagic fever in Thailand. Observations related to pathogenesis of a "new" dengue disease. *Amer. J. Publ. Health* **55**, 1386–1395.
Hammon, W. McD., Rudnick, A. and Sather, G. E. (1960). Virus associated with epidemic haemorrhagic fevers of the Philippines and Thailand. *Science* **131**, 1102.
Jusatz, H. J. (1972). Gegenwärtige Verbreitung des Dengue Hämorrhagischen Fiebers in Südasien. *Med. Klinik* **5**, 152–156.
Jusatz, H. J. (1975). The present distribution of dengue haemorrhagic fever in South Asia. *Appl. Sci. and Development* **6**, 119–126.
McDonald, W. W. (1956). *Aedes aegypti* in Malaya. *Ann. Trop. Med. Parasitol.* **50**, 385 ff.
Meade, M. (1976). A new disease in Southeast Asia: man's creation of dengue haemorrhagic fever. *Pacific Viewpoint* **17**, 2, 133–146.
Pant, C. P., Jatanasen, S. and Yasuno, M. (1973). Prevalence of *Aedes aegypti* and *Aedes albopictus* and observations on the ecology of DHF in several areas in Thailand. *Southeast Asian J. Trop. Med. Publ. Health* **4**, 113–121.
Rudnick, A. and Hammon, W. (1961). Entomological aspects of Thai haemorrhagic fever epidemics in Bangkok, the Philippines and Singapore 1956–61. *Proc. Thai Haemorrh. Fever Symposium SEATO Bangkok, Med. Res. Monograph* **2**, 24–29.
Smith, C. E. (1956). The history of dengue in tropical Asia and its probable relationships to the mosquito *Aedes aegypti. J. Trop Med. Hyg.* **59**, 243–251.
Surtees, G. (1971). Urbanization and the epidemiology of mosquito-borne diseases. *Abstracts on Hygiene* **46**, 2, 121–134.
Wellmer, H. (in press). Dengue Hämorrhagisches Fieber in Thailand 1970–79.

Primary health care and the epidemiological transition in Nepal

J. Anthony Hellen

Department of Geography, University of Newcastle upon Tyne, England

Nepal: the general background

The conventional division of Nepal into three landscape categories—mountains (15 per cent), hills (68 per cent) and *terai* (17 per cent)—is well known. Changes in the overall distribution and balance of the population influence and are influenced by this framework (cf. Hellen, 1981). Extending over 145,391 km² as a block roughly 800 by 175 km in size, Nepal has been described as forming a rugged staircase, rising from the low, alluvial plains (*terai*) between 90 and 300 m, through the Bhabar and Churia Hills or *inner terai* at 300 to 1800 m, to the sub-Himalayan and high-Himalayan areas between 1800 and 9000 m. In consequence of this three-dimensional range, Nepal presents remarkable environmental, climatic and ecological variations in any south–north transect. These variations affect not only the vertical zonation of agriculture and settlement forms, but also human disease and mortality patterns, yet in some places the Ganges plain and the central Himalayan chain are less than 150 km apart (Müller, 1981). Even in the case of one disease alone—malaria, formerly Nepal's main cause of death—the importance of topography and altitude in determining the extent of the hyper-endemic or hypo-endemic areas (areas above 1200 m being in general malaria-free) illustrates this complex relationship.

Although the four official development regions, first designated in 1978, have retained an almost constant share of the growing national population between the census years 1952–1954 and 1971, there has been a marked tendency for migration to move in the vertical dimension from mountains to hills and hills to *terai* rather than by traversing between

GEOGRAPHICAL ASPECTS OF HEALTH
ISBN 0 12 483780 8

Table 1. Population distribution by geographical and development regions

Region and sub-region	1952–1954	1961	1971	% increase over 1952–1954
Hills and mountains *Development region*				
Eastern	1,104,540	1,317,750	1,409,942	28
Central	1,296,205	1,747,178	2,095,517	61
Western	1,414,613	1,580,482	1,870,430	32
Far-western	1,515,712	1,698,083	1,834,128	21
Total	5,331,070	6,343,493	7,210,017	35
Terai *Development region*				
Eastern	825,968	955,746	1,387,558	68
Central	1,388,959	1,325,418	1,770,236	28
Western	364,578	418,181	595,110	63
Far-western	324,504	370,158	593,062	83
Total	2,904,009	3,069,503	4,345,966	50
Hills, mountains and terai				
Eastern	1,930,508	2,273,496	2,797,500	41
Central	2,685,164	3,072,596	3,865,753	44
Western	1,779,191	1,998,663	2,465,540	39
Far-western	1,840,216	2,068,241	2,427,190	32
All Nepal	8,235,079	9,412,996	11,555,983	40

Source: Central Bureau of Statistics, Kathmandu.

regions. The general shift from the hills and mountains to the *terai* has been rural to rural migration and, associated with such changes as malaria eradication in the *terai* after 1956, has allowed planned resettlement and unplanned squatting to combine with negative "push" factors in the hills and mountains.

Population distribution and demographic change

The broad details of Nepal's population distribution and growth, as well as its ethnic composition, are available in the literature, but the quality of information on fertility and mortality is at present inadequate for most of the demands placed on it by planners. Due to under-enumeration and misreporting little credence can be given to national censuses prior to that of 1952–1954, which suggested a national population decline from 5,639,000 to 5,535,000 between 1911 and 1930, and thereafter a steady increase to the 1971 total of 11,556,000 with a 1980 estimate of 14,250,000.

Even in 1971 difficulties surrounding population census-taking in Nepal include a complete absence of *panchayat*-level maps, which would have provided some reliability and comparability about the location and boundaries of enumeration districts.

Table 1 presents percentage increases in the four development regions, differentiated according to terrain areas. Thus between the first modern census of 1952–1954, taken on split dates, and the most recently published census of 1971, the *terai* population grew from 2·904 million to 4·346 million, that is by nearly 50 per cent against the national average of about 40 per cent. Discounting natural increase with estimated annual growth rates of 1·6 and 2·1 per cent respectively between the last three published censuses, over half that number represented unmonitored immigration to the *terai* zone. By contrast the hill and mountain region grew by only 35 per cent.

The components of population change

Fertility

Misreporting of age and omission of vital events were commonplace in attempts to establish levels and trends of fertility prior to the Nepal Fertility Survey of 1976 (cf. Goldman *et al.*, 1979). The Survey's findings established a benchmark for all subsequent investigations in an area previously characterized by uncertainty. Thus, among other data the long exposure of Nepalese women to childbearing is noteworthy: in the *terai* the mean age of first marriage was 14·7 years (against 15·3 years in the hills and 15·5 years in the mountains). The mean number of reported births by all ever-married women aged 45–49 years, that is approximately the completed fertility, was 5·7, adjusted to a total fertility rate of 6·5 births, or a crude birth rate of 44 per thousand—a marked contrast with the 1971 census figure of only 23 per thousand. However, the average woman had only 4 children alive at the close of her reproductive period, representing a 27 per cent loss of all live-births. Although many ethnic groups in Nepal practise child marriage, fewer than a quarter under 20 years of age were found to have produced children.

With such fertility levels over-population is now recognized as a serious problem. Family planning (FP) and any knowledge of contraception are matters of recent concern and an official FP programme began only in 1968 (Tuladhar *et al.*, 1979). Some ten years after this the Survey found that only 22 per cent of the sample knew of any method of

contraception, and a mere 4 per cent had practised it. Because contraception is increasingly seen in relation to health-care programmes, it is of
interest that relatively more women in the *terai* (29 per cent) than in the
hills (18 per cent) or mountains (11 per cent) reported any knowledge of
contraceptive methods. Educational differences accounted for much
greater discrepancies than physical isolation in the knowledge and use of
FP methods.

Mortality

Compared to fertility and migration little has been written, and less
seems to be known, about mortality as a component of population
change. Disease patterns and the medical geographical aspects of changing mortality, particularly regarding deaths by cause, will be discussed
below; here they are considered only as one aspect of demography.
Various authors have estimated total mortality using data from suc-
cessive censuses (cf. Gubhaju, 1972, 1975; Krotki and Thakur, 1971;
Vaidyanathan and Gaije, 1973; Tuladhar *et al.*, 1978). The difficulties
in calculating true mortality from census-reported data and life tables
appear in the general literature. Although Nepal still has one of the
highest crude death rates in Asia, the still limited evidence points to
a substantial decline between 1951 and 1961, followed by a further slight
drop in the period since 1961. As a rough indicator of health status the life
expectation at birth had increased from 25·6 years (male) and 25·7 years
(female) in 1952–1954 to 46 years (male) and 42·5 years (female) in
1974–1975, according to the Central Bureau of Statistics (CBS). Table 2
presents estimates from varied sources since the early 1950s when Nepal
began progressively to be exposed to direct outside influences.

More recently the 1977–1978 Demographic Sample Survey for Nepal,
based on a representative sample of 191 wards in 15 districts (mountains,

Table 2. Mortality estimates for Nepal, 1952–1978

	Vaidyanathan 1952–1954	Worth and Shah 1965–1966	1971 Census (corrected)	CBS Sample Surveys		
				1974	1976	1978
Crude death rate per 1000	30–37	27	23	19·5	22·2	17·1
Infant mortality per 1000 live-births	260–250	208	108	132·5	133·6	104·0

Sources: Authors as cited.

Table 3. Crude death rates in urban and rural areas

Area	1974–1975	1976	1976–1978
Urban	9·0	10·5	12·2
Rural	19·8	22·6	18·5
Nepal	19·5	22·2	17·1

Source: CBS (1978).

Table 4. Infant mortality rates per 1000 live-births by age and sex

Sample area	1974–1975			1976			1977–1978		
	Male	Female	Both sexes	Male	Female	Both sexes	Male	Female	Both sexes
Urban	55·2	59·2	57·1	55·3	50·2	52·8	72·8	60·8	67·2
Rural	143·9	124·9	134·8	130·7	140·6	136·1	110·0	99·1	105·1
Nepal	141·2	123·0	132·5	128·4	137·9	133·6	109·9	97·9	104·0

Sources: CBS Demographic Sample Survey Reports.

hills and *terai*), has amplified the information on basic mortality indicators for both rural and urban areas (see Table 3).

A clear measure of the uncertainty of these data is found in the CBS's own comment that

> the recorded and adjusted CDR of 22·2 seems to be an over-estimate. The increase of CDR in the urban areas . . . may really have been because of differences in the recording of deaths in urban areas

rather than because of any real increase in deaths. Nevertheless, on the assumption of accuracy in such estimates increasing from year to year and Nepal's CDR dropping from 30–37/1000 in 1954 to about half that level today, as well as the substantially lower urban as compared to rural rates, the tables indicate a rising health status and a death rate which

> has dropped dramatically to less than half the birth rate, though no organised health services reach the villages. *Judging from the present age distribution of the population, a dramatic fall in the death rate occurred in the previous generation, before the country opened to international contact and before health programmes were introduced* (Taylor and Taylor, 1976; my italics).

Sample surveys of infant mortality have paradoxically shown an increase in the IMRs in urban areas, which are generally lower than in rural areas (Table 4). Although extremely little is known about infant mortality in Nepal, the IMR none the less offers "a fairly sensitive index

Table 5. Adjusted age-specific death rates per 1000 person-years and age distribution by sex in 1977–1978 for Nepal

			Death Rates				Percentage share of total population	
	Urban		Rural		Total			
Age group	Male	Female	Male	Female	Male	Female	Male	Female
0 [a]	72·8	60·8	111·1	99·1	109·9	97·9	—	—
1–4	8·2	14·5	27·0	23·9	23·4	22·1	14·5	14·1
5–14	2·8	2·3	4·9	5·8	4·7	5·2	28·1	27·4
15–24	2·9	4·0	4·8	4·4	4·4	4·3	18·5	8·4
25–34	4·1	2·1	6·7	7·8	6·0	6·5	13·7	15·0
35–44	14·2	9·7	11·4	10·6	11·9	10·2	10·6	10·8
45–54	26·1	6·5	19·1	19·4	20·3	16·6	7·3	7·1
55–64	13·2	28·5	39·3	42·7	33·0	39·2	4·4	4·3
65–74	109·3	71·3	82·8	74·0	87·8	71·5	2·9 [b]	2·9 [b]
75+	157·1	97·0	145·6	145·7	145·7	129·0	—	—
Average	13·2	10·9	19·3	17·7	17·9	16·2	100·0	100·0

Source: CBS (1978).
[a] Rates per 1000 live-briths.
[b] Age group 65 years and over.

of mortality and is extremely valuable in assessing shifts in health status, modernisation and development in a country" (Tuladhar *et al.*, 1978).

Finally, for the purposes of later discussion, the adjusted age-specific death rates are given in Table 5. The rapid and generally regular fall-off of population in the upper age cohorts is apparent in the age–sex distribution for 1977–1978, with male–female percentages under 15 years being 42·6 and 41·4 respectively, 15–49 years being 46·3 and 47·6 per cent, and those over 50 years 11·1 and 10·9 per cent of the population respectively. When comparing urban and rural areas in the 1977–1978 sample the contrast is most marked in the first year of life, but also striking in the age group 1–4 years. This disadvantage persists for the rural male population up to ages of 35–44 years (thereafter reversing in favour of urban survivorship again). The rural areas are disadvantaged at all ages for female survival.

Migration

Population mobility, like the establishment of new transport networks, is clearly a major epidemiological and medical geographical factor in most developing countries. Nepal is distinguished by a very low rate of urbanization—in 1971 only 4 per cent of the total population were enumerated in urban *panchayats*—but the tradition of emigration to India dates from the mid-nineteenth century, and the country's population exports are reflected in India's own censuses—currently about half a million being Nepal-born migrants. Within the country the rural to rural migration affecting the movement from the hills to the *terai* has been particularly marked since about 1965, following the success of a malaria control programme in opening new land to settlement. The movement of hill peoples to "Nepal's economic frontier" (Weiner, 1973) has additionally been matched by substantial inflows from Indian areas like Bihar.

Apart from census figures there has been little information on migration flows to date. In the absence of compulsory registration of births and uncontrolled movements as well, it is small wonder that research findings are hedged about by *caveats*. Since 1969 the Centre for Economic Development and Administration in Kathmandu (CEDA) has conducted a number of migration studies, as in the Far Western Development Region (1977) and the Kathmandu area (Thapa and Tiwara, 1977). The latter showed that three-quarters of all migrants in a 7·5 per cent sample of the city's households fell into the 11–30 years age group and demonstrated a clear, inverse relationship between numbers and distance from the home district: 42·2 per cent originated from the Central Development Region, about 25 per cent from each of the Western and Eastern Regions, and a mere 6·2 per cent from the Far Western. In a 1979 household demographic survey of Kathmandu some striking contrasts with the generality of developing countries emerged, particularly the conspicuously low proportion of migrants to the capital city. In that 5 per cent sample, seven out of ten heads of household had been borne in Kathmandu, and only 15 per cent of the sample population were migrants in a city which numbered one-third of Nepal's total urban population.

> Apart from the weak 'pullforces' of urban areas, including Kathmandu, this is perhaps understandable in the light of the government's strategy of regional planning oriented towards agricultural expansion in the *terai*, horticultural development in the central hilly district, and livestock development in the upper mountainous regions (Rajbanshi, 1979).

Table 6 relates the regional variations in migrants' birthplaces for three distinct time periods (albeit ignoring factors such as mortality and return migration) to certain characteristics of the sending areas.

However, in the absence of reliable national data "internal migration generally seems to follow two patterns. One is the seasonal movement of hill people to the *terai* and the other is the permanent movement of population from the hills and mountains to the *terai*" (Nepal Fertility

Table 6. Source areas of Kathmandu migrant population in 1979 by region and period in per cent

Birthplace (development region)	Regional characteristics				Migration period			
	Share of national population	Proportion urban	Population living in hills and mountains	Density per km²	Before 1960	1960–1969	1970–1979	Total all periods
Central	33·45	7·58	54·2	137·1	75·2	52·2	58·3	59·8
Eastern	24·21	3·15	50·4	99·9	7·8	13·9	12·4	12·0
Western	21·34	2·32	75·9	67·5	7·4	12·2	12·8	11·5
Far-western	21·00	0·97	75·6	46·1	1·8	4·8	3·6	3·6
Total internal					92·2	83·1	87·1	86·9
Other countries					7·8	16·9	12·9	13·1

Sources: B. S. Rajbanshi (1979) and U.N. Cairo Demographic Centre: data on regional characteristics derived from 1971 Census and CBS, *Analysis of Population Statistics of Nepal* (1977).

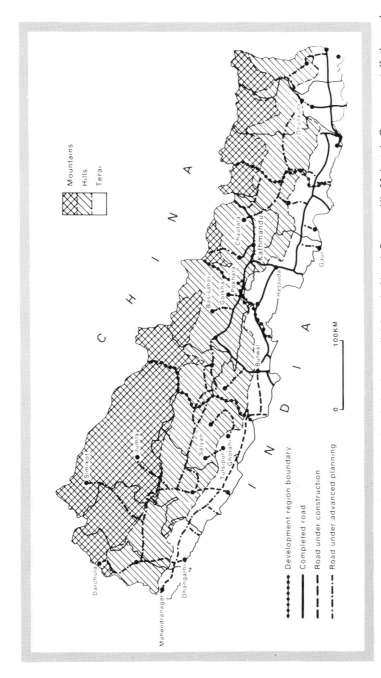

Figure 1. Existing and planned road network and main landscape divisions in Nepal. Source: His Majesty's Government, Kathmandu (1978).

Survey, 1976). At least Nepal is not yet faced by the health problems of squatter settlements found in so many cities in the developing countries.

Environmental changes

Population growth in Nepal has, like attempts at socio-economic development by the government, led to environmental changes in the widest sense. Some have been planned but many are the consequences of uncontrolled forces which threaten to do incalculable harm to the entire Himalayan ecosystem. In few countries of the developing world are the internal forces for change so limited, for reasons such as the low urban population, the low levels of literacy and schooling and the lack of an integrated national economy. "The factors at work elsewhere to accelerate social change—urbanisation, education, mass communications and transportation—are barely evident in Nepal except in Kathmandu Valley and in portions of the *terai*. Most but not all of the forces for change are external to the system" (Weiner, 1973). More recently Nepal's economic stagnation and environmental deterioration, particularly the increasing precariousness of the hill economy and the exhausting of the *terai*'s potential, have been interpreted in terms of dependency theory and the "natural" disasters regarded as visible symptoms of a much deeper-rooted crisis (Blaikie *et al.*, 1980).

Nepal's development planning experience has encompassed many of these changes over two decades (Bhooshan, 1979; see also Shrestha, 1974; Beenhakker, 1973). To forget that Nepal's modern era, like its scientific census-taking, dates back merely to the early 1950s is to fail to grasp the scale of radical changes which have occurred during this time-span. Five development plans have been implemented since 1956, and the sixth (1980–1985) is current: improvements in the transport and communications infrastructure are particularly striking and of obvious long-term importance both in migration and in the realization of government plans for "development corridors" and "growth axes". But in a country where agriculture accounted for 65 per cent of GDP and nearly 75 per cent of merchandise exports in 1978, it is not surprising that the *per caput* GDP is estimated at US $120 a year and that modernization is far removed from the remoter areas of the kingdom.

Urbanization

The very limited degree of urban development in Nepal has been noted, even though Kathmandu is unquestionably the primate city of a country

Table 7. Urban growth rates by size class

Size class	Growth rate (%)	
	1952/54–1961	1961–1971
5000–10,000	82·7	49·7
10,001–25,000	27·5	40·6
25,001–60,000	11·4	23·2
over 100,000	13·5	24·2

without a spatially regular hierarchy of central places (cf. Shrestha, 1973–74). "Nepal is a nation of more or less self-sufficient villages. The need for urban services is not great, and there are few urban places" (Karan, 1960). Statistical data on urban settlement may be limited by the absence of specifically urban information in censuses prior to that of 1952–1954, but an analysis of all Nepalese settlements of over 5000 inhabitants traces this urban growth from the original ten urban centres of 1952–1954 (Shrestha, 1974). Between this census and the 1961 and 1971 censuses growth by size class was higher for smaller towns than for larger towns, with the sole exception of Kathmandu (Table 7).

Nationally the urban growth rate was highest in the *terai* towns. In the Kathmandu Valley towns the growth rate was marginally lower (13·5 per cent) than the national population growth rate. Overall the urban population attained 5·5 per cent of the total over a period in which settlements of 5000 persons and upwards increased in number from 16 to 41. Using Shrestha's definition of urban settlements—the official one sets the lower threshold at 10,000 inhabitants—the Kathmandu Valley towns had a 64·9 per cent share (the eastern *terai* towns, 25·7 per cent of the remainder) in 1961; this had changed to 43 and 32 per cent respectively by 1971. However, the difficulties of reconciling arbitrary definitions of urban status are illustrated by the official view that a very much smaller population lives in the *nagar* or town *panchayats* than in the village *panchayats*. The 1971 census records in fact 253 localities having upwards of 5000 people, but only 16 were designated town *panchayats*. Indeed, if only those towns with more than 35 per cent of their labour force engaged in non-agricultural occupations are counted, the urban population of Nepal would fall from 461,938 to 340,450 persons, or merely 3 per cent of the national total (CBS, 1977).

From the aspect of health the national picture is one of unsatisfactory water supplies, sewerage and waste disposal in general, and although all but one urban centre have piped water systems the government admits that none of them is adequate in terms of quality or quantity, intermittent supply being commonplace. A major sewerage system is being installed in Kathmandu, but in 1981 the capital alone was served by a small system and that covered only the central area. Elsewhere water-borne sewerage is limited to hospitals, government buildings and private houses with septic tanks. In the absence of latrines indiscriminate defaecation on the ground is the norm. Likewise in 1981 there was still no organized system of solid waste collection or disposal in any town or village in Nepal. Kathmandu had instituted a pilot scheme in 1973 to cover seven city wards, but although effective this was abandoned due to lack of funds, and the problem continues to be inadequately solved by traditional sweepers who either sort the refuse near their homes or dispose of it in convenient rivers. Quite obviously the build up of solid wastes in the older town centres, where garbage is thrown into yards and lanes, creating breeding places for insects and rodents, constitutes a major public health risk.

Detailed survey data on morbidity and mortality rates arising from such circumstances are still unavailable, but the report by a British firm of consulting engineers in 1973 on water supplies and sanitation in Nepal reveals the broad extent of the problem of infectious and parasitic diseases, which can scarcely have improved since then (Table 8). Kathmandu itself illustrates the problems of the urban environment to an extreme degree in its core area of multi-storeyed, congested, over-crowded and archaic dwellings. In 1971 over 50 per cent of the core area's housing stock was more than 50 years old, compared to 28 per cent on the urban fringe (Bhooshan, 1979). A WHO worker commented,

> Though houses are fairly solidly built, individual rooms are small, dark and badly ventilated. People tend to crowd together especially for sleeping purposes. The lack of environmental sanitation, the habit of spitting, and the many dark, unventilated and overcrowded habitations contribute fundamentally to the dissemination of communicable diseases (Phelps, 1968).

Bhooshan's (1976) survey found that 98·6 per cent of Kathmandu's population had access to toilets and 90 per cent to water; elsewhere in the Kathmandu Valley such basic facilities were markedly less satisfactory, with only 40 per cent of Patan's households having access to toilets and 66 per cent to water, and Bhaktapur registering 18 and 78 per cent respectively. The *Physical Development Plan for the Kathmandu Valley* recorded that "during the Malla Period (*c.* 1768) an extensive drainage system was constructed and maintained. This system has gradually deteriorated since then because of lack of maintenance, particularly in recent years". By 1969 it was generally non-functional.

Although the *Physical Development Plan* had recommended basic research into the spatial characteristics of settlement, including gross and

Table 8. Water-borne diseases and other health problems

Disease	Kathmandu Bagmati	Biratnagar Koshi	Dharan	Pokhara Gandaki	Nepalgunj Bheri	Janakpur	Gorkha Gandaki
				Zones			
Typhoid	2	2	1	2	2	2	2
Amoebic dysentery	1	1	1	1	1	1	1
Bacillary dysentery	2	1	1	2	1	1	1
Giardia dysentery	2	2	N.D.	1	N.D.	N.D.	N.D.
Hookworm	1	2	4	2	3	1	1
Roundworm	1	2	1	2	1	1	1
Cholera	3	5	5	5	5	5	5
Malaria	5	4	5	4	5	5	5
Infectious hepatitis	3	4	5	4	4	3	5
Typhus	5	N.D.	5	5	5	N.D.	5
Schistosomiasis	5	5	5	5	5	5	5
Filariasis	3	2	3	5	2	2	5
Gastro-enteritis	1	1	1	2	2	1	1
Tuberculosis	1	1	1	2	1	1	1

Key: The numbers are based on subjective assessments of the relative importance of various health problems in the judgement of medical officers in charge of hospitals visited in the zones listed.
Codes: 1 = very common; 2 = common; 3 = some incidence; 4 = rare; 5 = no recent cases recorded; N.D. = not diagnosed.
Source: *Water Supplies and Sanitation in Nepal. Sector Study,* WHO/UNDP (Special Fund) Project—Nepal 0025 (1973).

net population densities, the area and location of built-up space, the spatial distribution of ethnic and caste groups, and the functional arrangement of the town, no substantive follow-up has been published. This is regrettable, given the Plan's example of Ward 7 in the city core where the net density (i.e. gross area less circulation area) was equivalent to 74,000 persons per km^2 in 1961; the net density of the entire city core was estimated at about 45,000 per km^2. Such conditions, it noted, reflect population pressures in the valley towns "scarcely known to Western industrial nations". The more recent CEDA study of in-migration to Kathmandu, based on the old ward boundaries, showed densities in 1971 of 365 persons per hectare in the southern core and 72 per hectare in the northern; not surprisingly the annual growth rates on the southern fringe (3·83 per cent) and northern fringe (4·58 per cent) were substantially greater than the already saturated southern core, 0·82 per cent (Thapa and Tiwara, 1977). Close investigation of health and disease variation is needed within this framework, which is further complicated by what Joshi (1972, 1973) has called the "socio-economic ecology" of the city.

Changes in the rural areas

Because Nepal's health problems are principally rural in setting, population increase is central to any discussion of health care or environmental changes. "The rural parts of Nepal represent one of the few areas of the world in which a traditional, pre-industrial ecological balance between man and his environment might be studied with modern investigational techniques" (Worth and Shah, 1969). The authors could scarcely have anticipated the scale of environmental degradation which population increase and commercial exploitation would occasion. Accelerating destruction of the once continuous forest belt in the Himalayan foothills and the resulting soil erosion, landslides and hydrological disruption now affect Nepal's neighbours in India and Bangladesh. Drastic landscape changes have been brought about by, for example, the movement of 50,000 migrants a year from the food deficit area of the hills and mountains since 1970 to the *terai* where legal and illegal forest clearance has amounted to 2 per cent of the stock annually over a decade (Bhattarai, 1979). The consequences of changes within these watershed run-off systems are of wide medical interest (cf. Rieger, 1975).

For the medical geographer changes in the equilibrium of existing ecosystems present fresh complications. For instance microclimatic modifications, vegetation change or the drying-out of soils may lead to changes in disease distribution by altering the living conditions of plant and animal communities. This area of possible future research into the natural nidality of disease, with its risk of creating man-made biotopes, might eventually be linked with the recent, and highly significant, *National Watershed Inventory* in Nepal, to provide map cover of watersheds and land systems (Nelson, 1979). Land systems have to date found their main applications in terrain evaluation and land management affecting activities like agriculture, forestry and civil engineering. There is undoubtedly scope for the employment of the ecological land units and land unit associations now being surveyed in primary health-care planning and for the control of actual or potential hazards such as transmissible diseases and malnutrition.

Disease patterns in Nepal

Writing as recently as 1951, Taylor could comment that "to the scientist today Nepal presents a field almost as untouched as Central Africa did to Livingstone a century ago"; in his view few countries had such a variety of diseases within so small an area (Taylor, 1951). Prior to the Nepal Health Survey of 1965–1966 there was no scientific baseline data available on a national scale, and even that survey (Worth and Shah, 1969) did not provide "the regional, socio-economic, geographic, demographic and innumerable practical considerations necessary for implementing a health programme" (Gautam, 1974). As recently as 1979 the Health Manpower Development Research Project (1973–1978), set up to develop an inventory of health manpower, to study the existing felt health and family planning needs of communities and *inter alia* to identify health problems, could report that

> government health services are currently meeting at most only 8 per cent of the estimated community health needs for curative services. . . . The over-riding factor determining the use of services is distance. Utilisation of services by households at a distance more than two hours walking is minimal (Shah *et al.*, 1979).

The altitudinal zonation of disease belts in Nepal is well-documented, not least because much of the early literature on disease is linked with climbing expeditions or the recruitment of Gurkha soldiers in the field (cf. Millar, 1957; Tokunaga, 1957; Dunn, 1962). The links between population mobility and epidemiology of medical geography have been barely touched upon. Nepal is

> one of the few remaining redoubts of pestilential disease, and the incidence of dietary deficiency disease is undoubtedly very high. Malaria, smallpox, cholera, tuberculosis, typhoid, dysentery, diarrhoea, as well as beri-beri

and other diseases of vitamin deficiency, are widespread throughout Nepal. There is no medical survey for the whole country, and the regional studies are limited in scope and number. In the past there has been no system of collecting vital statistics . . . analysis of the geographical distribution of disease is therefore extremely difficult (Karan, 1960, p. 74).

With the obvious exception of smallpox, this situation broadly persists, although vital registration began in 1977 for limited areas, and the situation remains one in which the great majority of fatal illnesses are untreated by modern medicine or practitioners. A malaria eradication project was launched in 1958, leprosy and tuberculosis control in 1964–1965, smallpox eradication in 1967–1968 and the Family Planning and Maternal and Child Health Project (MCH) in 1968. Some of the impacts of these official efforts are beginning to be reflected in mortality decline, and similarly the effect of the MCH programmes on the nutritional status and care of children may be inferred from tentative reports on birth rates and infant mortality levels. In the Western Region, changes among 4029 people in seven villages were monitored, and it was found that there was an apparent decline in CDR to 11·6 and IMR to 75 per thousand (under 5 mortality 29 per thousand) by 1977–1978, or half the national average, over a ten-year period (Harding, 1978).

The *Nepal Health Survey* itself was based on a very carefully constructed sample of 6321 people in 957 households in 23 villages in various regions throughout Nepal. The Survey gathered sample data on IMR and children surviving from each woman's total reproductive history in each of the three years preceding the enquiry. (Unlike census data collected mainly from male respondents, the Survey involved women-to-women communication.) It also recorded the total number of deaths in each household by age, over the previous year, plus the total number and ages of people surviving in them. The estimates of CDR and IMR, 27 and 150 per thousand respectively, were reflected in 37 per cent of all deaths being those of infants, and a further 19 per cent falling between the ages of 1 and 4. Deaths over this age were too few to allow calculation of anything but age-specific mortality rates, but on the basis of its more accurate registration of infant mortality the Survey interestingly found an actual population for Nepal apparently 3 per cent larger than the official census figure for 1961, due to the under-enumeration of infants and children below 5 years.

The Survey reports separately on various disease classes: nutritional and nutritional deficiency diseases, those transmitted by the direct route, those by the respiratory route, those by faecal contamination or by insect vectors, and other conditions including diseases of the lung and cardiovascular system, and diabetes. It found that the nutritional standard of the population compared well with FAO and WHO targets; directly transmitted diseases like leprosy and the venereal diseases were of low prevalence. Those of the respiratory tract were primarily governed by "the environmental variables of crowding within houses and ventilation of houses" and were associated with protein malnutrition. High age-specific rates for TB were found in Kathmandu and low ones in rural areas—suggesting a recent (i.e. 100 to 200 years) introduction of the disease. Diseases transmitted by faecal contamination may pass through the soil to skin or mouth, or by water supply, foodstuffs or flies: all the common intestinal parasites were found. The Survey commented

> As long as village water supplies are poorly protected, diseases transmitted by faecal contamination will contribute heavily to infant and child mortal-ity, to some extent to young mortality, to a continuous load of illness at all ages, and will set the stage for periodic disastrous local epidemics of cholera introduced from across the border. . . . The data support the general contention that protection of water supplies will probably yield quicker and more socially acceptable results in disease prevention than the socially difficult control of promiscuous defaecation (Worth and Shah, 1969, pp. 76–78).

Quantified evidence on mortality and morbidity is extremely hard to obtain: Nepal has as yet no separate Public Health Department, and an Environmental Health Division in Kathmandu was established only in 1979. It is, of course, possible to obtain information on the numerical growth of the health services, but epidemiological data are virtually unobtainable. Distortions inevitably creep into the national picture largely shaped by information gathered from 51 government and 15 other hospitals unevenly distributed between the regions in 1978. In the same year, of 257 government doctors 129 were in the Central Region alone. A similar number were in private practice, the Army, missions and health administration and so did nothing to correct the pronounced regional inequalities or the disproportionate medical services particu-larly in the Kathmandu Valley.

In 1979 the Ministry of Health published for the first time data based on 9188 in-patient discharges from nine hospitals over the period 1975–1976 (excluding normal deliveries), which ranked disease groups nationally. Although such figures are selective and distorted by factors such as distance decay in patient-usage of hospitals in remote areas, the rank order is interesting (Table 9).

Of the major causes of infant and child mortality the same source reported on 384 deaths in 10 hospitals for the year 1974–1975: the rankings for the first six causes of death were differentiated for the age groups of under one year and one to four years, and the obvious shifts

Table 9. Major disease groups among in-patients: 1975–1976

Rank	Disease group	Percentage
1	Infective and parasitic	28·9
2	Respiratory system	28·6
3	Symptoms and ill-defined conditions	10·9
4	Accidents, injuries, etc.	8·7
5	Genito-urinary system	6·1
6	Digestive system	4·2
7	Circulatory system	3·7
8	Complications of pregnancy	3·2
9	Nervous system and sense organs	3·0
10	Endocrinal, nutritional, metabolic	2·7

Source: *Nepal Health Profile* Kathmandu (1979), p. 271.

Table 10. Infant and child mortality by cause: 1974–1975

	Under 1 year			1–4 years	
Rank	Disease	(%)	Rank	Disease	(%)
1	Pneumonia	27·2	1	Enteritis etc.	21·6
2	Enteritis and other diarrhoeal	22·2	2	Symptoms and ill-defined conditions	16·8
3	Avitaminoses and other nutritional deficiencies	6·2	3	Pneumonia	11·2
4	Meningitis	6·2	4	Meningitis	8·0
5	Acute respiratory infections	4·9	5	Measles	4·8
6	Bronchitis, emphysema and asthma	3·7	6	Tetanus	3·2
Percentage of all deaths		70·4			65·6

Source: *Nepal Country Health Profile* (1979), p. 267.

from diseases of early infancy to childhood are apparent, as is the continuing role of gastro-enteritis in both groups. Clearly any improvements in housing, water supply, environmental sanitation and nutrition will immediately trigger reductions in the levels of most of the diseases in Table 10, but the secondary and later effects of childhood diseases upon adult morbidity should not be underestimated.

From this limited data the Ministry of Health has summarized that, in ten hospital returns for 1974–1975, infectious and parasitic diseases occupied first place in every age group. These were followed by respiratory diseases in second place for all ages up to 14 and over 45 years.

As with the radical improvement in fertility data brought about by the World Fertility Survey's work in 1976, so the recent completion of community or household surveys and health institution studies by the Institute of Medicine of Tribhuvan University represents a major advance in the collection of reliable data on health-care problems in four districts—Tanahu, Dhankuta, Surkhet and Nuwakot—as part of the *Health Manpower Development Research Project* between 1973 and 1978 (Fig. 2). Although those considered here for Tanahu (Western Region) and Dhankuta (Eastern Region) lack either maps or any other attempts to present their data in spatial or ecological frames, they provide information of great scientific merit. In the Tanahu Survey the data were related to four time–distance "strata" (i.e. households within one, or between one and three, hour's walk of Bankipur Hospital or a health post respectively). Information on all deaths showed that diarrhoea and gastro-intestinal disorders were the major causes in all ages above one year. Furthermore, the findings indicated very high levels of reported gross morbidity, as well as disability. Respiratory conditions, diarrhoea and general infections were the principal causes of a 40–50 per cent sickness level in the population at large. The survey suggested, moreover, that government health services were providing care for at most 10 per cent of sick persons seeking care, and only 3 per cent of all sick persons estimated to need care.

Some of the findings from the 77 tables of the Dhankuta District Survey are presented in collated form in Table 11. Conducted in a hilly region with no vehicular roads or communications with other districts, almost completely agricultural and one in which villages are connected by narrow tracks, the population was reported to have minimal awareness of hygiene, limited sources of good drinking water and neither sanitary drainage nor garbage disposal systems. Mortality data from the 601 sampled households showed that about 22 per cent of all deaths were attributable to each of the "fever" and "diarrhoea and gastro-intestinal disorder" groups, each of which is preventable. The CDR of 13·3 per thousand (IMR: 90 per thousand) was, remarkably, found to be lower than the national estimate.

Morbidity was measured in terms of "expressed problems" (i.e. signs and symptoms rather than by clinical diagnoses), and Table 11 emphasizes the variations in household levels of reported sickness in two main time–distance zones and contrasts these with sickness actually observed when villagers made use of three categories of health-care facility, including the folk medicine (*ayurvedic*) dispensaries. The average gross morbidity level was found to be 22 per cent over the fortnight recall period, with respiratory conditions predominating more or less uniformly in all households and all age groups, followed by parasites, gastro-intestinal conditions and diarrhoea/dysentery.

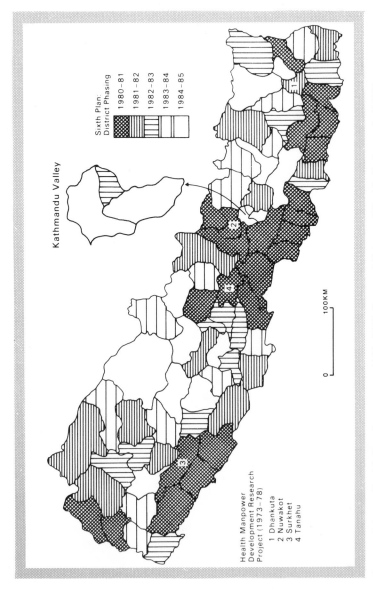

Kathmandu Valley

Sixth Plan:
District Phasing

1980–81
1981–82
1982–83
1983–84
1984–85

Health Manpower
Development Research
Project (1973–78)

1 Dhankuta
2 Nuwakot
3 Surkhet
4 Tanahu

Figure 2. Primary Health Care Programme 1980–1985. Source: Ministry of Health, Kathmandu (1979).

Table 11. Morbidity levels in Dhankuta District, Eastern Region, 1977

Conditions	Percentage distribution of all reported conditions for all ages derived from household surveys		Percentage distribution of morbidity in 24 days sample at various health care facilities		
	Households within 0–3 hours walking distance of hospital	Households within 0–3 hours walking distance of health post	District hospital	Health post	Ayurvedic dispensary
Fever only	4·7	5·0	2·7	3·2	5·9
Other general	8·0	3·5	3·8	7·8	2·9
Respiratory	40·0	34·4	27·7	27·9	26·8
Cardiovascular	0·7	0·2	0·3	0·2	0·1
Dental	1·8	2·8	—	—	—
Diarrhoea and dysentery	2·2	7·4	5·5	12·8	—
Parasites and other general infections	12·0	17·0	17·0	22·3	26·9
Genito-urinary (male)	—	1·4	0·7	0·1	1·6
Genito-urinary (female)	0·7	0·8	2·4	0·2	1·4
Skin	7·7	6·0	12·2	12·2	18·6
Musculo-skeletal	5·5	4·3	8·3	2·8	2·3
Eye	5·5	2·6	2·9	1·5	1·4
Ear	4·0	4·1	3·5	0·8	1·6
Other sensory and nervous system	1·8	4·1	0·2	0·1	0·8
Nutritional and weakness	1·8	1·8	2·5	2·5	0·8
Accident and injury	1·5	2·8	5·5	4·9	3·3
Specific infections	0·7	0·8	3·0	0·1	0·1
Others—unknown	1·1	1·1	1·8	0·6	0·1
Total cases and percentage	100·0 (274)	100·0 (605)	100·0 (1028)	100·0 (1422)	100·0 (689)

Source: Collated from Report of a Study in the Primary Health Care Unit of Dhankuta, Nepal, Kathmandu (1979).

Use of the curative services demonstrated a clear distance decay, with very low consultation rates for households further than one hour's walking distance from the one hospital: non-treatment or non-consultation rates increased from 53 to 82 per cent between the first and second strata (i.e. under one and over one hour's walking distance), and the rise in the case of health posts was from 61 to 75 per cent respectively. The survey usefully categorized "probably preventable" and "probably non-preventable" sickness, and estimated that 46 per cent of all expressed conditions were in the first of these categories, 72 per cent of which actually needed care. In the second category only 52 per cent of all cases needed care. Because only 17 per cent of all sick persons consulted any form of health service in Dhankuta, it was possible to estimate—on the basis of health service needs derived from survey data—that at most 27 per cent of the needs could be satisfied by the combined services, and that government health facilities actually met only 5 per cent of the medical care needs of the 121,945 people living in the district in 1977.

Primary health-care planning

Nepal's Sixth National Health Plan (1980–1985) has coincided with a growing world concern for primary health care as part of overall national and community development. The disease geography which has been described, along with the extent of preventable morbidity revealed in the Health Manpower Development Research Project surveys between 1973 and 1978, underline the significance of any attempt to deliver an effective rural health programme through a system attuned to the social and environmental conditions of a country manifestly unable to afford or instal a national system based on the Western model. In an overwhelmingly rural population the desirability of providing basic health services at the point of contact is clear. When Nepal began national development planning in 1956 the country had only 34 hospitals with 625 beds, plus 24 conventional and 63 *ayurvedic* (traditional) dispensaries. Today the national health policy covers such objectives as increasing the life expectation, the maintaining of a regional balance by providing at least minimal health services to the maximum number of people, the controlling of population growth, and the control, containment or eradication of communicable diseases through a radically re-oriented health-care delivery system.

The *Long Term Health Plan* (1975–1990) seeks to develop basic health services at the village level, and to establish 15-bed hospitals in every one of the 75 districts by the end of the current plan period in 1985. The egional distribution of health facilities in 1978–1979 is presented in Table 12 and in Fig. 3, and may usefully be compared with Shrestha's description of the facilities at the start of the decade, when there were still only 53 hospitals and a mere 189 health centres or health posts, yielding such extremes in service populations as one hospital bed per 44,000 population in Rapti Zone, one health post or health centre per 206,000 population in Bheri Zone, or one physician per 144,000 population in Sagarmartha Zone in 1970–1971 (Shrestha, 1972). Figure 3 illustrates the striking discrepancies between the four development regions, and in particular the concentration of both hospitals and physicians in the Central Region and the Kathmandu Valley area specifically. As recently as 1975 there were hospitals in only 31 of the 75 districts, and the majority of people depended upon health posts and centres. The figures for 1975 show that in remote areas health post service areas averaged 858 km^2, hose in the hills 392 km^2 and those in the plains 232 km^2. With accelerated construction in the Fifth Plan, remote areas raised their total by 118 to 168 posts, those in the hills by 143 to 299 and those in the plains by 88 to 233—a remarkable improvement as the average service area population dropped from 1 : 36,000 to 1 : 20,000. The average service area fell from 392 km^2 to 197 km^2 in the kingdom as a whole.

Given that the Sixth Plan's target is further to reduce these figures to 15,000 people and 131 km^2 per health post by 1985, the central role of health posts and centres in delivering preventive and curative medicine o the population at large is obvious. It is increasingly recognized that here will be insufficient physicians to meet various targets, particularly n the rural areas, and the use of paramedical workers is becoming central o the success of the primary health-care programme at community level. n the Nepali context the basic components of PHC include treatment of he common diseases, vector control, immunization, first-aid, referral, nutritional surveillance, maternity services and family planning. The Sixth Plan aims at a decentralized and community-based PHC infrastructure throughout the kingdom by 1985. Figure 2 summarizes the phasing of this programme over the quinquennium, with the apparent concentration initially upon the *terai* and the west–central core. Apart from provision of at least one 15-bed hospital per district, most interest deserves to be directed to plans to set up at least one health post in each of the nine *ilakas* into which each district is divided, plus the appointment of at least one village health worker (VHW) in each of the 2911 village *panchayats* and one voluntary ward-level *panchayat* health worker in the 26,199 wards (nine per *panchayat*) into which Nepal is divided. Despite contemporary interest in the role and potential of folk medicine in PHC programmes in some countries, Nepal's Rural Health

Table 12. Regional distribution of government health facilities and average service populations (S.P.) in 1978

Development region	Population	Zones	Districts	Physicians/ S.P.	Hospital beds [b]/ S.P.	Health centres and health post/S.P.	Ayurvedic dispensaries/ S.P.
Eastern	3,199,502	3	16	55/1 : 58,172	411/1 : 7785	120/1 : 26,662	17/1 : 188,206
Central	4,529,683	3	19	129/1 : 35,114	1443/1 : 3139	149/1 : 30,400	23/1 : 196,942
Western	2,841,286	3	16	37/1 : 76,791	335/1 : 8481	105/1 : 27,059	24/1 : 118,387
Far-western	2,850,813	5	24	36/1 : 79,189	220/1 : 12,958	137/1 : 20,808	18/1 : 158,379
Nepal	13,421,284	14	75	257/1 : 62,319 [a]	2409/1 : 8091 [b]	511/1 : 26,232	82/1 : 163,674

[a] In 1978 in addition to government doctors there were 75 full-time physicians in private practice, mainly in the Bagmati Zone around Kathmandu, 48 in the armed services and 50 expatriates. Of those in the latter group listed in the *Health Manpower Directory* the majority were accredited to hospitals such as the Shanta Bhawan in Lalitpur (10) and U.M.N. Hospital at Tamsen (5).
[b] Both government and mission hospitals are included here.
Source: Based on Ministry of Health records, Kathmandu (1979).

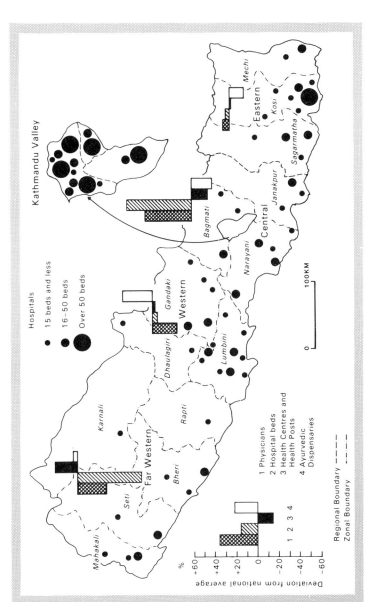

Figure 3. Regional share of health facilities and hospital distribution in Nepal, 1979. Sources: Ministry of Health, Kathmandu and Health Manpower Directory (1979).

Programme places a relatively modest emphasis upon *ayurvedic* medicines and traditional faith healers, apparently assuming this sector to be significant only in areas remote from government-run facilities. None the less, the Tanahu PHC Survey (1977) recorded that of the 26·4 per cent of all sick persons consulting any type of service in all households surveyed, 8 per cent used traditional faith healers. The Sixth Plan provides for the establishment of 50 more *ayurvedic* dispensaries between 1980 and 1985, and for the building of one *ayurvedic* hospital in each of the four regions.

This innovatory structure will ultimately be managed from 75 district health offices (there were 48 in 1979), but at the community level the ward-level volunteers will depend upon standard health manuals and receive 2–3 days training at local health posts. The community itself will be charged with deciding upon health priorities and identifying the "locally prevalent health problems". Among the general tasks of such paramedical staff will be not only first aid, malaria prevention, immunization and the referral of TB and leprosy cases, but also the maintaining of monthly returns of birth and death statistics in each ward and the promotion of health education and of family planning.

Whilst it would be unsound to accept that all plan targets can or will be reached by 1985 in a country which spends under 6 per cent of its GNP on health, around 13 rupees *per caput*, even slight improvements in overall living conditions and a modest general introduction of these simple health measures seem likely to lead to significant further declines in mortality over a short time period. In consequence the family planning aspect of PHC assumes a disproportionate importance. The current health plan envisages the existence of 240 family planning clinics and 1550 *panchayat*-based clinics, as well as mobile teams, capable of spreading family planning to 750,000 couples by 1985. The integration of all health posts with the home-visiting programme of the auxiliary health workers should mean that epidemiological transition becomes an aspect of population change under conditions where the transition from high to low mortality accompanies either social development or a combination of medical development and social change (Omran, 1971, 1977). Medical geographers appear to have disregarded the epidemiological transition model's value in conceptualizing the process whereby health and disease patterns have shifted from the stages of pestilence and famine through receding pandemics to degenerative and man-made diseases. If mortality is taken as the fundamental factor in population change, many of the demographic and social effects which follow are highly significant in development planning. Not only are such obvious alterations as life expectancy in general, or child survival in particular, important but a country like Nepal may be faced by problems for which it is little prepared in consequence of the timing and dynamics of the epidemiological transition. The social effects include a more healthy, and hence more efficient and productive labour force, the removal of what Omran has called the "complex social, emotional and economic rationales for high birth rates". This will involve the nuclearization of the family and destruction of group cohesion, an increase in demands for and cost of treatment of chronic ailments, the survival of the unfit and, most obviously, the problems of a growing number of dependent old people.

Trowell and Burkitt (1981) have recently collated evidence from a great range of developing areas which suggests that there is a definite sequence marking the onset and course of Western diseases which accompany the dietary, life-style, economic, environmental and other changes associated with development. Thus populations, once characterized by life-long low blood pressure, develop hypertension, followed by increased reporting of obesity, diabetes mellitus, coronary heart disease and other cardiovascular maladies. Similarly, surgical diseases of the large bowel and other related diseases may emerge and increase in prevalence over time and with increasing age in the sequence appendicitis, haemorrhoids, varicose veins, large bowel tumours, hiatus hernia, deep vein thrombosis, pelvic phleboliths and diverticular disease of the colon. Recent research in the islands of the Pacific has indicated some alarming consequences of the epidemiological transition where chronic degenerative diseases, although not fully manifested yet, *are appearing in earlier age groups than in most westernized countries* and may be—as in the case of such genetic susceptibility as a predisposition to diabetes which was once a survival factor in selecting those better able to store food as fat—unmasked by environmental changes and abandonment of traditional life-styles (Zimmet and Whitehouse, 1981). Of far-reaching importance for both public health costs and labour productivity in countries like Nepal, which have by no means experienced the full impact and severity of these shifts, is the authors' suggestion that "as a result 30–40 per cent of the workforce in certain developing countries may have one or several of these chronic diseases which could render them disabled and unable to work".

The changing incidence and levels of mainly infectious versus degenerative disease might be expected to be most apparent in urban areas of Third World countries, the onset of a transition being delayed in rural areas. Kathmandu, the city for which the best data are available, has not been beset by the worst problems of urbanization. It has slums but no squatter settlements so that expansion and suburbanization under conditions of very limited population increase has been possible. A recent

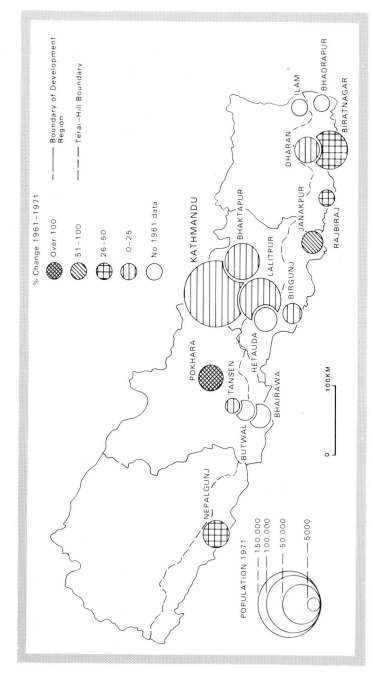

Figure 4. Urban population increase 1961–1971: Nagar (town) Panchyats. Source: Registrar General, Kathmandu (1978).

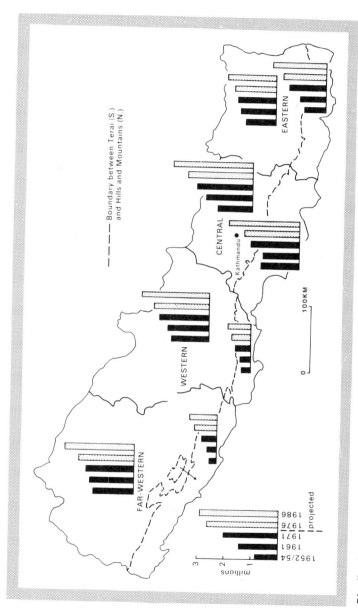

Figure 5. Distribution of population by development and geographical regions, 1952–1986. Source: Central Bureau of Statistics, Kathmandu (1977).

review of the prevalence of heart disease for the period 1969–1974, based on the analysis of 1788 cases of this sort out of a total admission of 12,315 persons (14·5 per cent) to the Bir Hospital may point to a long-term shift to degenerative disease (Pandey and Ghimire, 1975). The bulk of cases (46 per cent) were of pulmonary heart disease, a higher rate than elsewhere in the world affecting the 10–30 year age group (68 per cent of all cases) far more than the 31–50 year group (15 per cent) or those over 50 years (17 per cent). Factors associated with this steadily increasing disease were cited as smoking, overcrowding in damp and dingy surroundings and frequent attacks of respiratory tract infections in childhood (pulmonary lesions). Rheumatic heart disease fluctuated in incidence but paradoxically fell from 28·9 to 16·7 per cent of all cases over the period 1969–1974, this being accounted for by antibiotic treatment in childhood for respiratory tract infections or improved housing among those who might have developed the disease in adulthood. Ischaemic heart disease (8·1 per cent) was much lower in importance than in Western countries, although it rose steadily over the period. The authors attributed this to increased smoking, reduced physical exercise, changes in diet and stress. Hypertension (14·25 per cent) ranked third in the survey. No information on the extent of cancer, diabetes and other maladies of civilization was available in the medical literature.

However tentative these findings or uncertain the assumptions on which they are based, it is clear that intensified concern for the cause of death will need to match improvements in more general census data. Such data will preferably be not only epidemiologically-related (i.e. to abnormal incidence of disease in specific populations) but also be linked with changes in environment and life-style. The obvious variations in the built environment over short distances in places like Kathmandu lend support to the argument that a thorough understanding of the association of diseases with social and other variables will require a geomedical approach to the natural and social ecologies of mortality and morbidity. If an epidemiological transition is occurring, many of the changes may take place, as happened in developed countries, for non-medical reasons. The degree to which "development" outside the health services may lead to higher life expectancy without expensive medical or health service interventions has important implications when allocating scarce resources in any country. Nepal, like many other developing countries is paying increased attention to the collection of more comprehensive demographic data, and to improved epidemiological information services. There is a very strong case for monitoring the country's epidemiological transition within units more appropriate than census enumeration areas—such as ecological *nosochores* for rural areas and social areas for the towns (cf. Diesfeld, 1974; Diesfeld and Hecklau, 1978; Joshi, 1973).

Medical geography todays presents planners with a range of techniques and methods, which might arguably have had to be developed had they not already existed, to enable demographers and those engaged in epidemiology, public health and community medicine to cope with a new generation of tasks. Demography may have coped largely alone with the problems of fertility and nuptiality, but just as spatial considerations are an inescapable part of migration research so the unsolved problems of mortality and morbidity are indissolubly enmeshed in a geo-ecological and spatial plexus which require inter-disciplinary investigation and solution. Andrew Learmonth's perceptive comment à propos of malaria that "surely it is possible that geographical analysis may complement other approaches in elucidating problems that still remain of both academic and practical importance" (Learmonth, 1977) is increasingly true in the developing world. That this should be so is in no small part due to his own research in Nepal's southern neighbour, India, and to his ability to write for a constituency outside geography's narrowed confines.

Acknowledgements

Much of the fieldwork and archival research on which this paper is based was made possible when the author held a UNFPA consultancy in Nepal in 1979 and was engaged in working up household demographic survey material from that country at the U.N. Cairo Demographic Centre in 1979 and 1980. He is greatly indebted to the Centre's then Director, Professor S. A. Huzayyin. The opinions expressed are entirely the responsibility of the author.

References

Beenhakker, A. (1973). A kaleidoscopic circumspection of development planning with contextual reference to Nepal. Rotterdam.
Bhattarai, S. (1979). Human settlement and its impact on the mountain ecosystem. In *Journal of the Nepal Research Centre* (Ed. W. Voigt), **2/3**, 33–40. Kathmandu and Wiesbaden.
Bhooshan, B. S. (1979). *The Development Experience of Nepal*. New Delhi.
Blaikie, P., Cameron, J. and Seddon, D. (1980). *Nepal in Crisis: Growth and Stagnation at the Periphery*. Oxford.
Brown, M. L., Worth, R. M. and Shah, N. K. (1968). The nutritional state of the Nepalese people. *Am. J. clin. Nutr.* **21**, 875–881.
Central Bureau of Statistics (1977). *The Analysis of the Population Statistics of Nepal*. CBS, Kathmandu.

Centre for Economic Development and Administration (1971). Seminar on population and development. CEDA, Kathmandu.

Centre for Economic Development and Administration (1974). Proceedings of the seminar on regional planning. CEDA, Kathmandu.

CNRS (1969). *Bibliographie du Nepal. Sciences Humaines. References en Langues Européenes* (Eds L. Boulinois and H. Millot). CNRS, Paris.

Diesfeld, H.-J. (1974). Zur Methodik der Raumbezogenheit von Krankheitsvorkommen. In Fortschritte der Geomedizinischen Forschung. *Geographische Zeitschrift. Beiheft* **35** (Ed. H. J. Jusatz), pp. 126–141.

Diesfeld, H.-J. and Hecklau, H. K. (1978). *Kenya*. Geomedical Monograph Series. Heidelberg and Berlin.

Dixit, H. (1978). *A Medical Bibliography of Nepal*. Institute of Medicine, Kathmandu.

Donner, W. (1972). Nepal. Raum, Mensch and Wirtschaft. *Schriften des Institut für Asienkunde* **32**.

Dunn, F. L. (1962). Medical geographical observations in central Nepal. *Millbank Memorial Fund Quarterly* **40**, 125–148.

Flintoff, F. (1974). Solid waste management in Kathmandu. Assignment Report. WHO Project SEARO 0150, Kathmandu.

Gautam, P. S. (1974). Health problems in Karnali Zone. A hospital-based comprehensive survey. Remote Areas and Local Development Project, UNICEF, Kathmandu.

Goldman, N., Coale, A. J. and Weinstein, M. (1979). The quality of data in the Nepal Fertility Survey. *Scientific Reports* **6**. Internationalk Statistical Institute, Voorburg.

Gubhaju, B. B. (1972). *Fertility and Mortality in Nepal*. International Institute for Population Studies, Bombay.

Gubhaju, B. B. (1975). Fertility and mortality in Nepal. *J. Nepal Med. Assoc.* **13**, 5 & 6, 115–128.

Harding, J. W. R. (1978). Influence of a system of local M.C.H. clinic on nutritional status and birth and death rates in Western Hills. *J. Nepal Med. Assoc.* **16**, 3, 31–40.

Hellen, J. A. (1981). Demographic change and public policy in Egypt and Nepal: some long-term implications for development planning. *Science and Public Policy* **8**, 4, 308–336.

Institute of Medicine (1979). *Health Manpower Directory 1979*. Kathmandu.

Joshi, T. R. (1972). Exploration of the Socio-economic Ecology of Kathmandu, Nepal: A Factor Analysis Approach. Ph.D. thesis, University of Pittsburgh.

Joshi, T. R. (1973). Kathmandu, Nepal: A socio-economic ecology of the modernizing preindustrial city. *Proc. Assoc. Am. Geogr.* **5**, 126–130.

Kansakar, V. B. S. (1973–1974). History of population migration in Nepal. *The Himalayan Review* **6**, 5–6, 58–68.

Kansakar, V. B. S. (1977). Population censuses in Nepal and the problems of data analysis. CEDA, Kathmandu.

Karan, P. P. (1960). Nepal. *A Cultural and Physical Geography*. University of Kentucky Press, Lexington.

Karan, P. P. (1973–1974). Kathmandu-Patan. The twin cities urban system. *The Himalayan Review* **6**, 5–6 (plus map of 'Land use of the Kathmandu Valley').

Krotki, K. J. and Thakur, H. N. (1971). Estimates of population size and growth from the 1952–54 and 1961 censuses of the Kingdom of Nepal. *Population Studies* **25**, 1, 89–103.

Lang, S. and Lang, A. (1971). The Kunde hospital and a demographic survey of the Upper Khumbu, Nepal. *N.Z. Med. J.* **74**, 1–8.

Learmonth, A. T. A. (1957). Some contrasts in the regional geography of malaria in India and Pakistan. *Trans. Inst. Br. Geogr.* **23**, 37–59.

Learmonth, A. T. A. (1958). Medical geography in Indo-Pakistan: A study of twenty years' data for the former British India. *Indian Geog. J.* **33**, 1–2, 1–59.

Learmonth, A. T. A. (1977). Malaria. In *A World Geography of Human Diseases* (Ed. G. M. Howe), pp. 61–108. London.

Learmonth, A. T. A. and Learmonth, A. M. (1955). Aspects of village life in Indo-Pakistan. *Geography* **40**, 145–160.

Millar, W. S. (1957). Some aspects, mainly medical, of the Gurkha recruiting season. *Royal Army Medical Corps Journal* **103**, 147–154.

Ministry of Health (1979). Primary Health Care—Nepal. Position Paper (mimeo) Kathmandu.

Ministry of Housing and Physical Planning (1969). The Physical Development Plan for the Kathmandu Valley, Kathmandu.

Müller, U. (1981). Social and economic studies on a Newar settlement in the Kathmandu Valley. *Giessener Geographische Schriften* **49**.

Nelson, D. (1979). A national watershed inventory. In *Journal of the Nepal Research Centre* (Ed. W. Voigt), **2/3**, 81–96. Kathmandu and Wiesbaden.

Omran, A. R. (1971). The epidemiological transition: A theory of the epidemiology of population change. *Millbank Memorial Fund Quarterly* **49**, 4, 1, 509–538.

Omran, A. R. (1973). An appraisal of population theories, with an introduction to the theory of the epidemiologic transition. *Egyptian Population and Family Planning Review* **6**, 2, 75–93.

Omran, A. R. (1977). Epidemiological transition in the United States: the health factor in population change. *Population Bulletin* **32**, 2, p. 42.

Pande, B. R. (1978). Planned population to reduce pressure on resources in the hills. *J. Nepal Med. Assoc.* **16**, 3, 1–14.

Pandey, M. R. and Ghimire, M. (1975). Prevalence of various types of heart diseases in Kathmandu. *J. Nepal Med. Assoc.* **13**, 3 & 4, 37–46.

Phelps, D. R. (1968). Assignment report on tuberculosis and leprosy control pilot project, Nepal. WHO Project—Nepal 16, Kathmandu.

Rajbanshi, B. S. (1979). Dynamics of migration to Kathmandu City, U.N.-A.R.E. Cairo Demographic Centre, Seminar on Population Change and Development in some African and Asian Countries. Document CDC/S790/14 (mimeo).

Rajbanshi, B. S. (1982). Patterns of migration and labour force in Kathmandu City. Tribhuvan University, Kathmandu.

Rieger, H.-C. (1975). Himalaya Wasser. Literaturanalyse über die Frage der Auswirkungen von Entwaldung, Erosion und sonstigen Störungen in Einzugsgebiet des Ganges und des Brahmaputra. Süd-Asien Institut, Heidelberg.

Rieger, H.-C. (1978). Socio-economic aspects of environmental degradation in the Himalayas. In *Himalayan Mountain Ecosystems* (Ed. H.-C. Rieger), pp. 119–124. *Dialogue* 76/77.

Rieger, H.-C. (1979). An approach to the dynamic ecosystems model for a watershed. In *Journal of the Nepal Research Centre* (Ed. W. Voigt), **2/3**, 155–170. Kathmandu and Wiesbaden.

Schweinfurth, U. (1957). Die horizontale und vertikale Verbreitung der Vegetation im Himalaya. *Bonner Geographische Abhandlungen* **20**.

Schweinfurth, U. (1981). The vegetation map of the Himalayas 1957. A quarter of a century after. In *Documents de Cartographie Ecologique* (Ed. P. Ozenda), 29, 19–23. Grenoble.

Shah, M., Shrestha, M. and Parker, R. (1979). Rural health needs. Study No. 2. Report of the study of the primary health care unit (district) of Dhankuta, Nepal. Institute of Medicine, Kathmandu. (See also Study No. 1 (Tanahu District), 1977.)

Shrestha, B. P. (1974). *An Introduction to the Nepalese Economy*. Kathmandu.

Shrestha, C. B. (1973–1974). The system of central places in the Arnike Rajmarga area of Nepal. *The Himalayan Review* 6, 5–6, 18–39.

Shrestha, C. B. (1975). Urbanization trends and emerging pattern in Nepal. *The Himalayan Review* 7, 7, 1–13.

Shrestha, C. B. and Vaidya, K. L. (1978). Settlement patterns in the Kathmandu Valley. *The Himalayan Review* 10, 13–20.

Shrestha, R. M. (1972). The role of block grant funding from international and bilateral agencies in organizing basic health services for developing nations. *J. Nepal. Med. Assoc.* 10, 161–179.

Taylor, C. E. and Taylor, D. C. (1976). Population planning in India and Nepal. *Growth and Change* 7, 2, 9–13.

Taylor, C. G. (1951). A medical survey of the Kali Gandak and Pokhara Valleys of Central Nepal. *Geographical Review* 41, 4, 421–437.

Thapa, N. B. and Thapa, D. P. (1969). *Geography of Nepal*. New Delhi.

Thapa, R., Dixit, K. M. and Smith, D. L. (1979). Primary health care in the Nepalese context. *J. Inst. Med.* 1, 1, 27–50.

Thapa, Y. S. and Tiwara, P. N. (1977). In-migration pattern in Kathmandu urban areas. CEDA, Kathmandu.

Tokunaga, A. (1957). Experiences of medical survey in Central Nepal. *J. Indian Med. Assoc.* 29, 221–224.

Trowell, H. C. and Burkitt, D. P. (Eds) (1981). *Western Diseases: Their Emergence and Prevention*. Edward Arnold, London.

Tuladhar, J. M., Gubhaju, B. B. and Stoeckel, J. (1978). Population and family planning in Nepal, Ratna Pustak Bhandar, Kathmandu.

Vaidyanathan, K. E. and Gaije, F. H. (1973). Estimates of abridged life tables: corrected age-sex distribution and birth and death rates for Nepal, 1952–1954. *Demography of India* 11, 2, 278–290.

Voigt, W. (Ed.) (1979). The management of mountain ecosystems. *Journal of the Nepal Research Centre* 2/3 (Sciences). Kathmandu and Wiesbaden.

Usaid, X. (1975). *Nepal Nutrition Status Survey*. Kathmandu.

Weiner, M. (1973). The political demography of Nepal. *Asian Survey* 13, 6, 617–630.

World Fertility Survey (1977). Nepal Fertility Survey 1976, First Report, Kathmandu. (See also The Nepal Fertility Survey 1976: A summary of findings, International Statistical Institute, Voorburg, April, 1978.)

Worth, R. M. and Shah, N. K. (1969). *Nepal Health Survey 1965–1966*. University of Hawaii, Honolulu.

Zimmet, P. and Whitehouse, S. (1981). Pacific islands of Nauru, Tuvalu and Western Samoa. In *Western Diseases: Their Emergence and Prevention* (Eds H. C. Trowell and D. P. Burkitt), pp. 204–224. Edward Arnold, London.

Part three

Research design and methodological problems in the geography of health

Robert J. Stimson

School of Social Sciences, Flinders University,
Adelaide, Australia

Introduction

There is a disturbing tendency for researchers in medical geography and the geography of health care to pay insufficient attention to research design and questions to do with data reliability and problems of spatially aggregated data bases. Basic methodological problems are clearly evident in much of the published research, despite the fact that it is nearly 20 years since geography began to undergo the "quantitative revolution" and that scientific methods of hypothesis testing become widespread in the discipline. While many of the positive methodological gains coming out of this "revolution" have been incorporated in the research designs of medical geographers and those investigating the geography of health care, we continue to violate many basic tenets of scientific research. Greater care on the part of workers in medical geography and the geography of health care must routinely be directed to research design and methodology.

In particular we need to be more keenly aware of the inaccuracies, incompleteness and unreliability that characterizes the data sources we use; to refrain from implying cause–effect relationships where ecological or spatial associations between variables are all that can be statistically proved; to ensure that we use data disaggregated to the smallest possible level of scale and that we do not relate one data set to other data sets that are not scale and time compatible. This review of methodological issues is far from comprehensive, but it attempts to present a number of basic

GEOGRAPHICAL ASPECTS OF HEALTH
ISBN 0 12 483780 8

problems that researchers must be aware of. They must be satisfied that the research designs, methods of data analysis and inferences drawn from their data do not violate the assumptions of methods used and that they operate within the limitations of their data and the methods of analyses used.

Methodological and data problems typically encountered in medical geography and the geography of health-care research

The primary object of this essay is to discuss some of the major problems and pitfalls researchers face in pursuing the study of medical geography and the geography of health care. Methodological problems relating to general questions of research design, the mis-use of statistical methods of analysis, the problems of aggregated data bases, and data reliability problems are discussed in general terms. It will be evident that some of these problems are specific to a particular approach to research in medical geography and the geography of health care, but some problems may apply to any of the paradigms employed in the subject.

Data problems in cause-specific mortality and morbidity studies

It is seemingly simple to map cause-specific mortality data. The usual parameter for mapping is the standardized mortality rate (SMR), which makes allowance for variations in age and sex structure of local populations compared with a national population regarded as having a standard structure of age–sex groups. Ratio data (e.g. deaths or cases per 100 population) may be mapped using standard deviation classes or by examining scatter-of-values to produce choropleth map groupings. This is often the extent of analysis, and the patterns are simply described. There are major weaknesses in this method, especially if the aim of the research is as a step in aetiological enquiry where at least potential *why* and *where* questions are to be asked.

Major problems may be outlined as follows:

(a) Usually there is a great *variation in the gross population densities and in the size of spatial (administrative) units* for which vital and morbidity data are available. Techniques for mapping include assigning an area of map to each locality or area proportional to its population size, but this distorts geographical shape and continuity. We need to be aware of the problems arising from this lack of uniformity in the spatial units for which data are available.

(b) *Chance factors* affect all human activities, including mortality and morbidity statistics. Thus a *stochastic test* needs to be applied so that one can assert, within stated confidence limits, that a pattern is not due to chance. Detailed consideration has been given to this problem by McGlashan (1977). *Poisson distribution* and other tests may be used to establish confidence values, whereby the actual confidence level of each locality deviation of observed from expected numbers of, say, death by a specific cause for a specific age–sex group, is calculated, and a value, ranging from +100 through zero to −100, can be placed on each area. Thus, scores at either tail imply increased confidence that a score has not occurred by chance, whereas a score near to zero implies random fluctuation. *Isomell maps* are thus produced based on the Poisson (or other) distribution, these showing departure from the expected (normal) number of deaths (McGlashan and Harington, 1976). It is imperative that we perform these transformations to mortality and morbidity data in mapping their distributions.

(c) There still, however, remains the basic problem with most vital and morbidity data of *data not being available at a sufficiently disaggregated level of scale* to identify the areas of concentration of a phenomenon. Spatial distributions are typically *positively skewed*, and the level of skewness increases with increased spatial disaggregation. Thus, with large, heterogeneous spatial units we run into the problem of *regression towards the mean*, and must question whether within area variance is as great as between area variance where our spatial units are highly aggregated.

(d) A further common problem, especially with mortality data, relates to the *accuracy of statistics* in recording place of normal residence at time of death. Burnley (1977) cites instances for Australian data where nursing homes and mental hospital deaths were recorded as the locality of normal place of residence, and so was the hospital location for infant mortality. There is also the problem of accuracy of diagnosis in both morbidity and mortality statistics. Often death is a multiple cause event, but official recording methods force a single cause classification.

The aggregation problem is inevitable, in most instances, but it is imperative that all medical cartography studies adopt some form of stochastic adjustment procedure.

Associative studies, the ecological fallacy and causal relationships

The purpose of associative analyses in medical geography has been to introduce a degree of statistical understanding of relationships between incidence of morbidity or mortality and environmental or social phenomena. In using both simple correlation and multivariate statistical methods of analysis, all too often researchers have used the resultant correlation coefficients, coefficients of determination and regression equations to imply a *causative explanation* in the dependent variable which is a ratio measure of a disease morbidity or mortality statistic. This approach raises a fundamental question concerning the *ecological fallacy*, and may also be a root difficulty in comparisons of patterns of specific diseases with each other. For example, on pp. 349–360, McGlashan only considers which mortality patterns are alike *at significant levels*.

Three major problems are evident:

(a) The use of *correlation and regression techniques* in studying the relationship between ratio data variables, which themselves relate to sets of areal units that are usually both large (with possibly as much within area variance as between area variance in the data) and of varying size and density distribution, needs to be approached with the utmost caution. Cause and effect relationships *cannot* be inferred from such data, and all we can justifiably do in such analyses is point to the apparent strength of existence or non-existence of spatial association. It may be that there is a link between such location or area data and behaviour of individuals, but this cannot be statistically proved using aggregate ratio data analyses. This is one of the fundamental problems needing research in human geography as a whole. This problem was well spelled-out over 30 years ago by Robinson (1950), but too many researchers in medical geography appear to disregard it.

(b) It is necessary for the researcher to find out if his *independent variable(s) is (are) causal prior to the dependent variable*, and to demonstrate statistically that the *relationship hypothesized is not due to chance*. This requires clear specification of the hypothesized relationships by *testing the null hypothesis*. If the ecological association analysis appears to demonstrate a strong degree of spatial association, then it is incumbent upon the researcher to design a research strategy which will collect at the totally disaggregated, individual level measures on the dependent and independent data variables, and statistically to test for causality at that scale.

(c) Burnley (1977) has raised a yet further complication in using aggregate ratio data in associative analyses, especially when we are looking at what a specific mortality distribution may relate to. It is possible that a person who contracted a disease while engaged in one occupation or while living in a particular area was not in that occupation and no longer lived in that area at the time of death. Populations are increasingly highly *mobile* and have varying pathologies. After differential migration (or lack of it) within a city or country, morbidity and mortality data may exhibit cause–effect patterns which do not directly reflect residential or status characteristics of the *current* experience of people.

We must ensure, therefore, that in conducting associative studies and cause–effect relationships, data from which our variables are derived are compatible in time and space. All too often this is not the case and spurious relationships ensue.

Use of multi-variate methods to derive social well-being and health risk dimensions

In the derivation of social areas in cities and the identification of dimensions of social well-being and risk in territorial social indicator studies, geographers and other social scientists have typically employed *factor analysis*. Often the data sets are for relatively large and diverse spatial units, and invariably they comprise ratio data. Major problems are as follows:

(a) The data matrices contain variables that are characterized by *auto-correlation*, and the use of factor analysis (and related) methods is suspect as the data do not fit the requirements of the statistical technique.

(b) In territorial social indicator studies, which typically include a range of health statistics as data variables, not all sets of data variables relate to the *same time period*. Often high levels of aggregation are required because different agencies are responsible for collecting different set of data and use different spatial units for data collection.

This is not to say that factor analytic, and more particularly multivariate hierarchical classification procedures, are not useful for identifying broad dimensions and for stratifying areas to isolate the locations most *at risk*. However, there is a tendency to use these methods to do more than stratify areas for further in-depth survey analysis, and to build the results of these analyses into dubious cause–effect associations.

Some specific problems with diffusion studies

One of the more interesting methodological developments in medical geography has been the application of diffusion models, particularly to look at the spread of diseases and epidemics. Diffusion techniques allow for *stochastic modelling for purposes of prediction*, and it is in this regard that their use in medical geography has particular potential.

Infectious diseases, such as bronchitis, hepatitis and measles, may provide ideal material for diffusion modelling. There are, however, some problems in such uses of diffusion models.

It is important to recognize the requirements of spatial diffusion modelling (see Cliff *et al.*, 1981). These are:

(a) *Replicability*: In order to avoid one-shot phenomena reporting, and so as to permit repeated study of the spatial process, we need multiple-wave data.

(b) *Stability over time and space*: It is essential to know that waves that occur at different times or in different places are similar in all important respects.

(c) *Observability*: To study and model the process, we need to ensure that the process is observable both in principle and in practice, thus we need data on the diffusion phenomena which yields accurate observations at frequent intervals in both time and space. This again requires multiple-wave phenomenon that occur sufficiently often to enable several individual waves to be distinguished.

(d) *Isolation*: As the diffusion process is complex and multiple-waves may overlap with one another in either time or space, a very complicated and tangled picture often emerges, which existing models may not be able to cope with. Thus, we need data such that each wave studied has a distinct starting point in time and space and runs its course before the next wave begins.

While epidemics appear to be ideal phenomena for diffusion modelling, it is important that the data available meet these requirements, and many epidemics do not. Thus, with existing diffusion models (such as the Box-Jenkins time series model, the Kalman filtering model, the mixed-state generalized linear integrated models, the mixed-state Bayesian-entropy models, the Hamer-Soper model (both single and multi-region), and the chain binomial model) the actual nature of epidemics renders them difficult to model. This is because an epidemic, such as influenza, typified by virus changes, will make one diffusion and have a different attack rate from another wave. Also many epidemics do not meet the fourth requirement. Some infectious diseases have an endemic pattern with occasional peaks, while others are endemic in large communities but re-invade smaller and isolated ones as discrete waves.

Detailed, accurate, disaggregated data are needed for diffusion modelling of phenomena such as epidemics, and it is rare for such data to be available at a national level. Accuracy and completeness in reporting at all levels of scale present a problem. There is also the danger of ascribing deaths to a single cause (and not just with respect to epidemics).

Cliff and Haggett present a rigorous diffusion modelling study in epidemiology in their investigation of measles epidemics over a period of nearly 80 years in Iceland. The utility of a range of diffusion modelling strategies are tested on what is probably as good a data set as one can ever expect to work with (see pp. 335–348).

Diffusion modelling is one of the most important areas of research in human geography, but, especially with respect to health data, there is the basic problem of how a phenomenon originally located at one point becomes transferred to another location. Even allowing for the data deficiency problems, stochastic process modelling presents a rich field for research in investigating the spread of diseases, especially in developing countries, and these techniques have potential for assisting in policy formulation in public health. There are, however, great dangers in the simplistic approaches that have characterized much of the work on diffusion in medical geography which has been limited to descriptive cartographic and correlation analysis of the spread of diseases. Such approaches do not incorporate the all-important stochastic process element inherent in diffusion of a phenomenon. They cannot be predictive and should not be classified as modelling a spatial process.

Problems in locational analysis and modelling solutions

Spatial modelling has been widely used in the contemporary approach to the geography of health care. The major underlying premise in this broad area of research is that spatial models can be used to produce resource distribution solutions which satisfy stated criteria within the complex range of outcomes possible in the *equity-efficiency trade-off* situation. These models include *simple ratio solutions* (ensuring equality or stated minimum levels of service to population provision) on an area-by-area basis; the *gravity modelling* approaches for allocating potential consumers to service locations; *nested hierarchical solutions* of services ordered by threshold requirements (central place theory solutions); and *allocation-location and transport modelling solutions* which distribute services and allocate potential users on the basis of pre-determined aggregate travel levels and threshold size requirements. These models have been widely applied at all levels of scale, but particularly at the intra-urban level where *disaggregated data bases* are available.

There are a number of major problems which researchers need to be aware of in using these types of modelling approaches in investigating the geography of health care.

(a) The most obvious is the question of *level of spatial aggregation of the demand zones*. Far too often large and complex cities are subjected to complicated linear programming algorithm analyses to derive allocations of services to zones where the size of the zones is so large as to give rather generalized and even misleading solutions. The larger the zones used the less the internal homogeneity will be and the less the between-zone heterogeneity.

(b) Most location models provide a framework for examining aggregate *consumer behaviour without furnishing a theoretical base in behavioural terms*. For example, Morrill and Earickson (1969) in their study of patient-to-hospital flows in Chicago used a probabilistic gravity model, and found that while the model could empirically replicate, and even predict, actual flows, the model told nothing of the goal people had in undertaking their individual trips. These and the allocation–location type models are based on *normative behavioural assumptions*. Thus even within a probabilistic model framework solutions which seek to minimize travel, and other factors, such as quality of service, personal preferences and such-like, are invariate.

(c) The *demand* side of the question in location models presents a major problem. Stimson (1981) has summarized the *debate over demand and need* for health-care services. Most models take the approach that a *minimum standard* needs to be provided and that there will be a uniform preference function for all consumers with respect to a given service type. *Weighting population sub-groups,* according to known *propensities to use* services, may help overcome this problem. However, this begs the question whether some groups should be disadvantaged, and it will only replicate existing inequalities in potential consumer access to services if the purpose is to allocate additional facilities. Church and Stimson (1983) offer a possible solution to this problem.

(d) Similar problems exist with respect to the *supply* side of the allocation–location problem for health-care services. It is essential to understand the location strategies, and therefore motives, of fee-for-service practitioners. For all types of services, *variations in quality and the threshold level* of operation need to be determined. What actually constitutes the provision and accessibility of a service is a further problem. For example, Stimson (1980, 1981) has shown that service availability needs to be considered in both *time and space*, as a service only has utility if it is available at the time people need it.

(e) The above two problems highlight the necessity of conducting *allocation–location* analyses at a *highly disaggregated level of scale*. In cities the base unit for the population census is the most appropriate to use, and services location needs to be directly compatible to this digitized demand data. This involves considerable time and expense in developing the spatial data bases that are most appropriate to conduct such studies.

(f) These problems are further exacerbated by the proposition that any solution for one point in time is a *one-off best solution* approach. However, *people are highly mobile*, many health-care services are *privately supplied* and there is considerable freedom of *entry and exit* of the providers. Thus, location modelling needs to be undertaken in a *time–space* framework. It is difficult to update the required data bases frequently. In most countries new basic disaggregated census data is available only once in a decade. Much fundamental work remains to be done in this area of time–space allocation–location modelling, even assuming that we have solved the earlier problems relating to what constitutes demand and supply and how we measure it.

Beyond all these problems is one which involves a *political* consideration in the allocation–location modelling approach to health-care services provision and use. It is theoretically feasible to produce algorithms that will give any required solution, but the problem remains how we set the parameters in the equity-efficiency trade-off conflict. Rushton *et al.* (1976) have presented an interesting approach to this with respect to solving the allocation problem of primary care and dental clinics in Iowa State, USA. More work of this type is needed if we are to produce more realistic outcomes from our location models.

Consumer behaviour: how to quantify the variables?

Geographers investigating health care have contributed relatively little to the behavioural approach. Typically they have concentrated on analysis of *trade areas* of specific health-care service facilities, and derived *distance decay* functions for services in different levels of the hierarchy of health services. It has been relatively rare for behavioural data to be collected from the population of *potential consumers* of health services on a *random probability sampling basis*.

Other social scientists (including multi-disciplinary teams that contained geographers) have proposed elaborate models for investigating consumer health-care behaviour. Typical is this model by Gross (1972).

$$U = f(E, P, A, H, X) + \varepsilon$$

where

U = utilization rate of various services by the individual or family unit;

E = enabling factors, such as income, family size, occupation, education attained, insurance status;

P = predisposing factors, such as attitudes, values, knowledge;

A = accessibility factors, such as time/distance from facility, service availability, waiting time;

H = perceived health level (disability days);

X = individual and area wide exogenous factors;

ε = residual error term

The problem with such models is putting them into operation. Quantifying the variables involves extremely costly survey research and measurement of many of the non-economic and non-spatial variables is difficult. Once collected, data need to be aggregated so as to generalize and test hypotheses. The general paucity of behavioural data on the use of health-care services presents a fertile area of research for health-care geographers, but in my view it can only be conducted adequately by working in *multi-disciplinary teams*, and the major purpose of such studies need *not* necessarily be geographical. However, it would be interesting to study the spatial aspects of consumer health-care behaviour within the wide context of individual and household time–space activity budgets, and to look at things such as the use of health services as part of *multi-purpose trips*.

The problem of data reliability and validity

The final problem to be discussed is one which is common to all researchers working on health-related matters, and it is one which geographers apparently have not seriously considered. In this they are

Table 1. Under-reporting rate by number of weeks between using a health-care service and interview: USA data, household survey

No. of weeks	Hospitalization[a] % not reported	No. of weeks	Physician visit[b] % not reported
1–10	3	1	15
11–20	6	2	30
21–30	9		
31–40	11		
41–50	16		
51–53	42		

[a] From Cannell, Fisher and Bakker (1965).
[b] From Cannell and Fowler (1963).

not, however, alone. The problem is the general question of *how reliable and valid is the data* with which we work?

Reference has been made on numerous occasions in this chapter to the problem of *incomplete data* and to *inaccuracies* that may occur in data. There is, however, a tendency for researchers to accept official data as being perfect and to regard survey data as valid, assuming that rigorous *random probability sampling designs* have been used and *response rates* are high.

Increasingly social scientists are using survey methods to collect data from specific populations and from specific areas where official data are not available in disaggregated form. The social survey is also used to collect behavioural data (facts, attitudes and opinions) that are not available elsewhere. Individual surveys by questionnaire are also the basis of some case-control studies leading to relative risk evaluation.*

The questions of *error* and *bias* in surveys collecting data on health behaviour and the *reliability* and *validity* of that data have been the subject of almost 20 years of research by the Survey Research Center at the University of Michigan (see US Department of Health, Education and Welfare, 1975, 1977; Cannell and Fowler, 1963; Cannell *et al.*, 1965). It is now beyond doubt that the greatest error in survey data, collected using rigorous random probability sampling, is in *interviewer bias* and *mis-reporting* on the part of the respondent. Tables 1–4 illustrate the magnitude of the bias, and thus the concern about the reliability and validity of data that is collected in health surveys. These data were collected as part of a study for the US Department of Health, Education and Welfare in order to test the accuracy of data in its monthly household health

* See Giles (pp. 361–374) for one example of the use of disaggregated, questionnaire-based data.

Table 2. Under-reporting rate of chronic conditions, clinic patients: USA data, household survey

| By no. of days since last visit | | By no. of visits | |
No. of days	% not reported	No. of visits	% not reported
1–7	9	1	56
8–14	28	2	47
15–28	24	3	35
29–56	42	4–5	26
57–84	37	6+	14
85–112	42		
113–140	45		
141–168	46		
169–224	57		
225–280	52		
281–364	58		
365+	59		

From Madow (1967).

Table 3. Under-reporting rate of hospitalized patients by duration and number of weeks preceding the interview: USA data, household survey

| Duration of hospitalization | | Duration of hospitalization and number of weeks preceding interview | | | |
| Duration in days | % not reported | No. of weeks hospitalization preceded interview | Days duration and % not reported | | |
			5+	2–4	1
1	26	1–20	5	5	21
2–4	14	21–40	7	11	27
5–7	10	41–52	22	34	32
8–14	10				
15–21	6				
22–30	2				
31+	8				

From Cannell, Fisher and Bakker (1965).

Table 4. Under-reported rate of hospitalized patients by diagnostic threat rating: USA data, household survey

Diagnostic rating	% not reported
Very threatening	21
Somewhat threatening	14
Not threatening	10

From Cannell, Fisher and Bakker (1965).

survey, which is used as the basis for policy decision making. The data come from a random sample of persons interviewed in the monthly health surveys who had been hospitalized and who had seen a doctor. Thus, the actual behaviour of the respondents was known, and it was possible to determine the degree of misreporting. The tables present data which should have a sobering effect on researchers who blindly accept the accuracy and completeness of official and survey data!

From Table 1 it is apparent that the rate of under-reporting of hospitalization increases at an increasing rate as the period of recall increases. More disturbing is that 15 per cent fail to report a doctor visit made within the last week, and this increased to 30 per cent for visits made within two weeks. Table 2 indicates the magnitude of non-reporting of chronic conditions, this rate increasing from 9 per cent within 7 days, to 28 per cent within 8 to 14 days, and to 59 per cent for over one year. The percentage of under-reporting for chronic conditions by number of visits to the doctors' clinic decreased markedly as the number of visits increased, changing from 56 per cent for 1 visit, to 35 per cent for 3 visits, but then declined after ⩾6 visits to 14 per cent. Table 3 shows that under-reporting of hospitalizations decreased as the duration of hospitalization increased, changing from 26 per cent for 1 day to 2 per cent for 22 to 30 days. Under-reporting of hospitalization increased with the lapse of time since hospitalization, but it decreased as the duration of hospitalization increased. Table 4 shows that under-reporting increases substantially as the diagnostic threat rating increases.

These data exemplify a real problem, which must put in question the reliability and validity of data collected in health surveys, especially because of the *ex post facto* nature of many of the questions, and because as recall time increases, accuracy of reporting decreases.

Conclusion

This chapter has raised a number of the major problems that are evident in the literature in medical geography and the geography of health care. The review is deliberately selective in choosing a range of methodological problems relating to data deficiencies and reliability, spatial disaggregation, and the wider question of research design, especially in the context of testing hypotheses, establishing cause–effect relationships and making statistical inferences. The plea is for researchers to be more keenly aware of the limitations of the data with which they work and to refrain from going beyond the limitations of their data in drawing conclusions and inferring explanations.

Bibliography

Burnley, I. H. (1977). Mortality variations in an Australian metropolis: the case of Sydney. In *Studies in Australian Mortality, Environmental Studies Occasional Paper 4* (ed. N. D. McGlashan), pp. 29–61. University of Tasmania, Hobart.

Cannell, C., Fisher, C. and Bakker, T (1965). Reporting of hospitalization in the health interview survey. In *Vital and Health Statistics*, Series 2, No. 6. US Public Health Service, Washington, D.C.

Cannell, C. and Fowler, F. J. (1963). A Study of Reporting of Visits to Doctors in the National Health Survey. Survey Research Center, University of Michigan.

Church, R. and Stimson, R. J. (1983). Modelling spatial allocation–location solutions for GP medical services in cities: the equity-revenue maximizing conflict case. *Regional Science & Urban Economics.*

Cliff, A. D., Haggett, P., Ord, J. K. and Versey, G. R. (1981). *Spatial Diffusion: An Historical Geography of Epidemics in an Isolated Community*, Cambridge University Press, Cambridge.

Gross, P. F. (1972). Urban health disorders, spatial analysis and the economics of health facility location. *International Journal of Health Sciences 2.*

Learmonth, A. (1978). *Patterns of Disease and Hunger*. David and Charles, Newton Abbot.

Madow, G. W. (1967). Interview data on chronic conditions compared with information derived from medical records. In *Vital and Health Statistics*, Series 2, No. 23. US Public Health Service, Washington, D.C.

McGlashan, N. D. (1977). Spatial variations in cause-specific mortality in Australia. In *Studies in Australian Mortality, Environmental Studies Occasional Paper 4* (Ed. N. D. McGlashan), pp. 1–28. University of Tasmania, Hobart.

McGlashan, N. D. and Harington, J. S. (1976). Some techniques for mapping mortality. *The South African Geographical Journal 58*(1), 18–24.

Morrill, R. L. and Earickson, R. J. (1969). Problems in modelling interaction: the case of hospital care. In *Behavioral Problems in Geography: A Symposium* (Eds K. R. Cox and R. G. Golledge), pp. 254–276. Northwestern University Department of Geography, Research Studies No. 17.

Robinson, W. S. (1950). Ecological correlations and the behavior of individuals. *American Sociological Review 15*, 351–357.

Rushton, G., Dueker, K. J., Hillsman, E. L., Kohler, J. A. and Meneley, G. J. (1976). *A Statewide Plan for Regional Primary Medical & Dental Care Centers in Iowa.* Institute of Urban & Regional Research & Health Services Research Center, University of Iowa.

Stimson, R. J. (1980). Spatial aspects of epidemiological phenomena and of the provision and use of health care services in Australia: a review of methodological problems and empirical analyses. *Environment & Planning A 12*, 887–907.

Stimson, R. J. (1981). The provision and use of general practitioner services in Adelaide, Australia: application of tools of locational analysis and theories of provider and user spatial behaviour. *Soc. Sci. Med.* **15D**, 27–44.

US Department of Health, Education and Welfare (1975). *Advances in Health Survey Research Methods: Proceedings of a National Conference*, NCHSR, Research Proceedings Series, DHEW Publ. No. (HRA), 77–3154.

US Department of Health, Education and Welfare (1977). *A Summary of Studies of Interviewing Methodology*, Data Evaluation & Methods Research, Series 2, No. 69, DHEW Publ. No. (HRA) 77–1343.

Changing urban–rural contrasts in the velocity of measles epidemics in an island community

Andrew D. Cliff and Peter Haggett

Department of Geography, University of Cambridge,
England and Department of Geography, University
of Bristol, England

Introduction

The speed with which viruses are passed through a human population in the form of an epidemic wave has attracted both theoretical and empirical studies. Mollison (1972) has considered the limiting conditions under which an epidemic will be propagated as a continuous wave form, rather than as a series of broken, spatially irregular outbreaks. Other studies have tried to establish how the speeds of transmission are related to the distribution of the susceptible population. For measles, Black (1966) has studied monthly records of reported cases for 18 islands over a 15-year period. When small outbreaks involving less than 100 reported cases were eliminated, a consistent inverse relation was found between the duration of an epidemic and population spacing on the island: *ceteris paribus*, epidemics of equal severity appeared to be shorter on the high-density islands than on the low-density ones. A parallel study of weekly measles records for an English county found statistically signifi-cant differences between the behaviour of epidemic waves in high- and low-density districts (Haggett, 1975). Measles outbreaks were slightly briefer in duration and more sharply peaked in form in the 17 urban districts as compared with the 10 rural districts with much lower popula-tion densities.

In this essay, we test the hypothesis that measles epidemics move at different relative speeds through populations of different densities by examining one of the islands in Black's original study, Iceland, but over a longer time period.

GEOGRAPHICAL ASPECTS OF HEALTH
ISBN 0 12 483780 8

The regional setting

With an area of 39,800 square miles, Iceland is approximately the same size as the state of Indiana. Lying just south of the Arctic circle and with seven-eighths of its land surface covered with tundra, lava fields or ice, it has a very low population density. In 1901, Iceland's total population was 78,500, with 6680 (9 per cent) in the only major city, the capital, Reykjavík. In 1973, its population was 213,000, with 86,800 (41 per cent) in Reykjavík. The distinction between the capital city and the rest of Iceland is crucial in terms of the susceptible population; outside the Reykjavík area, the largest settlement had only 13,384 people in 1973 and most of the inhabitants were scattered in small farming and fishing communities around the coast or on offshore islands. In this chapter, a simple distinction will be drawn between urban Iceland (the Reykjavík medical district) and rural Iceland (the rest of the country).

Method of analysis

Data sources

The measles records for Iceland have been analysed at length by Cliff *et al.* (1981) in their monograph on the spatial diffusion of epidemics; they are summarized in a statistical appendix to that volume. The monthly records go back to 1896 in an unbroken sequence and are available for more than 50 small geographical areas. Although the reporting rate can only be established indirectly, it appears to be substantially better than that of England and Wales or the United States over comparable time periods (Cliff and Haggett, 1979). Certainly Black adjudged Iceland as among the best recorded of his 18 islands. None the less, it seems likely that the accuracy of reporting has changed over the 70-year period; standards of diagnosis have improved and the number of physicians has increased. In Iceland the ratio of doctors/population has grown by around 2·5 times since 1900. Thus in selecting indices to describe the velocity of spread of epidemic waves (see below) we have chosen measures which are independent of reporting rates over the long run. In the short-term, we assume comparable reporting rates in urban and rural areas over the lifetime of an epidemic, i.e. up to a maximum of 27 months.

Over the period, some 90,000 cases of measles were reported by Icelandic physicians to their central public health office. These data are published by month for medical districts: both the time and spatial scales

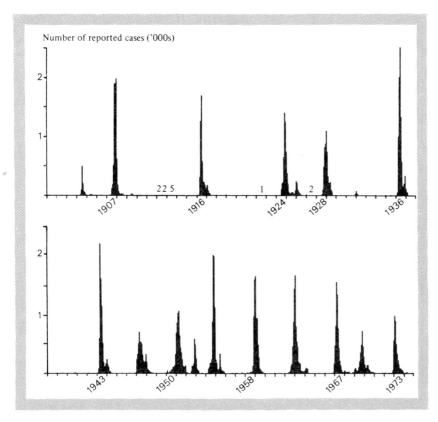

Figure 1. Time-series of reported cases of measles in Iceland, 1901–1974. (Numbers inserted between major outbreaks indicate sporadic case levels too small to be shown at the scale of the diagram.)

are highly aggregated. Ideal data based on patient or school records are not available for the period considered. Of the reported cases, all but a few occurred in 16 clearly separated discrete waves or epidemics (see Fig. 1); the epidemics ranged in size from 822 to 8408 cases and lasted as unbroken records of infection ranging in length from eight to 27 months (Table 1). Gaps between waves averaged around three years. In the 304 epidemic months, the reporting rate averaged 294 cases per month; in the remaining 584 non-epidemic months, the rate averaged only two measles cases per year. These sporadic outbreaks usually occurred in a fishing port with overseas contacts, and stand apart from the major epidemics. They are, therefore, not included in the analysis which follows. In countries such as the United Kingdom, the endemic nature of measles

Table 1. Velocity characteristics for 16 measles epidemics, Iceland 1896–1975

Wave	Years	Total cases (n)	Cases/1000 population	Duration, months (T)	Gap between epidemics (months)	Velocity parameters			
						$\bar{t}$	b_2	s	$\hat{b}$
I	1904–1905	822	11	8		4·53	4·03	1·23	—
II	1907–1908	7398	89	16	29	7·05	5·84	1·52	—
III	1916–1917	4944	55	14	91	4·80	5·09	2·46	0·86
IV	1924–1926	6130	61	26	84	7·61	4·77	5·22	0·37
V	1928–1929	5317	51	17	23	6·15	3·71	2·45	0·82
VI	1936–1937	8408	72	14	73	5·41	5·54	2·14	1·03
VII	1943–1944	7155	57	16	70	5·74	5·50	2·67	0·82
VIII	1946–1948	4791	35	22	29	8·42	3·04	3·74	0·59
IX	1950–1952	6645	45	27	16	15·45	4·86	3·52	0·56
X	1952–1953	1872	13	10	3	5·22	3·52	1·77	1·23
XI	1954–1955	7787	50	21	10	9·05	5·98	2·92	0·65
XII	1958–1959	7102	42	22	27	11·29	5·58	2·03	0·83
XIII	1962–1964	7405	40	26	27	10·54	7·58	3·54	0·55
XIV	1966–1968	6152	30	22	29	5·85	11·76	2·40	0·57
XV	1968–1970	3625	18	27	1	13·32	3·97	3·96	0·50
XVI	1972–1974	3953	18	16	21	6·46	5·19	2·33	0·95

means that cases are reported in every week of the year; this poses the usual problems of deciding when an epidemic starts and finishes. In contrast, the non-endemic nature of the disease in Iceland means that, as we have noted, periods of infection are separated by generally long periods when no cases are reported, leading to the 16 self-evident, "naturally" defined epidemics used here.

Measures of velocity

If the diffusion of an epidemic is conceived of as a simple spatial process with a well-defined wavefront, then the physical concept of distance travelled over time (for example, miles per month), may be an appropriate measure of velocity of spread. Where, as in the case of the Icelandic measles outbreaks, the spread is complex and where the susceptible population through which the epidemic moves is both discontinuous in space and has sharp variations in density, then an alternative definition of velocity must be sought. We have chosen to adhere to classical statistical measures based upon the frequency distribution of cases against time shown in Fig. 1. Four indicators were used; they are summarized here and discussed at length in Cliff and Haggett (1982).

(a) Average time lag, $\bar{t}$

Suppose we conventionally code the first month in which measles cases are reported in any given epidemic as $t = 1$, and subsequent months as $t = 2, 3$, and so on. Let T denote the duration of the epidemic in months, x_t denote the number of reported cases in month t, and n be the total number of cases reported in the whole epidemic. Then the quantity,

$$\bar{t} = \frac{1}{n} \sum_{t=1}^{T} tx_t$$

gives the average time at which cases occurred in that epidemic; that is, $\bar{t}$ gives the average or expected time to infection of an individual in the epidemic. All other things being equal, we should expect a rapidly moving wave to have a small value for $\bar{t}$, and a slow moving wave to have a large value for $\bar{t}$.

(b) Standard wave duration

The standard deviation of the frequency distribution of cases against time is a measure of the spread of cases about the mean, $\bar{t}$. Statistically, it is defined as

$$s = \sqrt{m_2}$$

where

$$m_2 = \frac{1}{n} \sum_{t=1}^{T} (t - \bar{t})^2 x_t$$

Epidemics in which cases are concentrated around $\bar{t}$ have small values for s, and are likely to be characteristic of rapidly moving waves and/or highly infectious epidemics. An epidemic in which cases are drawn out or spread over a long period of time, as in a slow moving wave, will have a large value for s. Thus, whereas $\bar{t}$ represents the centre of gravity of a number of cases in the epidemic, s represents the spread around that centre of gravity.

(c) Wave kurtosis, b_2

If an epidemic moves rapidly, we would expect the number of cases to be heavily concentrated in the few months of the wave around $\bar{t}$; the wave should be sharply peaked. A statistical measure which compares the degree of concentration of cases in the peak months with the spread over the duration of the epidemic is the kurtosis. This is defined as

$$b_2 = \frac{m_4}{m_2^2}$$

Here, m_2 is specified above and

$$m_4 = \frac{1}{n} \sum_{t=1}^{T} (t - \bar{t})^4 x_t$$

Epidemics in which cases are highly concentrated in time have large values for b_2; an epidemic which is dissipated over a long period of time will have a low value for b_2. Unlike $\bar{t}$ or s, b_2 is, by construction, dimensionless—independent of t and therefore of the duration of the epidemic. This makes interpretation simpler.

Use of these measures is justified by the simple biological model underpinning the various threshold theorems for measles epidemics (see, for example, Kendall, 1957). The population at risk, of size S, is assumed to build up by births over a period of time to a critical level. Infection is introduced into the population and disease runs through the population. In the case of measles, immunity is conferred, S falls, and the disease dies out because S is not large enough to support it. The S population then builds up again by births and, in the absence of

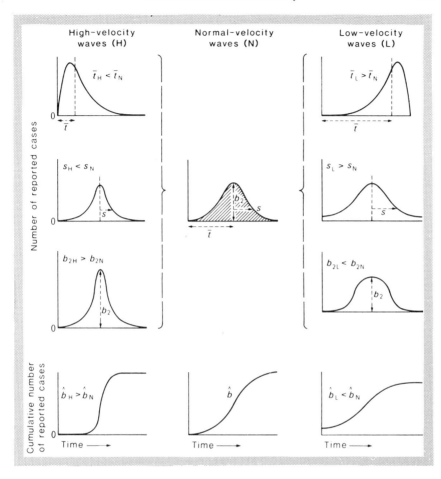

Figure 2. Graphical definition of $\bar{t}$, s, b_2 and $\hat{b}$ for a "normal" epidemic.

vaccination, the cycle repeats itself. This pattern produces the typically bell-shaped curves of reported cases against time for any given epidemic and the characteristic cycles of epidemics and non-epidemic interludes shown in Fig. 1. For such approximately bell-shaped epidemic waves, the proposed measures (a)–(c) are valid descriptions of curve shape and summarize the properties indicated in Fig. 2. If the curve is perfectly bell-shaped and fits the statistically normal distribution, we know for measure (c) that $b_2 = 3$. When $b_2 > 3$, the distribution is more sharply peaked than a normal distribution, and when $b_2 < 3$, the curve is flatter than the normal distribution.

(d) Diffusion coefficient, $\hat{b}$

If the plot of cases against time is approximately bell-shaped, a graph of
the cumulative number of cases against time will be S-shaped, with the
point of inflection corresponding to the epidemic peak. Such sigmoidal
growth curves are widely described by the logistic model in the biological
literature (Pielou, 1969). The model is given by

$$p_t = \frac{1}{1 + e^{a-bt}}$$

where p_t is the cumulative proportion of cases up to time t, e is the base of
natural logarithms, and a and b are parameters. Rearranging terms and
taking natural logarithms yields the equivalent linear regression form,

$$\ln\left(\frac{1}{p_t} - 1\right) = a - bt$$

so that b represents the average rate of growth in $\ln (1/p_t - 1)$ with time.
A rapidly moving wave will have a large value for b and a slow moving
wave will have a small value for b. We denote the ordinary least squares
estimate of b for real-world data by $\hat{b}$ (see Fig. 2).

   Study of the histograms of reported cases against time for each
epidemic and area (Cliff and Haggett, 1981, pp. 63–87) showed some
variations from the bell-shaped epidemic curve. While all the plots for
Reykjavík had a single peak, four of those for the rest of Iceland were
bimodal; a second, much lower, peak followed the first with a time lag of
nine to 12 months. The causes of the secondary peak are unclear, but
generally relate to a delayed surge of new cases in separate regions of the
island. In one of these (wave IV), there is historical evidence of a
secondary and external introduction of the disease into a remote eastern
part of the island. To sum up, most of the epidemic waves studied were
unimodal and likely to be economically described by measures (a) to (d);
a few were regional in character.

Regional application

Results

The values obtained for the four velocity parameters, $\bar{t}$, s, b_2 and $\hat{b}$ for the
separate epidemics are shown in Figs 3 and 4. Waves which affected only
parts of Iceland (waves I, II and X in Table 1) were eliminated from the

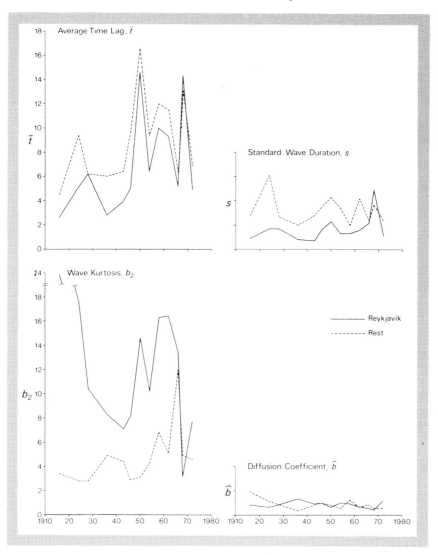

Figure 3. Values of the velocity parameters $\bar{t}$, s, b_2 and $\hat{b}$ for measles epidemics affecting Reykjavik and the rest of Iceland, 1910–1974.

analysis and we concentrated on those which engulfed most communities on the island. These remaining 13 epidemics were separated into records for urban Iceland (Reykjavík) and rural Iceland (the rest of the country). The velocity parameters were computed for both sectors. In Fig. 3, we have plotted the values obtained against time. The diagram

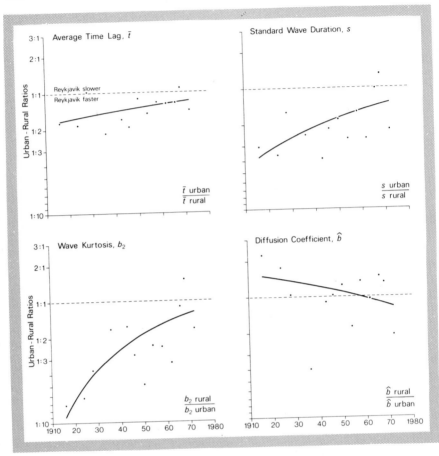

Figure 4. Trend lines and values of urban/rural ratios formed from velocity parameters *t*, *s*, *b₂* and *b̂* for measles epidemics affecting Reykjavík and the rest of Iceland, 1910–1974.

makes clear the fact that the average time to infection ($\bar{t}$) is generally longer in rural than in urban Iceland, that the epidemics are more spread out over time (bigger *s*) and that they are less sharply peaked (smaller b_2) in rural than in urban areas. Taken together, these results imply that, over the study period, epidemics have tended to move relatively more slowly through the rural hinterland than through the main urban area of Iceland. This coincides with Black's findings reported in the introduction. Additionally, the $\bar{t}$ graph shows a fairly clear trend, in both sectors, of increase in average time to infection over the period. The b_2 graph hints at different time trends in peakedness as between urban and rural Iceland. Peakedness has tended to decrease in Reykjavík and to increase in the rest of Iceland. No clear patterns emerge from the diffusion coefficient graph.

Because the values in Fig. 3 could reflect, in part, unknown changes in reporting rate, it is useful to gauge velocity differences between urban and rural sectors in a way which is independent of such temporal trends. Figure 4 plots for each epidemic the ratio of the urban and rural parameters; because a higher or lower reporting rate is likely to inflate or deflate the parameters in a given epidemic in a roughly similar way, the ratio may be regarded as a stable historical measure. A logarithmic rather than an arithmetic scale has been adopted in Fig. 4 to give equal weight to ratios above and below one. Simple regression methods were then used to calculate the linear trend lines relating ratio values to time. These trend lines are plotted and appear as curves because of the log scale. For $\bar{t}$, s and b_2, the trend lines all move with time up the "Reykjavík faster" part of the chart towards the equal velocity line. This points to a growing uniformity of behaviour with time between the two sectors of the country. The positions of the trend lines imply, bearing in mind the results from Figure 3, that this growing uniformity has been achieved by (1) a slow-down in velocity in both Reykjavík and the rest of Iceland over time, and that (2) this decrease in velocity has become more marked in Reykjavík than in the rest of Iceland over the study period; that is, epidemics in Reykjavík have become slower by a larger amount. As in Fig. 3, the diffusion coefficient, $\hat{b}$, is less helpful. The trend to uniformity again appears, but the trend line moves down the "Reykjavík slower" part of the chart.

Finally, we note that, as might be expected from such aggregated data with problems of under-reporting, possible mis-diagnosis and a study period occupying three-quarters of a century, the sequence provided by the results is noisy and by no means unambiguous. However, an interpretation that epidemic behaviour has changed through time is reinforced by Table 2, which compares the characteristics of measles epidemics in earlier and later periods for Iceland as a whole. Student's t-test for differences between two means has been used to determine whether there is a significant difference on the particular characteristic before and after 1945, the break point year suggested by Fig. 1. From Table 2, the attack rate, death rate and time gap between epidemics have all declined significantly on the basis of the t-test. The results for $\bar{t}$ and CV also indicate that the decrease in velocity is statistically significant.

Table 2. Comparison of epidemic wave characteristics, 1916–1944 and 1948–1977

Characteristic (averages)	Summary parameter	Cases		Student's t-test value
		1916–1944	1948–1974	
Cases/1000 population		59·14	32·42	4·01 [a]
Deaths/1000 cases measles		8·42	0·66	2·71 [a]
Time gap between waves (months)		68·20	18·11	5·02 [a]
Duration (months)		17·40	21·44	1·36
Velocity	$\bar{t}$	5·94	9·51	2·21 [a]
	s	2·99	2·91	0·14
	b_2	4·92	5·72	0·65
	CV	49·40	32·40	3·18 [a]

Number of waves, 1916–1944 = 5; 1948–1974 = 9.
[a] Significant at $p < 0.05$ level (1 tailed test) on 12 d.f.
Figures in the table give the average characteristic or parameter value over the $n = 5$ waves, 1916–1944, and the $n = 9$ waves, 1948–1974. $CV = 100\,s/\bar{t}$.

Discussion

The data presented indicate that the rate of spread of major measles epidemics in Iceland during this century has gradually decreased, and that this decrease has been more marked in the urban than in the rural sector of the country. This trend in spatial behaviour has to be set alongside the more well-known phenomena of decreasing death rates and attack rates, and the change from a pattern of large and infrequent epidemics to smaller and more frequent epidemics.

Given the available data and the highly aggregated scale of analysis the reasons behind the velocity changes remain obscure. Among the known facts that may be linked to the trends are the following:

(i) Transport changes since 1945 have reduced both internal and external isolation in Iceland, resulting in increased mixing of infectives and susceptibles. Cliff *et al.* (1981) have mapped the known movements of index cases as reported in doctors' records over an 80-year period. At the turn of the century, the Icelandic population was dominated by small fishing and farming communities strung necklace-like around the coastline. The main links between settlements were by boat and, in a sub-arctic environment, these links were frequently broken by bad weather or winter pack ice. The main month for measles transmissions was May and most index cases moved by coastal shipping. Today Iceland has a complete round-the-island road network and the most heavily-used (in terms of passenger miles per 1000 residents) domestic airline system in Europe.

These improved internal transport links may be related to the increasing homogeneity of epidemic velocity in the different sectors of Iceland. In addition, international airline travel has bonded Iceland increasingly to Europe since 1945. If this has enhanced the chance of re-introduction of the disease into a country where it is not endemic, it may help to account for the observed decrease in the interval between epidemics since 1945.

(ii) Educational reorganization in Iceland this century has had a particularly dramatic effect on rural areas. The ambulatory system in which a teacher visited outlying farms for a few weeks each term is now confined to the most remote areas. In its place have come larger boarding schools at which farm children live during the week. Within Reykjavík itself, a rapidly growing population of schoolchildren has meant the creation of new primary schools. Thus in urban Iceland, educational changes have tended to fragment the school population into more separate spatial units, while in rural Iceland the same vulnerable school-age population has become more concentrated and accessible to virus movements. To confirm the impact of such institutional changes on measles transmission would require detailed school-level data, but the directions of the educational changes are consistent with the interpretation we have placed upon Figs 3 and 4.

(iii) The historical evidence of physicians' reports in Iceland points to external sources for the virus. The origins of 11 of the 16 waves can be traced (Cliff *et al.*, 1981, p. 90); almost all were from the crews of fishing vessels and nine of these came from other Scandinavian countries. Since the mid-1960s, the weight of international air traffic using the main Icelandic airfield at Keflavík has introduced a new potential source of infectives and the official accounts of each epidemic no longer identify the source. Given the continuing gaps between epidemics (see Table 1) and the small size of the resident population, it seems unlikely that the measles virus remains in permanent residence in Iceland (see Fig. 1).

(iv) As noted earlier, the number of doctors per head of population has increased by about 2·5 times in Iceland this century, with a more than proportionate increase in the Reykjavík area. How far the relative increase in medical manpower in urban Iceland as opposed to its rural areas over the 70-year period has affected the extent and speed of measles spread in the two sectors is impossible to measure, but as with educational changes, the directions are consistent with the velocity contrasts reported. Fraser and Martin (1978, pp. 2–3) discuss the relative importance of medical care and dietary change in reducing measles mortality.

The striking role of measles vaccinations in reducing morbidity in the United States is not replicated in Iceland in the period studied. The pattern of vaccinations in the period 1965–1975 was small in total number (c. 6000 recorded in the Public Health statistics) and sporadic in geographical distribution, reflecting the judgement of individual parents and physicians rather than a co-ordinated countrywide vaccination policy.

The links between these facts and observed epidemic behaviour remain to be tested systematically. If they can be shown to exist, then the Icelandic pattern may well be repeated in the records of measles outbreaks in other, less isolated, populations. This will have wider implications for understanding how infections are passed through populations with different geographical structures (Yorke *et al.*, 1979).

References

Black, F. L. (1966). Measles endemicity in insular populations. *J. Theor. Biol.* **11**, 207–211.

Cliff, A. D. and Haggett, P. (1979). Geographical aspects of epidemic diffusion in closed communities. In *Statistical Applications in the Spatial Sciences* (Ed. N. Wrigley), pp. 5–44. Pion, London.

Cliff, A. D. and Haggett, P. (1982). Methods for the measurement of epidemic velocity. *Int. J. Epidem.* **11**, 82–89.

Cliff, A. D., Haggett, P., Ord, J. K. and Versey, G. R. (1981). *Spatial Diffusion: An Historical Geography of Epidemics in an Island Community*. Cambridge University Press, Cambridge.

Fraser, K. B. and Martin, S. J. (1978). *Measles Virus and its Biology*. Academic Press, London and New York.

Haggett, P. (1975). Simple epidemics in human populations: some geographical aspects of the Hamer-Soper diffusion models. In *Processes in Physical and Human Geography* (Ed. R. F. Peel), pp. 373–391. Heinemann, London.

Kendall, D. G. (1957). La propagation d'une épidémie ou d'un bruit dans une population limitée. *Publ. Inst. Statist. Univ. of Paris* **6**, 307–311.

Mollison, D. (1972). The rate of spatial propagation of simple epidemics. *Proc. 6th Berkeley Symp. Math. Stats. Prob.* **3**, 579–614.

Pielou, E. C. (1969). *An Introduction to Mathematical Ecology*. Wiley, New York.

Yorke, J. A., Nathanson, N., Pianigiani, G. and Martin, J. (1979). Seasonality and the requirements for perpetuation and eradication of viruses in population. *Am. J. Epidemiol.* **109**, 103–123.

The use of cluster analysis with mortality data

Neil D. McGlashan

Department of Geography, University of Tasmania,
Hobart, Tasmania, Australia

Introduction

Among the problems which routinely face medical geographers is the question of what next to do *after* having defined the spatial pattern of a disease. Whether the mapped portrayal of a mortality distribution is by dot or by incidence rate, by age-standardized mortality ratio or by some stochastic means there is often a sense of "so what?" about the result.

Among answers frequently given are, first, to change the scale of the analysis and so to "zoom in" upon local areas showing particular deviation (in high or low tail) from the geographical pattern or incidence rate looked upon as normal. At a more local and detailed scale the explanation may be more easily observed. A second technique is to approach explanation by looking for other similar patterns in the environment. This may be by time-based similarities; for instance, a regular pattern of outbreaks of vector-borne disease after the seasonal rains. Alternatively correlation may be sought on a spatial basis; the localities of disease may be dominantly those of poorest living conditions or those furthest from clinical assistance.

Data clustering

This essay is concerned, on an overtly experimental basis, with another conceptual approach altogether, namely, clustering of data into classes either by causes of death or by places where death occurs. A hierarchical

GEOGRAPHICAL ASPECTS OF HEALTH
ISBN 0 12 483780 8

clustering procedure has been used previously for producing taxa of areas on the basis of defined health service criteria in West Virginia (Harner and Slater, 1980) but not to date, it is believed, for the purposes of geographical pathology. At the most basic, the clustering approach requires a matrix of information built up of disease occurrence information on one axis and location on the other. Taxonomic method requires that all data items within such a matrix be of similar quality. This underlying assumption is hard to satisfy with mortality incidence rates because their dependability varies with the numbers of death recorded and the population size involved as well as with diagnostic variables. Random fluctuation will be likely to reduce confidence when small numbers are involved.

For example, two deaths in 10 people is more affected by chance than 200 deaths in 1000 persons or 2000 in 10,000. Ordinary rate calculations give an appearance of direct comparability and yet lose this valuable information concerning scale of numbers involved. For this reason stochastic tests should usually be employed to ascertain which localities deviate at selected significance levels in either tail of the distribution, high (above normal) or low (below normal), from the national or regional norm (McGlashan and Chick, 1974). For the purposes here of displaying the clustering method, significance testing has been omitted and the patterns are compared directly on the basis of mortality incidence rates in each case. With this *caveat* then two modes of question can be asked about the full data set.

(a) Can the diseases be shown to exhibit any similarities or dissimilarities when viewed across the set of places? (In cluster taxonomic jargon this is the R-mode.)

(b) Do certain of the places exhibit similar or inverse total constellations of death to others? (Q-mode.)

No doubt even this information will imply other questions. On the other hand some modest advance in understanding may be gained. For example, in the R-mode, to find that a number of infectious diseases display comparable patterns across space may imply something about the activity of their vectors. Alternatively, in Q-mode, to find that several places are alike for total patterns of death, but unlike others, equally might stimulate further enquiry.

A mathematical approach to data sets

Several mathematical approaches may be employed to establish a means of achieving these aims (see Everitt, 1974). In this essay only one method is used and two deliberately disparate data sets are demonstrated in order to obtain maximum contrast. The first data set refers to cancer mortality (only) over a 16-year period, 1964–1979, among African goldminers recruited from ten diverse home territories and employed in the South African gold-mining industry. The South African miners' (SAM) ages at recruitment and at death are unknown so the cells of the matrix contain Crude Mortality Rates (CMR), which are uncorrected for age. The causes of death are certified in excellent industry-wide hospitals and those utilized here include only the ten most common sites of cancer (Table 1) (Bradshaw et al., 1981).

The second data set (CARIB) refers to certified mortality in ten island territories of the ex-British Caribbean with ten age-corrected causes of death for males and 12 causes for females for a five-year period around 1977 (McGlashan, 1981, 1982). These sets can also be amalgamated to give 22 causes of death for persons. In each sector of these three data matrices, male, female or persons, the numbers in the cells are Standardized Mortality Ratios (SMR) and so represent an improvement of information compared with SAM matrix where ages were unknown.

From each mortality-against-place matrix a triangular Pearson Correlation Matrix was computed of each disease against every other and of each place against every other (Tables 2 and 3). This pair was then fed into various options of the CLUSTAN program (Wishart, 1978). Because no cluster solution is uniquely correct, several were investigated and considered (Everitt, 1974) before it appeared that, in this instance, hierarchy complete linkage (furthest neighbour) provided an intelligible means of turning the correlation values into taxonomic pictorial form as dendrograms. In earlier runs further options within the CLUSTAN package were explored in order to establish one method of choice for this specific problem. For example, one option could be used to produce similarity matrices directly from the raw data but the output of this led to serious difficulties. Interpretation proved to be obscure because values of similarity seemed not to be related to the underlying data. With only small matrices, such as these 10 by 10 SAM or CARIB data sets, this two-step method, correlation matrix plus cluster algorithm, retained for the researcher a direct touch which seemed impossible when the program itself acted as a "black box" coming between him and his data. In this regard "furthest neighbour"* has the advantage of being most directly comparable with the correlation matrix.

---

* "Furthest neighbour" refers to the classificatory procedure whereby a new member joins a taxon by comparing its value with the most dissimilar individual already in that cluster. This contrasts with a new link being forged by the new member's value being compared either with the most similar existing member of the class (nearest neighbour) or with a mean or mode value calculated for each class.

Table 1. SAM matrix of crude cancer mortality rates

	Liv	Oes	Resp	Blad	Lymp	CoRe	Leuk	Stom	Panc	Bucc
Mozambique	56·9	1·1	1·7	4·3	2·0	0·6	0·8	0·5	0·9	0·4
Cape Province	11·9	14·4	4·7	0·5	1·0	1·1	0·9	1·4	0·9	1·1
Lesotho	4·9	2·2	2·0	0·4	0·6	1·1	1·2	1·0	0·8	0·5
Malawi	8·5	2·0	0·6	1·6	1·1	0·7	1·8	0·7	1·1	0·0
Northern	13·1	1·4	0·5	1·8	3·6	0·0	2·4	0·0	0·0	0·0
Botswana	3·3	2·6	1·3	1·0	0·4	0·8	1·1	1·1	0·4	0·8
Transvaal	9·0	8·6	7·2	1·4	2·1	1·0	0·5	1·0	0·5	1·0
Orange	2·4	9·4	4·1	0·6	1·2	0·0	0·0	0·6	0·0	0·0
Natal	23·9	10·6	12·0	0·7	2·6	2·6	0·9	4·2	2·6	2·6
Swaziland	8·9	1·0	2·0	1·0	2·4	0·0	0·0	0·0	0·0	0·0

Abbreviations: Liv, liver; Oes, oesophagus; Resp, respiratory; Blad, bladder; Lymph, lymphoma; CoRe, colon-rectum; Leuk, leukaemia; Stom, stomach; Panc, pancreas; Bucc, buccal cavity.

Table 2. SAM mortality rates: R-mode

Pearson Correlation Matrix

	Liv	Oes	Resp	Blad	Lymp	CoRe	Leuk	Stom	Panc	Bucc
Liver		-0·154	0·080	0·856	0·333	0·137	0·013	0·117	0·356	0·175
Oesophagus			0·728	-0·466	-0·114	0·479	-0·336	0·566	0·361	0·599
Respiratory				-0·307	0·212	0·781	-0·355	0·859	0·685	0·878
Bladder					0·312	-0·224	0·161	-0·307	-0·032	-0·242
Lymphoma						-0·074	0·201	0·009	0·017	0·068
Colon-rectum							0·036	0·949	0·932	0·942
Leukaemia								-0·059	0·113	-0·095
Stomach									0·904	0·952
Pancreas										0·831
Buccal cavity										

Table 3. SAM mortality rates: Q-mode

Pearson Correlation Matrix

	Moz	Cap	Les	Mal	Nor	Bot	Tvl	OFS	Ntl	Swz
Mozambique		0·552	0·886	0·972	0·958	0·751	0·577	0·069	0·842	0·954
Cape Province			0·799	0·631	0·537	0·921	0·921	0·850	0·815	0·593
Lesotho				0·900	0·837	0·906	0·826	0·423	0·968	0·879
Malawi					0·966	0·810	0·608	0·173	0·822	0·925
Northern						0·715	0·506	0·097	0·775	0·959
Botswana							0·821	0·635	0·878	0·730
Transvaal								0·812	0·894	0·690
Orange									0·499	0·197
Natal										0·879
Swaziland										

Disease and space dendrograms

The full SAM raw data set of CMRS (Table 1) was first turned into two correlation matrices; one disease oriented (Table 2) and one place oriented (Table 3). These become, in R-mode, the disease dendrogram (Fig. 1) and, in Q-mode, the place dendrogram (Fig. 2). Certain selected examples can be pursued through the method from the tables to the figures to illustrate what is happening. For example, liver and bladder cancers show similar patterns across the territories. Note especially that each of these conditions occupies first rank by CMR among Mozambique miners (Table 1) and they then show a high correlation value ($r = 0.856$, $p < 0.01$) in Table 2. Finally, the pairing of these two sites of cancer, liver and bladder, occurs at junction 3 in Fig. 1. One may also observe that the junctions of taxa can be followed in the dendrogram to any desired level

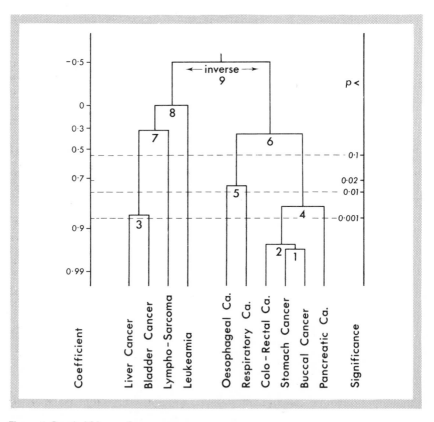

Figure 1. South African miners: cancers.

of significance (depending on n) which has been superimposed by hand on the figure. The dendrogram has also been redrawn by hand from the computer plotter against a logarithmic vertical axis of r values (with significance indicated) to give emphasis where it is needed—in the parts where higher statistical significance lies.

The dendrogram suggests that cancers of the buccal cavity, stomach, colon-rectum and pancreas occur similarly at junctions 1, 2 and 4. Here one has three sites in the alimentary tract and one associated physiologically with it. Existing literature suggests some degree of causative effect in common among these anatomic sites by some known carcinogens (e.g. betel nut).

The second group, bladder and liver cancer at junction 3, are also likely to be organs open to the effects of chemical agents in common and, in the third group, respiratory system and oesophageal tumours at junction 5, tobacco (for one) is a known agent in both sites (Schonland and Bradshaw, 1969).

A methodological problem arises in portraying a dendrogram containing an inverse relationship, that is a correlation where high incidence of Disease X is associated with a low incidence of Disease Y. It might prove

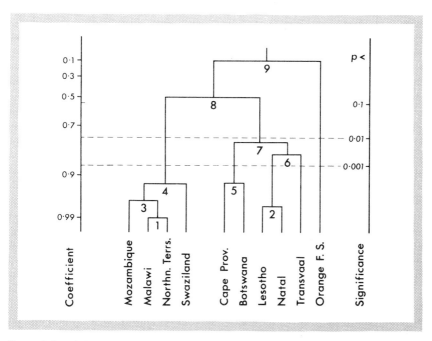

Figure 2. South African miners; homelands.

appropriate to devise a form of third dimension to show the inverse taxa
or, alternatively, to show them above the dendrogram as if the tree were
"branching" above the tree "root" system.

In the Q mode the dendrogram (Fig. 2) has recognized a cancer
constellation typical of a group of four territories whose climatic characteristics have much in common, namely, the hot humid lowland association. The analysis groups Malawi and other Northern Territories with
Mozambique and then with Swaziland. Natal and Lesotho show similar
patterns possibly related to recruiting in the higher, colder inland areas.
A third locational group but with a less close similarity of total cancer
mortality is Cape Province (where the miners are drawn mostly from
Transkei and Ciskei) with Botswana.

Turning now to the CARIB SMR data matrices, six dendrograms can be
prepared; diseases and places (where the units are the individual island
territories) for each of males, females and total persons. As an example
closest to the goldminers, Fig. 3 shows CARIB male deaths as a dendrogram based on Table 4. The format differs from SAM in two respects.
First, not all of these causes of death are cancers; diabetes, ischaemic
heart disease and motor vehicle fatalities are included together with five
sites of cancer. Secondly, a sub-total "all cancer deaths" (including all
other unspecified sites of cancer) is given in the matrices but not in the

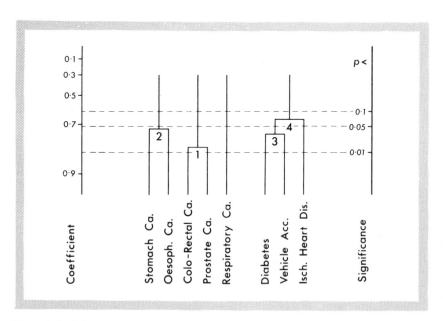

Figure 3. Caribbean male causes of death.

Table 4. CARIB male mortality rates: R-mode

Pearson Correlation Matrix

	Oes	Stom	CoRe	Resp	Pros	All Ca	Diab	Isch. H.	Vehi	All D.
Oesophagus		0·722	0·282	−0·167	0·258	0·766	0·077	0·020	0·055	−0·177
Stomach			0·220	0·016	−0·010	0·734	0·036	−0·128	0·007	−0·126
Colon-rectal				0·283	0·808	0·496	0·339	0·058	0·079	0·154
Respiratory					0·326	0·423	0·189	0·409	0·357	0·335
Prostate						0·538	0·211	−0·038	0·143	−0·123
All cancers							0·123	0·086	0·203	−0·057
Diabetes								0·677	0·754	0·277
Ischaemic heart									0·682	0·714
Vehicles										0·078
All deaths										

dendrograms. There is also a grand total "all deaths" in the data which is excluded from the dendrograms. The reason for these exclusions is that the CLUSTAN program assumes that each parameter represents an independent data-set.

In this dendrogram each of the groups has significance $p < 0.1$. One suggests similar patterns for prostate and colo-rectal cancers, another links oesophagus and stomach cancers and the third brings together diabetes mellitus and vehicle accidents, and then heart disease. These three non-cancer causes made up only 15·4 per cent of all male deaths, and all cancers together a further 11·4 per cent.

Figure 4 employs the CARIB SMR data for both sexes together to assess inter-island similarities. The most extreme position is occupied by Trinidad and Tobago, quite dissimilar to all others in its death patterns. The remaining territories fall into three groups; where Antigua and

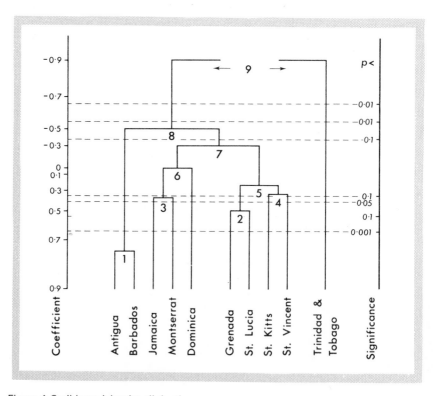

Figure 4. Caribbean Islands: all deaths.

Barbados are most alike. Jamaica belongs to a second taxon with Montserrat (junction 3) and Dominica (junction 6). A final cluster groups St. Lucia with Grenada (junction 2) and St. Vincent with St. Kitts (junction 4) and all four islands together at junction 5.

A final potential use of these analyses can be considered. Does any disease regularly closely cluster with "all deaths"? Or, any single cancer with "all cancers"? If such a single condition were to exist it might act as a surrogate measure for the grouped causes of death.

In Table 4, of CARIB male causes of death by SMR, ischaemic heart deaths correlate significantly ($r = 0.714$, $p = 0.02$) with all deaths and oesophagus with all cancers ($r = 0.766$, $p = 0.01$). Only a small part of this correlation can be auto-correlation since only 8.7 per cent of all male deaths are ischaemic heart and only 4.8 per cent of all male cancers are of the oesophagus. This pairing is corroborated among females: 7 per cent of all female deaths are ischaemic heart (correlating with all deaths at $p = 0.026$) and only 2.3 per cent of all female cancers are oesophageal (correlation with all cancers, $p = 0.002$). This at least suggests that these two single causes of deaths provide surrogate measures for the totality of deaths and for all cancers respectively.

Conclusions

The overall purpose of the cluster approach investigated here has been to assess the intuitive idea that some diseases have similar distribution patterns to each other and that some places experience similar cause-of-death constellations. Further, whilst intuition suggests that some amongst these patterns will be more alike than others, there may be little *prima facie* notion of how many members of groups or of how many clusters will emerge. For this reason selected significance levels of cut-off of the clustering process are helpful (Barker, 1976).

In conclusion it seems reasonable to suggest that these methods could be used on larger geographical data sets, which might also possibly be of stronger statistical validity, in order to test relationships implied by these two sets. Larger numbers of deaths, available perhaps for more populous regions, might yield either corroboration or rebuttal of ideas about distributional similarities either between the patterns of individual sites of cancer or between specific types of geographical regions. By such means taxonomies of geographical pathology might be refined in order further to explore aetiological relationships both between disease syndromes and between culpable environments.

Acknowledgements

The data set for South African goldminers has been provided by the Chamber of Mines through Dr J. S. Harington of the Cancer Research Department of the National Cancer Association of South Africa and that for the Caribbean territories in cooperation with Dr P. J. S. Hamilton, Director of the Caribbean Epidemiology Centre of the Pan-American Health Organization at Port-of-Spain. The assistance of Medical Officers in both areas is most gratefully acknowledged as is a Commonwealth Foundation Bursary for research travel in the West Indies in 1980.

Dr David Barker and Dr Paul Mather have kindly provided many appreciated and most useful ideas during the compilation of this essay.

References

Barker, D. (1976). Hierarchic and non-hierarchic grouping methods. *Geografiska Annaler* **58**, Ser. B1, 42–58.

Bradshaw, E., McGlashan, N. D., Fitzgerald, D. and Harington, J. S. (1982). Analyses of Cancer Incidence in Black Gold Miners from Southern Africa, 1964–1979. *British Journal of Cancer* **46**, 737.

Everitt, B. (1974). *Cluster Analysis*. Social Science Research Council. Heinemann, London.

Harner, E. J. and Slater, P. B. (1980). Identifying medical regions using hierarchical clustering. *Soc. Sci. Med.* **14D**, 1, 3–10.

McGlashan, N. D. (1981). Cancer mortality in the Commonwealth Caribbean. *West Indian Medical Journal* **30**, 142–148.

McGlashan, N. D. (1982). Causes of death in some English-speaking Caribbean countries and territories. *Bull. PAHO* **16**, 212–223.

McGlashan, N. D. and Chick, N. K. (1974). Assessing spatial variations in mortality: ischaemic heart disease in Tasmania. *Australian Geographical Studies* **12**, 190–206.

Schonland, M. and Bradshaw, E. (1969). Smoking patterns in Africans and Indians of Natal. *International Journal of Cancer* **4**, 743.

Wishart, D. (1978). CLUSTAN Version 1C Release 2. Inter University Research Councils' Series No. 47, London.

The utility of the relative risk ratio in geographical epidemiology: Hodgkin's disease in Tasmania 1972–1980, a case-control study

Graham G. Giles

Royal Hobart Hospital Clinical School,
University of Tasmania, Hobart,
Tasmania, Australia

Introduction

Starting in the late 1970s a growing enthusiasm began in medical geography for a disaggregate approach to disease ecology especially in regard to cancers (Armstrong, 1976). This movement has been highlighted by a few recent reviews of the spatial analysis of cancer occurrence which have brought medical geographical thought much closer to mainstream epidemiology (Glick, 1980). In the past much medical geography has been limited to the areas of geographers' competence; mapping and the manipulation of spatially-based statistics. Traditional geographical methods using data aggregated at scales ranging from international comparisons to those of small census districts, have produced striking, often statistically significant, variations in disease patterns. These patterns have been used to generate hypotheses that have been tested by correlating the variations in disease levels with their respective local variations in human-ecological and environmental factors. The associations revealed by such analyses have commonly been left for others to follow up at the level of the individual. Geographers have no proprietary claim to the former methodology other than their special interest in maps and spatial patterns. Geographical pathology has long

GEOGRAPHICAL ASPECTS OF HEALTH
ISBN 0 12 483780 8

been a preliminary exercise of epidemiological method and a fruitful source of leads for more rigorous epidemiological investigation.

Much overlap exists between modern medical geography and epidemiology. Given this overlap, where can geographers make the most meaningful contribution to an understanding of disease ecology especially in regard to chronic diseases and cancers? There are probably three main areas of development within the subfield; in the maintenance of the strong tradition of mapping and the aggregate approach to associative occurrence, in the acquisition of biometric and epidemiological skills needed for disaggregate studies, and in the development of spatial analysis at different scales. The last mentioned would include research into the problem of modifiable units and spatial autocorrelation (Glick, 1979). Overshadowing these methodological trends is the continuing need for geographers to join their efforts with multidisciplinary teams. The subsequent cross-fertilization of ideas will undoubtedly be blessed with hybrid vigour. As a team member the geographer's expertise would lie firmly in the domain of spatial analysis, an area not without sufficient problems of its own!

Spatial analyses of disease patterns, especially those of chronic diseases like cancer, present several problems. These include data availability, data quality, disease latency, population mobility, ecological fallacy and the acquisition of representative controls. Historically, the data used for geographical and distributional analyses of cancer occurrence have been mortality statistics; hardly any morbidity incidence data have been available on a population basis. Mortality data have known limitations and geographical analysis is usually limited to the information included on death certificates. As the accuracy and completeness of these records is extremely variable, maps of cancer mortality variations across space may, in reality, show very little. Many patterns can be obtained by chance, others can be due to regional variation in diagnostic habit or frequency of autopsy. In the highly mobile populations of most western countries the meaningfulness of cancer death maps dwindles especially if based upon residence at death. Population mobility may make nonsense of hypothesizing from spatial patterns of cancer deaths. Many cancers have a latency period of 20 years or more between the initial insult and the manifestation of malignancy. Survival from onset is also variable in many tumours and is often related to socio-economic and geographical factors affecting life-style, symptom recognition and access to medical care.

Many of the difficulties associated with mortality data are removed when morbidity data are considered instead. Their use is not problem free; there is the nuisance arising from the latency period and from population mobility within that time and although it is relatively easy to fix the time of death it is not so easy to determine the moment when onset occurs. Notwithstanding these limitations, morbidity data provide the best estimate of disease generation within a community. As population-based registries become more prevalent cancer mapping should become more meaningful and revealing. The problems of latency and mobility can be overcome by the collection of historical data particularly upon residence and occupation (King, 1979). The collection of this kind of information makes a case-control design mandatory because such historical details are not usually available for the base population. Census data are meagre in this regard.

Medical geography and case-control studies

Within medical geography the aggregate and disaggregate approaches should not be seen as separate. They are in fact complementary and sequential; the aggregate approach being a convenient and cheap first approximation at pattern identification and hypothesis generation and the disaggregate approach applying more efficient methods of hypothesis testing. Case-control studies have been rare in the medical geography practised by medical geographers. This has been due in part to the lack of good quality biostatistical data. However, the value of case-control studies exemplified largely by the work of one geographer has stimulated a new growth in geographical epidemiology (Armstrong, 1978).

Armstrong's work on nasopharyngeal carcinoma (NPC) in Malaysia grew from antecedent work at both the international and intra-national scales (Armstrong et al., 1974). The state of Selangor was selected for disaggregate analysis because, of all the Malaysian states, it provided the best opportunity for estimating the incidence of NPC. It possessed modern, reliable detection and reporting services and conditions were favourable for follow-up and interviewing. Living NPC patients were matched with adult controls from randomly selected households in the same area. The major concept was to compare the self-specific environments of cases to those of controls. This entailed detailed interviews on a variety of social and cultural habits and daily activity patterns.

One very geographical outcome of the study was a comparison of the time spent in various census districts by cases and controls. Cases spent more time in the older and low-lying, riverine districts that contained more housing of low socio-economic status and industrial sites than controls. Case-control pairs were matched on all or some of the following for various analyses based on the individual and his family: ethnic group, sex, age, socio-economic status, census district of residence and household type. NPC was found to occur more often in Chinese who were more traditional in life-style, who lived under poorer circumstances in older housing in districts with more industry, traffic and less green space and who ate less fresh foods and had little dietary variety.

Questions arising from the results of this study might relate to the different relative risks obtained when the unit of comparison was modified from that of the individual to that of the family/household. Also the use of only live patients may have introduced a bias toward those patients with a higher host-resistance, lower genetic susceptibility and/ or smaller environmental insult that resulted in a better prognosis and delayed death. The current activity patterns may have had little to do with the causal factors acting some years before. Latency has not been dealt with satisfactorily. "An important unanswered question is whether the association between NPC and socio-economic variables in Selangor is an association with poor conditions at the time of the study, or with poor populations over a long time" (Armstrong, 1978).

Given sufficient historical data upon the residence of cases and controls, cancer mapping and geographical analysis can progress further than the level of standardized mortality/morbidity ratios and the probability mapping conducted to date. It is possible to map the relative risks of persons with cancer having resided in a particular location compared to their controls. This essay will demonstrate the use of residential risk ratios with a population-based series of Hodgkin's disease (HD) and age–sex matched controls. This approach removes the spatial noise due to disease latency and population mobility. The maps will be compared to those produced by standard methods.

Hodgkin's disease in Tasmania 1972–1980

The data upon Hodgkin's disease (I.C.D. 201) incidence used here are taken from a large population-based study of the entire spectrum of myeloproliferative and lymphoproliferative disorders occurring in Tasmania between 1972 and 1980 (Lickiss *et al.*, 1977). Because of unusually high cooperation between the university, hospitals, oncology clinics, pathologists and physicians throughout the state, it is believed that case acquisition is almost total. Tasmania's size and population distribution, 402,868 at the 1976 census midpoint of the study period, render it an ideal laboratory for detailed case-control studies. From each case and control the data obtained includes a complete residential and occupational history in addition to clinical and pathological verification and genealogical information. Depending upon age, the controls were selected randomly either from the electoral rolls or from school health records.

The nature and cause of HD have been a source of controversy since its first description in 1832 (Ultmann *et al.*, 1966). The question of whether it is a true neoplasm or an unusual response to an infection persists to this day. Many features of the disease are consistent with a viral aetiology (Gallo *et al.*, 1981). The epidemiology closely resembles that of poliomyelitis with age peaks in incidence becoming older as living conditions improve. Risks, though always small, are increased for high social class and small family size (Gutensohn and Cole, 1981). Added to this are the sporadic reports of clusters of HD (Vianna *et al.*, 1971). There is some evidence of increased HD among people who have had infectious mononucleosis (Munoz *et al.*, 1978). This suggestion that the Epstein-Barr Virus is involved in HD parallels the association of that virus with Burkitt's Lymphoma in Africa (Miller and Beebe, 1973).

During the nine-year study period there were 84 cases of HD detected in Tasmania; of these, 52 were male and 32 female, giving a masculinity ratio of 163 : 100. The crude rate for males was 2·87 per 100,000 per annum and the corresponding rate for females was 1·77 per 100,000 per annum. When directly adjusted to the World Standard Population (Doll, 1976) these rates were reduced a little to 2·77 and 1·67 respectively. The cumulative incidence (Day, 1976) to age 75 was 0·27 per cent for males and 0·14 per cent for females. These figures compare well with other Australian states (Ford, 1981; South Australian Health Commission, 1980; Cancer Council of Western Australia, 1981). From Table 1 it can be seen that Tasmanian values are closest to those from New South Wales. South Australia possessed the highest values and Western Australia the lowest. The Western Australian rates were arrived at after pathological and diagnostic review and this might explain some of the disparity between their rates and those of the other states.

Table 1. The incidence of Hodgkin's disease in Australia

	Males			Females		
Rate	Crude	Standard	Cumulative	Crude	Standard	Cumulative
Tasmania (1972–1980)	2·87	2·77	0·27	1·77	1·67	0·14
South Australia (1977–1979)	3·20	2·90	0·31	2·10	1·80	0·22
Western Australia (1966–1969)	1·95	2·00	0·19	1·27	1·26	0·12
New South Wales (1975–1977)	2·80	2·70	0·23	1·84	1·60	0·15

Graham G. Giles

The age–sex specific incidence curves in Fig. 1 demonstrate a bimodal distribution with a peak in young adulthood and a rising trend thereafter with age. The bimodal nature of the incidence can be interpreted as demonstrating the action of two separate aetiologies; an infectious aetiology in the young adults and a typical neoplastic aetiology in the

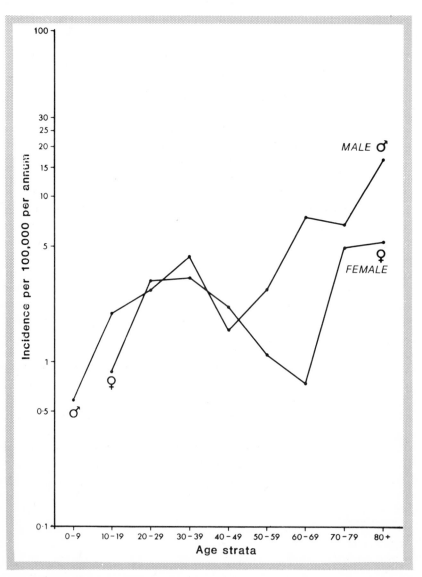

Figure 1. Hodgkin's disease in Tasmania, 1972–1980. Age–specific incidence. Rates per 100,000 *per annum* for males and females.

ageing population. Good reasons can be put forward for examining the two peaks separately and also for treating the two sexes and the four histological subtypes separately, but it was felt that the numbers were too small to subdivide at this level of analysis. No significant temporal variation in incidence was observed, neither was any space–time clustering detected using either Knox's (1964) or Mantel's (1967) methods.

Methods and maps

The intention here is to examine the data at different levels, using a variety of analytical methods in order to compare the results obtained by standard practices with those obtained by estimates of relative risk applied on residential criteria. It is proposed first to calculate standardized incidence rates adjusted for age and for sex for each region within Tasmania. Secondly, the significance of these ratios will be assessed using an appropriate probability model. Thirdly, the full benefit of the control series will be illustrated in two maps; one of the relative risk of residence at diagnosis and one of the relative risk of ever-residing in a given region.

Residential information was available in four different forms; by degree of urbanization, by postcodes, by local government areas (LGAs) and by a system of grid co-ordinates. For this analysis, the map of Tasmania was divided, *a priori* of any examination of spatial patterns, into nine regions. These regions comprised clusters of contiguous LGAs. LGAs were used as the base units for aggregation because of the availability of census details from the 1976 census in this form. The regions were based largely upon natural boundaries of watershed, geology, vegetation, land-use and urbanization (Fig. 2a). Two of these were the metropolitan areas of Hobart (140,000) and Launceston (60,000). The others were rural with the exception of the north-west coast which contained two towns of 20,000 population each.

Hobart is the largest urban area in Tasmania and is the state capital. In addition to the high-level service functions of a regional node, it has a busy port and a good mix of manufacturing and retailing activities. Its principal industries include Electrolytic Zinc, paper, food and textile manufacturing. Launceston also serves as a port and is the location of some light industry but has fewer service and government functions than Hobart. The north-west coast contains the remainder of the urban population of Tasmania. It is dominated by the coastal, industrial towns that serve as ports and processing centres for the rich agricultural hinterland where dairy, beef and vegetable farming provide the raw

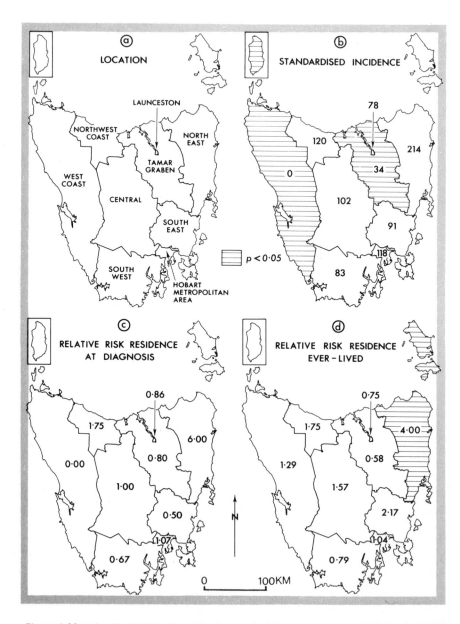

Figure 2. Mapping Hodgkin's disease in Tasmania. (a) Location of nine major regions. (b) Standardized incidence ratios of Hodgkin's disease by regions. (c) Regional variation of relative risk of residence at time of diagnosis. (d) Regional variation of relative risk based upon having ever lived in a region, with probabilities at $p < 0.05$.

materials for the canneries and cheese factories. It also contains a sizeable paper manufacturing facility.

The other regions are predominantly rural. The west coast is in large part concerned with mining except in the far north-west, where dairy and vegetable farming come to the fore. The area is covered in temperate rainforest and experiences the highest rainfall in the state. The north-east is drier but very similar to the west coast with mining, logging and farming setting the land-use pattern. The central area is mainly occupied by pastoral and logging interests and experiences the most extreme climate found in these parts. The Tamar Graben is also dominated by pastoral activity especially sheep grazing. There is some heavy industry at the mouth of the Tamar; a paper mill and an aluminium smelter. Both the south-east and the south-west are similar though the east is drier. Mixed farming, orcharding, logging, market gardening and fishing describe the major activities in these areas.

Standardized incidence

Using five-year stratified, sex-specific rates, the expected number of events for each region was calculated by the indirect method. Dividing the observed number by the expected number and multiplying by 100 gave the standardized incidence ratio (SIR) for each region (Fig. 2b). An SIR of 100 indicates an incidence equal to that expected. It was observed that most regions obtained SIRs of about 100 ± 10. The north-east displayed the highest value—214, over twice the cases expected. The west coast with no cases had an SIR of zero and the Tamar Graben with an SIR of only 34 possessed little more than a third of the cases expected from its population structure.

The map is based upon morbidity data and is therefore of far better quality than a comparable map of mortality rates. Its shortcomings are due to the limitations of data utilized. The locational data are those of residence at diagnosis, the only biases that have been adjusted are those due to gross variation in age–sex structure from region to region. A further refinement is to assess the statistical significance of the differences revealed.

Probability mapping

The confidence limits of an SIR can be calculated using established methods (Fisher, 1956), but when small numbers are involved it is preferable to re-examine the observed and expected frequencies in light of an appropriate statistical model. These occurrences of HD are sufficiently rare events to be modelled adequately by the Poisson distribution, after the method first described by Choynowski (Choynowski, 1959). The confidence limits for the observed frequency at a selected p value can be calculated or obtained from tables. If the expected value is contained within these limits the SIR can be rejected at the given level of significance.

The regional values were examined in this manner and the results were overlaid on Fig. 2b. The high SIR in the North-east was found to be insignificant but the two low SIRs, the West Coast and the Tamar Graben, were significant at $p < 0.05$. The establishment of statistical significance, however, did not change the meaningfulness of the map. The patterns, significant or not, might have been due to a variety of factors totally unrelated to aetiology. The major oncology centres were located in Hobart and Launceston and the deficit of cases on the west coast could be explained by a differential access to diagnostic facilities. This explanation was not supported by the excess of cases in the almost equally isolated north-east. The low values in the Tamar Graben were particularly disquieting because of the proximity of an oncology clinic at Launceston, the regional node. Because of the location of the facility in Launceston, Launceston's value would have been expected to be high but this was not so, its SIR was below 100.

Case-control comparisons

Both of the methods described above use the total state population as a control for age–sex variation across space. This approach is intuitively satisfying because the incidence can be viewed as the output generated by the aetiological process(es) acting within the population. Unfortunately, the historical data available upon a population basis are scarce compared to those which can be obtained from patients. Figure 2b can show nothing more than the pattern found at diagnosis. It can be adjusted neither for population mobility nor for disease latency. To overcome these problems it is necessary to suffer some loss of information by ignoring the total population and to introduce a probabilistic dimension to the investigation by sampling. Given a population-based series of patients it is possible to select a random sample of population-based controls.

A control series was selected from electoral rolls and school health records. Because of the age–sex structure of the incidence data it was decided to match upon these two variables. Residence was not a matching criterion because variations in residence between cases and controls was of interest. When the residences of the controls (at the time of their respective cases' diagnoses) were mapped and compared to their expected frequencies from Fig. 2b, a fair agreement was observed except in the Tamar Graben where only one control resided compared to 11 expected. On the same level, only four cases were found to reside there. This area was significantly low in both cases and controls at the time of diagnosis. In the north-east where six cases resided at diagnosis, only one control shared this locality.

These observations, although interesting, do not tell very much. To gain the maximum from the case-control design it is necessary to follow prescribed methods (Breslow and Day, 1980). The appropriate unit of analysis is not individuals or groups but the matched pair. Analysis proceeds to sort out the differential exposure status of each pair. Here, the exposure of interest could be residence in a particular region at time of diagnosis. A pair will fall into one of four categories: (a) both exposed, (b) case-exposed, control not, (c) control-exposed, case not, and (d) neither exposed. Categories (a) and (d) are not important because they contain no useful information. What is of interest is the ratio of discordant pairs, a measure known as the odds ratio and a maximum likelihood estimate of relative risk. The data are customarily arranged in a four-fold table. The relative risk estimate is merely (b)/(c) and its significance can be evaluated by McNemar's test (McNemar, 1974), chi-squared with one degree of freedom. When (b) or (c) are small, significance is better established by using the tail probabilities of the binomial distribution (Breslow and Day, 1980).

Figure 2c illustrates the regional variation of relative risk of residence at time of diagnosis. Values range from zero on the West Coast to six in the north-east with most areas being close to unity. None of the estimates shown in this map have any statistical significance. Again, this analysis is based on residence at diagnosis and this is unlikely to be very revealing. The final analysis attempts to go beyond this and tries to account for mobility and latency. The design looks at where the cases had ever lived throughout their lives. The risk estimates are based upon having ever-lived in a region. This allows for mobility and sets latency at a maximum from birth to diagnosis. The results are given in Fig. 2d. Comparing Figs 2c and 2d, the risks in the latter occupy a much smaller range. This is probably due to an effect of mobility evening out the differences between regions. Most estimates continue to be close to one with the exception of the two eastern regions, both with risks greater than two The West Coast's zero risk is removed but the Tamar Graben's risk remains low. The North-east with a risk of ever having lived there of four, reaches statistical significance, $p = 0.035$, and deserves closer examination.

Discussion and follow-up

The high relative risk of residence found in the North-east was based upon 12 case-control pairs being discordant in favour of the case's exposure compared to only three pairs being discordant in favour of the control's exposure. The sensitivity of the risk estimates can be enhanced by considering only those cases that meet some arbitrary minimum residential period. If an environmental agent is culpable for the increased risk, it follows that the longer the period of residence the greater the chance of an individual being exposed or accumulating a sufficient dose. When a five-year minmum period was introduced into the analysis the $12:3$ ratio was increased to $10:1$ giving a revised relative risk of 10, $p < 0.01$.

The obvious follow-up was to undertake a detailed investigation of these ten cases who had spent at least five years in the North-east region. It was of interest to try to discover whether the cases could support a theory of case-to-case transmission *vis-à-vis* a common environmental insult. To look at this question the residential history of each case was reviewed on a much finer scale than that of region. Other factors that needed to be considered included the possibility of the regional concentration being due to familial clustering of cases in close relatives living in the same area and also the possibility of common occupational exposures.

No known case-to-case contact could be established between the ten cases who had spent at least five years in the North-east region. This included possible contact at schools and other institutions. Upon reviewing the residential histories, it was discovered that five of the ten cases were born in the locality compared to none of the controls. Two cases and two controls were born outside Tasmania. The five local births all occurred in tiny isolated hamlets rather than in the towns of the region and were all well separated both in time and space. The circumstances of birth may have played an important role in the aetiology of HD in this area but it seems unlikely that a horizontally transmitted agent was involved.

At present, 10 out of the 84 cases of HD are known to have at least a second degree relative with either a lymphoproliferative or a myeloproliferative neoplasm. Among ten cases one would, therefore, expect at least one familial case on average. Actually, two out of the ten were familial cases. This is an interesting but statistically insignificant trend. The ascertainment of familial cases is grossly underestimated, based only upon the verification of evidence supplied by a respondent (usually the patient). Given a more aggressive genealogical approach, more familial cases will undoubtedly be detected. At the moment, although a fifth of the cases are familial, the case for genetic segregation contributing to an excess of cases in the north-east is weak.

In many ways the ten cases differed little from their matched controls or from the rest of the HD cases. For example, nothing unusual could be seen in the time of birth, time of diagnosis, the sex ratio, the mean age or in other previous residences. An examination of lifetime occupation, however, was revealing. (In the case of children, the parents' occupations were looked at.) Eight out of the ten at one time had been occupied in primary industry; one miner, two foresters and five farmers. In the control group only two have been involved in such employment; both were farmers. The relative risk of HD due to having farmed in this area was calculated to be four but because of the small numbers this was insignificant. No other occupations demonstrated any excess.

Summary

The analysis presented above was an elementary one. It examined residential risk for Hodgkin's disease in Tasmania but did not purport to be a thorough investigation of this disease and its environmental and residential associations. It merely attempted to illustrate a method in action and the utility of that method when high quality data are available. Used on larger data sets it will undoubtedly produce worthwhile advances in geographical epidemiology. On this small data set the limited follow-up of the extreme patterns of residential relative risk has produced some new leads for further research, especially in regard to the events surrounding birth and the hazards surrounding the farmyard.

References

Armstrong, R. W. (1976). The geography of specific environments of patients and non-patients in cancer studies, with a Malaysian example. *Econ. Geogr.* **52** (2), 161–170.
Armstrong, R. W. (1978). Self-specific environments associated with nasopharyngeal carcinoma in Selangor, Malaysia. *Soc. Sci. Med.* **12D**, 149–156.

Armstrong, R. W., Kannan Kutty, M. and Dharmalingham, S. K. (1974). Incidence of nasopharyngeal carcinoma in Malaysia: with special reference to the state of Selangor. *Br. J. Cancer* **30**, 86–94.

Breslow, N. E. and Day, N. E. (1980). *Statistical Methods in Cancer Research*, Vol. 1. International Agency for Research on Cancer, Lyon.

Cancer Council of Western Australia (1981). *Leukaemia and Allied Disorders in Western Australia: Diagnostic Incidence 1960–1969*. Cancer Council, W.A., Perth.

Choynowski, M. (1959). Maps based on probabilities. *J. Am. Statist. Ass.* **54**, 385–388.

Day, N. E. (1976). In *Cancer Incidence in Five Continents* (Eds J. Waterhouse, C. Muir, P. Correa and J. Powell), pp. 443–445. International Agency for Research on Cancer, Lyon.

Doll, R. (1976). In *Cancer Incidence in Five Continents* (Eds J. Waterhouse, C. Muir, P. Correa and J. Powell), pp. 453–459. International Agency for Research on Cancer, Lyon.

Fisher, R. A. (1956). *Statistical Methods and Scientific Inference*. Oliver and Boyd, London.

Ford, J. (1981). Unpublished data. N.S.W. Cancer Registry.

Gallo, R. C. and Gelmann, E. P. (1981). In search of Hodgkin's disease virus (editorial). *N. Engl. J. Med.* **304**(3), 169–170.

Glick, B. J. (1979). Distance relationships in theoretical models of carcinogenesis. *Soc. Sci. Med.* **13D**, 123–130.

Glick, B. J. (1980). The geographic analysis of cancer occurrence: past progress and future directions. In *Conceptual and Methodological Issues in Medical Geography* (Ed. M. S. Meade), pp. 170–193. University of North Carolina at Chapel Hill, Department of Geography, Chapel Hill, N.C.

Gutensohn, N. and Cole, P. (1981). Childhood social environment and Hodgkin's disease. *N. Engl. J. Med.* **305**(3), 135–140.

King, P. E. (1979). Problems of spatial analysis in geographical epidemiology. *Soc. Sci. Med.* **13D**, 249–252.

Knox, G. (1964). Epidemiology of childhood leukaemia in Northumberland and Durham. *Br. J. Prev. Soc. Med.* **18**, 17–24.

Lickiss, J. N., Baikie, A. G. and Panton, P. (1977). Lymphoproliferative and myeloproliferative disease in Tasmania. *Nat. Cancer Inst. Monogr.* **47**, 37–39.

Mantel, N. (1967). The detection of disease clustering and a generalized regression approach. *Cancer Res.* **27**, 201–220.

McNemar, Q. (1974). Note on the sampling error of the difference between correlated proportions or percentages. *Psychometrika* **12**, 153–157.

Miller, R. W. and Beebe, G. W. (1973). Infectious mononucleosis and the empirical risk of cancer. *J.N.C.I.* **50**, 315–321.

Munoz, N., Davidson, R. J. L., Witthoff, B., Ericsson, J. E. and de-The, G. (1978). Infectious mononucleosis and Hodgkin's disease. *Int. J. Cancer* **22**, 10–13.

South Australian Health Commission (1980). *Cancer in South Australia*, Vol. II. Government Printer, Adelaide.

Ultmann, J. E., Cunningham, J. K. and Gellhorn, A. (1966). The clinical picture of Hodgkin's disease. *Cancer Res.* **26** (1), 1047–1060.

Vianna, N. J., Greenwald, P. and Davies, J. N. P. (1971). Extended epidemic of Hodgkin's disease in high school students. *Lancet* **1**, 1209–1211.

Subject index

Statistical methods index

SOCIAL SCIENCE LIBRARY

Manor Road Building
Manor Road
Oxford OX1 3UQ
Tel: (2)71093 (enquiries and renewals)
http://www.ssl.ox.ac.uk

This is a NORMAL LOAN item.

We will email you a reminder before this item is due.

Please see http://www.ssl.ox.ac.uk/lending.html
for details on:

- loan policies; these are also displayed on the
  notice boards and in our library guide.

- how to check when your books are due back.

- how to renew your books, including information
  on the maximum number of renewals.
  Items may be renewed if not reserved by
  another reader. Items must be renewed before
  the library closes on the due date.

- level of fines; fines are charged on overdue books.

Please note that this item may be recalled during Term.